THE APPETITES OF MAN

SALLY DEVORE and THELMA WHITE are professional nutrition guidance counselors in San Diego, California. Together, they prepared the exhibit upon which this book is based for the Museum of Man in San Diego. For over two years, the exhibit set attendance records at the museum, after which it was donated to the Price-Pottenger Nutrition Foundation. In the years to come this foundation will be making it available to nutrition conferences and museums throughout the country.

THE APPETITES
OF MAN

An Invitation to Better Nutrition
from 9 Healthier Societies

SALLY DeVORE and THELMA WHITE

Originally published under the title *Dinner's Ready!*

ANCHOR BOOKS
ANCHOR PRESS/DOUBLEDAY
GARDEN CITY, NEW YORK
1978

The Appetites of Man was originally published in a hardcover edition, with the title *Dinner's Ready!* by Ward Ritchie Press in 1977.

Anchor Books edition: 1978

To Bob and John
and
The Klee Wyk Society

Acknowledgments

We would like to gratefully acknowledge the help and encouragement of the following people: D. P. Burkitt, M.D. F.R.C.S.E., Medical Research Council, London; D. R. Brothwell, Senior Scientific Officer, Anthropology, British Museum (Natural History) London; Robert Fletcher Allen, *Let's Live* magazine; Robert Rodale, Editor, *Prevention* magazine; the staff of the San Diego Museum of Man; the staff of the Price-Pottenger Nutrition Foundation, San Diego; Granville F. Knight, M.D., President, Price-Pottenger Nutrition Foundation; Consulate General of Japan, Los Angeles; Embassy of the Democratic and Popular Republic of Algeria, Washington, D.C.; Jay Milton Hoffman, Ph.D.

The evaluation of protein qualities used in this book is based on figures found in *Diet For a Small Planet* by Frances Moore Lappe (Ballantine Books, 1971).

The Agriculture Handbook No. 8, United States Department of Agriculture, provided information on nutrient composition for most of the foods described in the book.

Contents

Foreword ix

The First Course 1

The Marquesans' Island Paradise 8

The Nomadic Tuareg of the Sahara 31

Hunza in the Himalayas 56

The Digueños of Southern California 83

The Gandans of Lake Victoria 110

The Eskimos of the Pacific Coast 135

The Chinese, Relentless Survivors 161

Japan, A Land of Harmony 198

Mexico, A Land of Contrasts 227

Healthy Cultures in the United States 258

Simple Rules for Good Nutrition 261

The Great Snack Food Ripoff 282

Science of Health 295

Have a Care 326

Index 355

Foreword

Granville F. Knight, M.D.
President
Price-Pottenger Nutrition Foundation

In recent years the subjects of "ecology" and "good nutrition" have become common topics of discussion in most households. Unfortunately, many writers have jumped on the bandwagon and ridden off in all directions—espousing the values of this vitamin or that mineral—until the average reader is thoroughly confused. Scientific treatises on these subjects are technical and limited. Since nutrition is often equated with dietetics in the minds of physicians, and medical journals parrot the fallacy that malnutrition in the United States is almost impossible, it is not surprising that most doctors are indifferent to the question of proper nourishment.

It is, therefore, an event of great importance when women like Sally DeVore and Thelma White decide to write a book to simplify the basic facts of good nutrition. Their observations are an extension of the fundamental truths expounded in an excellent exhibit, "Nutrition: The Appetite of Man," which was on display for more than two years at the Museum of Man in San Diego, California. This exhibit was conceived by Sally DeVore and erected by members of the Klee Wyk Society—the women's auxiliary to the museum with the help of members of the Price-Pottenger Nutrition Foundation. (The exhibit has since been donated to the Foundation for future showings.)

The theme of the exhibit at the Museum of Man was a comparison of the foods of primitive and semiprimitive cultures with those of our own. The exhibit and this book graphically illustrate the penalty civilized countries are now paying in tooth decay and degenerative diseases for failing to learn and abide by Nature's immutable laws.

The authors were stimulated by the work of Dr. Weston A. Price, as reported in his classic and profusely illustrated book, *Nutrition and Physical Degeneration* (San Diego: Price-Pottenger Foundation, 1970) first published in 1939. Dr. Price, a dentist blessed with great imagination and drive, had enough horse sense to study the dietary customs and health of fourteen primitive tribes before and after they contacted "civilization." The contrast was startling, and is preserved in hundreds of striking photographs.

In 1969, Mrs. Price assigned the rights to Dr. Price's book and all his materials to the Price-Pottenger Nutrition Foundation. The New Heritage edition of the book appeared in 1970.

Dr. Price found that even though native diets differed markedly, they had one thing in common—an intake of relatively unprocessed foods from native soil that provided at least four times the water-soluble, and up to ten times the fat-soluble, vitamins recommended for our daily consumption. Dr. Price's findings are being substantiated by others. Sally DeVore and Thelma White's book provides documentation of these facts.

Their book is written in a concise, readable, and persuasive style. It contains material of practical value for every man, woman, and child. The importance of their message cannot be overestimated. It should be widely read—and acted upon—to help stem our national malnutrition.

The First Course

You are cordially invited to dinner, one you've probably never had before. Unless you're an ardent and adventurous traveler, it is unlikely that you have enjoyed a bowl of *couscous* and some lamb (or goat) in the tent of a friendly Tuareg family. If you've missed this experience, you can prepare the same meal for your own family or friends and savor at least some of the Tuareg way of life by using recipes in this book. You may not be able to duplicate the atmosphere of a desert oasis, but the couscous will be the same.

The delicate elegance of a Japanese meal can also be re-created in your home. To make the experience complete, you should use chopsticks. You'll even find instructions on how to get the food from dish to mouth; it's actually rather simple.

The island paradise of the Marquesans tends to make them pretty casual about meals. Bananas grow everywhere, coconuts abound, and fish are plentiful. However, when the Marquesans decide to have a feast, no one can resist an invitation to that dinner. Prepared in your kitchen, it can be just as tempting. The Marquesans have developed a diet that is unique, different from that of their Hawaiian or Polynesian kin.

In fact, all the national food preferences described in the pages ahead are unique. Over thousands of years these peoples evolved basic diets so distinctive that their foods serve as a means of national or cultural identity. Because their diet provided all the elements needed for good health and a vigorous life, these groups survived and grew.

Primitive people ate everything and anything, a lack of prejudice that generally filled their vitamin and mineral requirements. As palates grew more sophisticated and processed food became available, the taste of the food became more important than its quality. The body's energy requirements were satisfied before vitamin and mineral requirements were met. Dr. Weston A. Price, a dentist and dedicated scientist, was a pioneer in observing the correlation between diet and physical deterioration. He noted that: "No era in the long journey of mankind reveals in its skeletal remains such a terrible degeneration of teeth and bones as this brief period of modern civilization records."

The people described in the following chapters have stayed with their ancient ethnic diets and have largely escaped the degeneration Dr. Price found throughout the world among people who had replaced their traditional foods with modern, refined products.

All the cultures examined have a lesson to teach. Each is different yet they have a basic similarity. The good and infinitely varied foods that we find growing and living on our beautiful planet provide us with everything we need for a healthy life. How that food is prepared and served may seem strange and unfamiliar. By sharing the meals of other cultures, we can overcome national barriers. To make the occasion even more complete, the food should be presented, served and eaten in the same manner as the people whose recipes you are following. Of course, some modifications will have to be made. Apartment dwellers might have difficulties preparing a Marquesan *imu*, or fire pit, but substitutes are suggested and the meal will still be authentic. You will have a chance to visit and dine with families of Chinese, Eskimos, Japanese, Marquesans, Tuaregs, Hunzas, Mexicans, Gandans of the Lake Victoria area, and even a trip back in time for a meal with the Digueño Indians of Southern California. It is hoped that these visits will expand your knowledge and understanding of our neighbors.

Unlike the often-primitive cooking areas used by the majority of the people described, the American kitchen is the product of engineering genius. As skillfully planned as the assembly line of a modern factory, it is time-saving, space-saving, and step-saving. From electric can opener to mixer and blender, from electric fryer to microwave oven, every conceivable device is designed to make meal preparation a cinch. Of course, if the electricity goes off, starvation is a serious possibility.

The sad fact is that some rather inferior food often emerges from these marvelous kitchens. One of the most serious defects in our diet is that we habitually eat too much in quantity and too little in quality.

The following meal is typical of that served in millions of American homes on any given night. It's not a bad meal; it's just a typical meal. In fact, many people would say it's a very good dinner. With a few minor variations it will consist of: salad made with one-sixth head of iceberg lettuce, two cherry tomatoes, a few cucumber slices and about two tablespoons of french dressing; one four-ounce ground beef patty; one medium potato, pan-fried; about one-half cup of canned green beans; a white dinner roll with

NUTRIENTS FOUND IN THE TYPICAL AMERICAN MEAL					U.S. Gov. R.D.A.* of each Nutrient for an adult male living in U.S.A. weighing 150 lbs.
% of R.D.A.*	25%	50%	75%	100%	
Protein	////////////////				68 GRAMS
Fat	//////////////////////////////////				80 GRAMS MAX.
Carbohydrate	//////////				350 GRAMS
Calories	/////////////////				2400
Vitamin A	///////////				5000 UNITS
Vitamin B₁	/////////				1.2 MG.
Vitamin B₂	//////////				1.3 MG.
Niacin	/////////////////////////				16 MG.
Vitamin C	/////////////////////////////////				45 MG.
Calcium	///////				800 MG.
Iron	//////////////////////////////				10 MG.
Fiber	/////				15 GRAMS MIN. (NO R.D.A.)

*R.D.A. is the recommended daily nutrient allowance intended to meet the needs of a *healthy* individual.

two pats of butter; and, to top it off, one-sixth of an eight-inch frozen pie, usually apple.

The chief sources of nutrients in a typical American meal are:

PROTEIN	hamburger
FAT	hamburger fat and pan-fried potatoes
CARBOHYDRATE	potatoes
CALORIES	pan-fried potatoes
VITAMIN A	tomatoes and butter
VITAMIN B_1	potatoes
VITAMIN B_2	hamburger
NIACIN	hamburger
VITAMIN C	potatoes
CALCIUM	green beans and potatoes
IRON	hamburger
FIBER	potatoes

What's wrong with that meal? The chart shows that it is far too high in fat and far too low in most of the vitamins and minerals. And while it's not so hot nutritionally, it's also dull. How much more fun it would be to prepare and serve a Ugandan meal! To enhance the enjoyment of your dinner, the chapter on the Gandans describes the people as well as their social and historical background. Why do they use mashed bananas instead of a grain in making their *matoke?* It happens that bananas grow very well in Uganda, an example of environment directly influencing diet.

Along with a description of the particular people, their health, and their food, each chapter presents a complete dinner menu, with recipes, plus a number of other healthful and interesting dishes from that country. The Westernized versions of the recipes all serve four and, while the quantities of food seem to be greater than in a typical American meal, their calorie content is lower. In addition, a comparison of the nutrients in each meal with those of the typical American meal will show that the ethnic meals are far more nutritious.

Desserts are rarely included because the cultures described generally do not use them. In many cases the basic meal consists of a stew made with almost any available vegetable, a little meat, poultry, or fish, and generally some variety of legume, all accompanied by grains or other high carbohydrate food. While the preparation of the stew follows a basic pattern, there is no specific recipe. All the foods should be seasoned to taste, so don't worry about careful measurements. Any green leafy vegetable, broccoli, or combination of greens may be used in place of the greens specified. Likewise, any other whole grain or whole grain product like tortillas, sourdough rye bread, or chapattis may be substituted for the grain called for in the recipe. Be careful about substitutions. For instance, if one source of calcium is removed from the recipe, an-

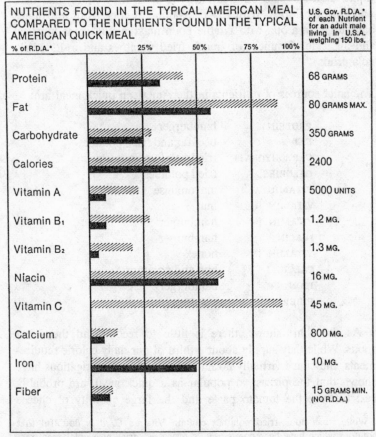

NUTRIENTS FOUND IN THE TYPICAL AMERICAN MEAL COMPARED TO THE NUTRIENTS FOUND IN THE TYPICAL AMERICAN QUICK MEAL					U.S. Gov. R.D.A.* of each Nutrient for an adult male living in U.S.A. weighing 150 lbs.
% of R.D.A.*	25%	50%	75%	100%	
Protein					68 GRAMS
Fat					80 GRAMS MAX.
Carbohydrate					350 GRAMS
Calories					2400
Vitamin A					5000 UNITS
Vitamin B₁					1.2 MG.
Vitamin B₂					1.3 MG.
Niacin					16 MG.
Vitamin C					45 MG.
Calcium					800 MG.
Iron					10 MG.
Fiber					15 GRAMS MIN. (NO R.D.A.)

*R.D.A. is the recommended daily nutrient allowance intended to meet the needs of a *healthy* individual.
   Diagonal lines represent the American meal.

other should be included. Use the recipes as a guide. Feel free to express yourself and enjoy flexibility in the amounts and the sorts of foods used. Above all, have fun trying out new foods and novel meal patterns.

To make between-meal eating a guilt-free pleasure, directions on how to make dozens of delicious snacks are included. They too reflect national origins, and they differ from American snacks in two major areas—they are inexpensive and they are nutritious.

Almost as ubiquitous as the snack in American society is the fast meal. Usually eaten during the middle of the day, when nutritional intake should be greatest, it is often little more than bulk and empty calories. With few exceptions, it consists of a 3 ounce hamburger in a bun with 1 tablespoon mayonnaise, some mustard and a pickle, 5 ounces of french fried potatoes and a 12 ounce cola drink.

The chief sources of nutrients in the American quick meal are:

PROTEIN	hamburger
FAT	beef fat and fried potatoes
CARBOHYDRATE	fried potatoes and cola
CALORIES	fried potatoes
VITAMIN A	mayonnaise
VITAMIN B_1	bun
VITAMIN B_2	hamburger
NIACIN	hamburger
VITAMIN C	none*
CALCIUM	bun and potatoes
IRON	hamburger
FIBER	potatoes

As the chart shows, there is little to recommend these fast foods. While they supply about a third of our daily calorie requirements, they have virtually no nutritional value. Investigations have shown that the pizzas, so popular as a quick meal, are probably best because the tomato paste and the large quantity of cheese

* While fresh home-fried potatoes contain Vitamin C, it is doubtful that potatoes which have been commercially processed, fried at a quick-meal restaurant, and perhaps held under a heat lamp for a long time would contain even a trace of Vitamin C.

used in their preparation are both fairly high in nutritional quality.

Those cultures that do include a fast meal in their daily diet usually eat leftovers from a previous meal. A Hunza fast meal is a couple of chapattis and some dried fruit and nuts. In Mexico, beans wrapped in a tortilla provide a quick bite that is both filling and nutritious. Americans can "brown bag" a delicious meal, one that is superior in every way to the fast foods shoveled out by the ton at franchised stands. Some of these exotic fast meals will raise a few eyebrows and a lot of questions from friends and coworkers, but you could probably take a trip to Hunza or Mexico or Japan or any of the other countries with the money you'll save.

In the meantime, take a trip to the nine different countries through knowledge of their foods and their cultures. Be a pioneer in the kitchen and put together a meal like none you've ever eaten before. Go ahead, take a chance. You've everything to gain and nothing to lose but your food prejudices. These people consume the foods their ancestors consumed, they cling to their old customs and methods of preparation and, in most cases, they are healthier than we.

The Marquesans' Island Paradise

The modern-day Garden of Eden was a group of small islands located in the South Pacific and known collectively as the Marquesas.

The first European visitors to this Polynesian paradise found the inhabitants beyond question the healthiest, happiest, and handsomest people in the world. They had come to terms with their environment in a manner not duplicated anywhere else on earth.

Lying a few degrees south of the equator, these formidable volcanic outcroppings presented a challenge to their inhabitants. There were no broad, shallow lagoons typical of the coral atolls, so the sea broke unrestrained on their shores. The mountains, rising precipitously to an altitude of 5,000 feet, tended to isolate the various villages that were home to a population estimated at about 120,000 in the late eighteenth century. Marquesan villages were generally in deep inland valleys. Because of the rich volcanic soil, these valleys produced an abundance of nutritious foods, and the Marquesans simply built their homes adjacent to the food supply.

Life in these villages was joyous and uninhibited, although there were often battles between neighboring settlements in which the losers ended up serving as supper for the victors. Frequently there was a religious ceremony connected with this cannibalism, but early chroniclers of the islands reported that the Marquesans simply liked the taste of "long pig," human flesh. However, it was a very minor part of their diet and strictly taboo for women.

The Marquesan men (the native name for their islands is "The Land of Men") were unusually tall, the average height being about six feet. Extremely strong and agile, they were wonderful athletes. The women were smaller, slender and well formed, and the outstanding feature of both men and women was their gorgeous teeth —white, even, and perfect. Herman Melville wrote in 1841:

Nothing in the appearance of the islanders struck me more forcibly than the whiteness of their teeth, they were more beautiful than ivory itself. The jaws of the oldest greybeards among them were much better garnished than those of most of the youths of civilized countries; while the teeth of the young and middle aged, in their purity and whiteness, were actually dazzling to the eye. This marvelous whiteness of teeth is to be ascribed to the pure vegetable diet of these people and the uninterrupted healthyness of their natural mode of life.

Melville goes on to write:

I was especially struck by the physical strength and beauty which they displayed; in beauty of form, they surpassed anything I had ever seen. Not a single instance of natural deformity was observable in all the throng.

The Marquesans were superb swimmers. The children swam before they could walk. Their island home provided them with such an abundance of food for the taking, about the only exercise they got was swimming. Not much energy was spent on the cultivation of crops. But in an example of perfect attunement to their environment, they ceremoniously planted a breadfruit tree each time a child was born, thus ensuring a future food supply. Breadfruit is seedless so a new tree must be grown from a slip. All the other vegetation on the island was self-perpetuating and grew rapidly in the rich volcanic soil with no assistance from the Marquesans.

The social structure of the villages consisted of the chief, a religious leader, and warrior ranks made up of young males. Marquesan sexual habits were casual and uninhibited; a man often took new partners and a woman would invite another man to come live in the household. This arrangement provoked neither jealousy nor quarreling; sex was too unimportant to fight about.

The islanders doted on their children, never leaving them alone for a second during their early years. A child was breast fed until three or four and, during this time, was constantly supervised by his mother or some other member of the household. If a baby started to cry, the entire family would stop what they were doing to console the unhappy child. Such devotion and love produced extremely happy, well-adjusted children and adults.

The Marquesans were devoted to tattooing and carried it to the height of an art form before it was outlawed by the French, who governed the islands. Each village had an expert in tattooing who would decorate the arms and legs of his neighbors with elaborate drawings of fish and plants in beautiful designs. The quantity and quality of these decorations indicated the status of the owner. It certainly indicated his bravery since the tattooing was an extremely painful and bloody process.

The making of tapa cloth was another accomplishment of the island artisans and, although the Marquesans rarely wore clothes, they used the tapa cloth as a covering at night and as a cape at ceremonial gatherings.

One of the favorite pastimes of the Marquesans was massaging each other with coconut oil. They would spend two or three hours at a time rubbing the oil into their bodies. The act was a sign of friendship or devotion and again demonstrated their perfect balance with nature. They spent so much of their time in the water, the oil was needed to keep their skin moist and to serve as protection against the tropical sun. It also allowed rainwater to roll off their bodies so they were dry minutes after a shower. When the missionaries insisted that the Marquesans wear clothing, this natural protection was lost. The clothes simply wouldn't dry between the frequent rains and, as a result of wearing damp clothes all day, the Marquesans began to develop pneumonia and other respiratory ailments, diseases heretofore unknown in their island paradise.

Living for centuries in isolation, the Marquesans had never developed natural immunities to disease. There was no known sickness on the islands, no poisonous snakes or insects and, barring accidents or warfare, nothing to cause premature death. Because of their near-perfect diet and isolation from disease, these island people lived amazingly long lives. It was not uncommon to see an old man or woman whose teeth had been ground to stubs from nearly a century of chewing.

Meals were eaten when hunger dictated; no special time of day was set aside. They considered no day complete without a nice long swim, possibly around the island, over to a particular cove a few miles from the village, or just out to sea and back. They often carried food along on these excursions—a few bananas, steamed breadfruit wrapped in leaves, or a coconut—the whole thing tied to a pole which they dragged along as they swam. When they were hungry, they would tread water while enjoying their meal. Both men and women swam great distances, treating the sharks that infested their waters with an indifference that bordered on the foolhardy. If any of their population was lost to shark attacks, it must have been rare, for they certainly paid little attention to this danger.

There were fifty-two varieties of breadfruit growing on the islands and this starchy vegetable was their staple food. Prepared in a number of ways, frequently the large lumpy fruit was simply peeled and mashed into a paste and then steamed. The mortar used for the pounding process was an elaborately carved stone, an object of respect and honor, handed down through the family. As the breadfruit was being pounded, one of the men would grate coconut meat into it. When the mixture reached the consistency of library paste, it was ready to cook. The flavor is mild with a slight tang, considered quite palatable even to sophisticated tastes, although foreigners have difficulty getting the stuff into their mouths without making an awful mess. Like *poi*, it is eaten with the fingers.

Another method of cooking the breadfruit was steaming it in a ground oven, a pit filled with stones. This was a major project so the men took charge. They started a wood fire, gathered the stones and placed them into the flames. These were the porous lava stones, found all over the islands, which can be heated white hot with no danger of exploding. Each family had its own stone supply, often very old, used and reused through the years. When the stones were hot enough, they were rolled into the pit, covered with a layer of gravel; woven mats were spread on top to hold the food.

Now into the pit went a whole pig or goat, if the occasion warranted. The breadfruit, bananas, a large fish, or any other food that was handy, was wrapped in breadfruit leaves. More mats were placed on top of the food, the pit was filled with dirt, and the wait began. Neighbors would gather because this *imu*, or fire pit, was quite an event. After a few hours, the pit would be uncovered, and the feast would begin.

While cooking in this fashion is probably impractical for most people, especially apartment dwellers, it is certainly one of the most nutritious ways to prepare food. Because it is wrapped in leaves and steamed, the food is not exposed to light and great heat. Thus it retains most of its vitamins and minerals. A crock pot could substitute nicely; slow cooking at low temperatures over a long period of time duplicates as nearly as possible the imu. This is the least destructive method of cooking protein foods.

The balance of the Marquesan diet consisted of taro root, coconut, any of the thirty varieties of bananas found on the islands, mangos, fish, and shellfish. The favorite way to eat fish was right out of the sea, dipped in lime juice and consumed on the spot. The men were skilled fishermen, but fishing with hook and line was taboo for the women, so every day they would wander down to the tide pools and deftly catch the tiny fish and crustaceans found in abundance there. Amid laughter and joking they would grab the flashing fish and pop them into their mouths. Foreign visitors to the islands soon became accustomed to this and ended up preferring a raw fish to one cooked.

Because of the generally mild climate that ensured a year-round food supply, little in the way of food preservation was developed by the Marquesans. One notable exception was their method of preserving the breadfruit, their staff of life. In times of drought, breadfruit will not produce, so during bountiful seasons, huge pits, some measuring thirty to forty feet in length and ten feet in depth, would be dug. This was a community effort with everyone helping. In preparation, they lined the pit with the broad leaves of the breadfruit tree. Then they peeled the breadfruit, cut it in half, wrapped it in leaves and placed it in the pit. When a sufficient quantity had been stored, the pit would be covered with dirt and the breadfruit allowed to ferment. After removal from the pit, the fermented breadfruit, a dark brown, soggy mass, was placed in a mesh bag, soaked in sea water and, still in its bag, kneaded by hand to remove the moisture. It was then combined with coconut cream and baked in a ground oven. During the baking process, it rose like leavened bread. The resulting food was quite good and still very nutritious, as all fermented foods are. Breadfruit that had been stored for as long as ten years was still edible and the Marquesans seemed to prefer it this way, the older the better.

Coconut was consumed in a variety of ways. The immature nut was cut open and the rich, creamy albumen was the first diet supplement of the children. Coconut cream, an ingredient of many

Marquesan dishes, was extracted from the fresh-grated nut meat; the grated meat was also used in combination with other foods. The ubiquitous breadfruit, which supplied so many of the nutrients in the Marquesan diet, was lacking in Vitamin A. This shortage was partly augmented by the many varieties of bananas found on the islands. The small, fat, red species, their favorite, is especially high in Vitamin A. Bananas were a part of the daily diet and no Marquesan home was complete without a huge hand hanging from the ridge pole. As is customary, they were picked green and allowed to ripen.

The main protein source of the Marquesan diet was seafood, frequently eaten raw usually after being marinated in a combination of seawater and lime juice or raw coconut milk. A great favorite was soft-shelled crabs. During the moulting season, these delicacies would be gathered from the rocks and tide pools and everyone would get together for a feast. The crabs were consumed live, whole and raw, and it must have been a bit unnerving to see a young man or woman biting into the soft-bodied animal while its legs were still wildly waving. Not surprisingly, crabs are an outstanding source of Vitamin A.

Another seasonal favorite was the coconut crabs, who left the protection of the coconut trees during their mating season. The Marquesans would tie a ring of grass around the trunk of the tree, about fifteen feet above the ground. As the crabs made their way down the tree, they would come to the grass ring and, thinking they had reached the ground, let go of their hold on the tree. Meantime, a fence had been erected around each tree and, when the stunned crab revived, he was neatly penned. Preparations for the crab roundup took very little time and needed no supervision at all—certainly a perfect example of food literally dropping into people's laps. The crabs were force-fed coconut meat until they burst their shells and were then roasted. This migratory meal was another occasion for a feast.

The idyllic Marquesan life ended when foreign traders began making regular stops at the islands for copra. In exchange for copra, the traders gave the islanders whiskey, sugar, cloth, white flour, and canned goods. They also gave them syphilis, smallpox, tuberculosis, diphtheria, and leprosy. The Chinese merchants came soon after the copra traders and set up their shops along the waterfront, where they sold canned food, candy, white bread, sugar, and polished rice. For the increasing Chinese population, the sea captains added opium to their list of trade items. The Marquesans began to abandon their traditional diet and buy food at the Chinese markets. They felt that eating the European foods increased their status. It showed their neighbors how successful they were because they could afford to buy the white bread and canned peas. These strange foods must have taken a lot of getting used to.

The missionaries came next, bringing rules and religion. Ancient traditions were banned, cultural heritage forbidden, tattooing declared sinful, nakedness became a disgrace, and singing was intolerable. The relaxed and casual attitudes about sex were radically altered; monogamy was enforced.

Then came the French to rule the islands by military force, putting rebellious villages to the torch. The last straw was a horrifying disaster that struck in 1894. A sea captain abandoned a boatload of sailors stricken with smallpox on one of the islands. With the Marquesans' low tolerance to disease aggravated by the poor diet they had begun to follow, there was little hope for many of the islanders. Before the epidemic ran its course, more than half the natives had died. Some islands lost their entire populations and remain to this day uninhabited, overgrown relics of an ancient and proud people deceived and destroyed by civilization. By 1920, there were only about 1,000 Marquesans left, their spirits broken, waiting sullenly for death. Suicide among the survivors was commonplace. In one of the villages, no children had been born in twenty-five years, due mainly to the appalling incidence of venereal disease.

The copra traders stopped coming to the islands. There weren't enough able-bodied men to load the ships, let alone produce the copra. The missionaries gave up in despair, many suffering severe emotional breakdowns as they viewed the results of their efforts. Stating that the Marquesans were doomed, the French departed, leaving a nominal head of government and a couple of gendarmes. Relics of this once happy people stoically awaited their fate.

During the next thirty years, the few miserable survivors clung to life. With no money, they couldn't buy food at the Chinese stores. They had to eat what the island provided. The island provided what it had always provided—breadfruit, bananas, coconut, mango, wild pigs, and fish in abundance—everything needed for good health and vigor. The Marquesans began eating the foods of their ancestors and, for the first time in over half a century, their birth rate began to exceed the death rate.

The islanders' attitude underwent an astonishing change. These sullen, quarrelsome people began to smile and sing and flirt and joke. Their distrust of foreigners, although understandable under the circumstances, did not extend to treating them rudely; they just played rather wicked jokes on them. A group of anthropologists visiting the islands in 1958 found the people genial and happy, but not inclined to cooperate. The Marquesans were concerned because one of the scientists was trying to learn their complicated language. They felt this was an intrusion on their privacy. Very politely they told the scientist the Marquesan words for bread, water, house, fire, and other objects. It wasn't until months later that the poor anthropologist realized he'd been "had." Each term was actually the word for a very personal reproductive function or organ. As he was smugly asking for a piece of bread, he was actually requesting something far more ribald. One can hardly blame the Marquesans for trying to retain their identity by denying their language to foreigners.

Unless the Marquesans are "discovered" again, things look promising indeed for these happy people. In 1962, the first significant rise in population was noted. By 1967, the population stood at 5,175 with more than 3,000 of that total under twenty years of age; and in 1973, there were over 6,000 Marquesans in the archipelago. This is truly exciting and encouraging news.

Deep in isolated valleys, new villages are flourishing. Typical of these villages is one in the valley behind the main seaport town of Taiohae. It is run by a vigorous 95-year-old patriarch who remembers the old days and is dragging his village back to the era of the *poi poi* pits of fermenting breadfruit, to the raising of taro plants, to the ground oven, or imu, method of cooking. He enforces strict rules about food and eating habits. All kids love candy, but every child who returns to the village from the coastal town is searched and any candy seized and thrown into the privy.

The old leader will not let the women go to the government hospital to have their babies; they are delivered in the village by midwives. A recent comparison of birth weights between the town and village children showed that those born in the villages and whose mothers ate the traditional foods weigh two to three pounds more at birth than the city-bred infants. During their first thirty-six months of life, the village children are healthier, learn faster, walk sooner, and have better tooth development than their counterparts in the waterfront towns. In addition, the city children suffer more frequently from meningitis, tuberculosis, pneumonia, and malnutrition. After a year or so of breast feeding, the village mother supplements the infant diet with a sort of porridge made from the albumen of the immature coconut and starch from grated native arrowroot. A nutritionist who visited the islands analyzed the chemical composition of the coconut through its various stages of development and discovered that the very young nut is low in calories, which increase as the coconuts mature. They are extremely rich in phosphorus, iron, thiamine, riboflavin, niacin, ascorbic acid, and Vitamin E, and, when eaten in combination with breadfruit, taro root, or other starchy vegetables, provide the major portion of nutrients needed for good health. Village babies get a marvelous start in life with this simple diet.

The favorite sweetener of the Marquesans is wild honey gathered from hives far back in the valleys. Mixed with hot water and lemon, it is also used medicinally for any number of benefits—from a good night's sleep to treating burns effectively. A free, never-ending supply of sweets comes from the sugar cane fields and all the Marquesans chew on a length of raw cane frequently. Raw cane is a fine source of energy and is not harmful to the teeth of a healthy person when its fibers are also chewed. The children carry several pieces of sugar cane to school for snacks.

In the open-air mission schools, these healthy, happy youngsters, lightly dressed and barefoot, eat simple nutritious foods prepared by the native cooks—fish, vegetables, taro, fresh fruits. No tinned meat, polished rice, and white bread for these children.

Life in the villages is actually better now than it was before the civilized invasion. Communal gardens of sweet potatoes, watermelons, peanuts, tomatoes, corn, carrots, and other vegetables, are flourishing in soil so rich it needs no fertilizers. Good nutritious foods, unknown to the ancient Marquesans, are now part of their descendants' daily diet. Education, too, is part of their lives; but singing, dancing, and swimming are still their favorite pastimes.

The Marquesans have a new lease on life and the future promises well for them. Truly, a rare instance of paradise regained.

FOODS OF THE MARQUESANS

The foods available to the early Marquesans were fairly limited in variety; however, they had developed so many ways for preparing these foods, their menu was rather extensive. Breadfruit was their staple, supplying more than half their calorie intake. They evolved dozens of ways to serve this starchy plant.

CHIEF SOURCES OF NUTRIENTS IN THE MARQUESANS' DIET

PROTEIN	seafood
FAT	coconut oil
CARBOHYDRATE	breadfruit
CALORIES	coconut
VITAMIN A	mango, red banana, greens, raw whole seafood
VITAMIN C	breadfruit, mango, greens, coconut sap
VITAMIN B₁	breadfruit
VITAMIN B₂	seafood
NIACIN	seafood
CALCIUM	bones
IRON	bones
FIBER	coconut and breadfruit

Breadfruit

The breadfruit comes from a handsome tree with large, smooth leaves. There are over fifty varieties growing on the islands. It is generally seedless so shoots are planted. The fruit is about the size of a cantaloupe and has a rough lumpy skin. When ripe it is a yellowish green or brown. The shape varies widely; it can be round or long, symmetrical or lopsided. Eaten in large enough quantities to satisfy caloric needs, breadfruit furnishes enough, or most, of all nutrients required to support life except Vitamin A.

The Marquesans preferred the flavor of the slightly immature breadfruit, which is fairly bland compared with the sweet taste of the ripe fruit. *Kon* was the most popular method of preparing this staple. The procedure was long and tedious and began with peeling the breadfruit and cutting it into sections. These were wrapped in banana leaves and placed in the ground oven. Through an opening in the top of the bundle, water was poured to create steam; the hole was then sealed and the breadfruit allowed to cook for about two hours. After the cooking was done, the men took over. Using a coral rock, they pounded the fruit and formed it into a loaf weighing about eight to ten pounds. The loaf was divided into small pieces, wrapped in leaves, and stored. Kon was the mainstay of the diet. It traveled well in its leaf wrapper and provided a fine meal when combined with dried fish or fruit. Breadfruit was also peeled and roasted or baked like a potato.

Being a seasonal plant, it had to be preserved for future use. One method consisted of soaking the peeled fruit in salt water, covering it with leaves, and allowing it to ferment, which took about forty-eight hours. It was then squeezed to a doughy mass, sprinkled with fresh water, and placed in a leaf-lined pit. In three weeks the breadfruit was ready to prepare, but it could be kept for up to two years by changing the leaf covering from time to time. The poi-poi pit was for long-term preservation. Tossed into this pit, the whole unpeeled breadfruit remained edible for up to ten years.

Taro

Taro is the starchy corm (main root stalk) of an attractive plant with large heart-shaped leaves. It grows in abundance throughout the South Pacific. While it is the staple food of many islanders, it wasn't too popular with the Marquesans; they usually ate it only between breadfruit seasons. The nutrients in taro are similar to those in the potato. The calcium, iron, and phosphorus are easily assimilated and the starch grains are small, making them easy to digest. Unlike the sloppy poi prepared by many Pacific islanders, taro as prepared by the Marquesans is grated, mixed with coconut oil, and baked into a cake. The leaves of the taro plant are edible and occasionally the Marquesans ate them raw; but their favorite method was to chop them up, mix them with coconut cream, and bake them in the ground oven. The plant's leaves are rich in Vitamins A and C, calcium, and iron.

Coconut

The coconut is the most versatile food found on the islands, and was eaten at all stages of its development. The immature nut, with its soft, jelly-like consistency, was fed to babies. The milk in the mature nut was a favorite drink, pure and refreshing. Men of the Marquesas grated the coconut, using an apparatus that looked something like a saw-horse. It had an extension with a shell grater attached on one end. The men would straddle the saw-horse and grate the meat from the nut with the shell attachment. The grated coconut would then be mixed with water to make coconut cream, pressed into oil, or mixed with other foods.

In making coconut oil, the grated meat was first dried, mixed with finely chopped leaves, tied in a mesh bag, and the oil then extracted by a press. It was the chief source of fat in their diet. Coconut oil has the most saturated fat of all oils. It contains 86 percent saturated fat compared with butterfat, which is 57 percent saturated. The Marquesans used the oil in cooking and also rubbed it on their bodies every day. The blossom of the coconut tree was also a favorite food source for the Marquesans. For about three weeks the blossom gives off sap, called *jekamai,* and by tapping its base, they collected the sap. Most Marquesan families had about three blossoms at a time going all year round. The sap was heated to prevent fermentation and this sweet syrup was then added to many dishes. While the coconut is not particularly high in nutritive value, the sap of the blossom contains the same amount of carbohydrate and about half the Vitamin C found in orange juice.

A special treat awaited any sharp-eyed Marquesan. This was the discovery of a sprouted coconut. The milk of a sprouted coconut condenses into a snow-white, spongy ball. This soft, sweet food was usually consumed on the spot. Coconuts were the main source of fat in the Marquesan diet. They also contain iodine and Vitamin D, a nutrient rarely found in natural foods. It is believed that raw coconut meat has the ability to destroy tapeworm.

Bananas

Many varieties of bananas grow on the Marquesas. They were consumed raw in great quantities and provided the islanders with a small amount of high quality protein, easily assimilated carbohydrate, and most vitamins and minerals. The favorites were the redskinned bananas, which fortunately have three times more Vitamin A than the yellow. The Marquesans prepared bananas by steaming them in a ground oven; for special occasions, they would be peeled, seasoned with lime juice, mixed with grated coconut, and baked.

Mangos

Mangos were the favorite fruit of the Marquesans. They were also their main source of Vitamins A and C. The mango is about the size of a large apple; the skin is yellow with a red blush and, when ripe, is somewhat speckled. Fully ripe they are extremely sweet and taste like a combination of pineapple and apricot. They contain a large flat seed to which the flesh clings. They can be sliced but are best when eaten whole, over the sink, as they are very juicy.

Sweet Potatoes and Yams

The Marquesans weren't very fond of sweet potatoes or yams. Like taro, these were usually eaten when the breadfruit became scarce. The usual way of preparing them was to roast them in the ground oven. Sometimes they would toss a few sweet potatoes into their imu to steam. Occasionally the tubers would be grated, mixed with coconut cream, and steamed. While most people regard sweet potatoes and yams as similar, they are from entirely different botanical families. They are also dissimilar in food value. Sweet potatoes contain 8,800 units of Vitamin A and 21 grams of Vitamin C per 3½-ounce serving, while yams contain almost no Vitamin A and only nine units of C. Both contain a small amount of good quality protein and are easily digested. What are called yams in our vegetable markets are really a variety of sweet potato.

Arrowroot

The arrowroot is a perennial herb with large leaves and a tuberous root system. The Marquesans gathered the arrowroots to make into a flour used in cooking as a thickener or shaped into balls and baked. In making arrowroot flour, the tubers were peeled and ground into paste. This paste was then put into a coconut cloth bag and hung over a container of salt water. The water was repeatedly poured over the paste and allowed to drip into the container, leaching all the starch out of the grated arrowroot. The residue in the bag was discarded and the starch in the salt water settled to the bottom. When the water was poured off and the starch allowed to dry, it was ready to use. Arrowroot is similar to cornstarch and is used in the same way. It is very easy to digest and a source of calcium and other minerals. It was, not surprisingly, fed to Marquesan babies.

Seafood

Fish constituted the main protein source of the Marquesans and the only nonvegetable protein the women ate. Frequently the small whole fish—including head, scales, bones, and internal organs—was devoured fresh from the sea. After the women caught the fish, they usually marinated them in a mixture of seawater and lime juice or coconut milk. Larger fish were gutted, wrapped in leaves, and baked in the imu. They were also dried for future use. Analysis of the quality of fish found in the Marquesan waters shows that they have a higher calcium, phosphorus, and protein content than the same species found elsewhere.

The Marquesans were extremely fond of eel, and it is interesting to note that eel have a higher fat and Vitamin A content than most other seafood. This is an important factor because breadfruit is low in both these nutrients.

Pork and Goat

There were a few wild pigs on the islands, but they were seldom eaten. For very special occasions, they were roasted whole in the imu. The women were never allowed to eat this meat. In later years, goat became fairly popular and was also part of a feast menu. The head of the goat was presented as a gift to someone very special, a bridal couple or an honored guest. It was usually eaten as dessert.

DINING WITH A MARQUESAN FAMILY

Marquesan villages, nestled in deep valleys at the foot of steep mountains, were as beautiful and graceful as the people who lived in them. The homes, about twelve feet wide and twenty feet long, were built on raised stone foundations. The sturdy corner posts, roughly six feet tall on the wide front of the house and twelve to fifteen feet high at the back, supported a roof of palm fronds. Thin sticks placed an inch or two apart made up the walls. In the center of each home was a *fata* pole, a beautifully carved post with pegs jutting out that held the utensils used in cooking, the ever-present hand of bananas, and string bags of food. About a foot above the floor, a concave disk, eight inches in diameter, served as a guard to keep rats and other pests from the food.

The houses were placed in a rather random fashion, wherever the owner happened to decide to build. Meals were pretty random, too. The Marquesans ate whatever suited them whenever they felt hungry.

But on special occasions, and these could occur at any time, an imu would be planned. At this event everyone ate together and celebrated with singing and dancing and story-telling. The men did all the cooking, while the women made arrangements for the dinner. They would spread woven mats of coconut leaves on the ground for a table. Flowers of every imaginable variety would decorate the makeshift table and coconut shells, spoons and ladles made of seashells, and knives fashioned of bamboo would be set out. The spoons were only for dishing out the food, for everything was eaten with the fingers of both hands.

After the pit, filled with the food for the feast, was opened, everyone happily stuffed and gorged himself into a stupor. The individual food was served on a banana or breadfruit leaf, while liquids were served in coconut shells. Often a finger bowl was brought at the end of a meal.

But the imu pit was not a frequent event and the daily fare of the Marquesans was far simpler. Roasted breadfruit, fish and bananas, all prepared a number of ways, were the usual meal. One great favorite was *ror*. Making *ror* begins with roasted breadfruit, mashed and mixed with coconut cream. About five taro leaves are broken into small pieces and arranged so they cover the palm of the hand. A blob of breadfruit, about one half cup, is then placed in the center of the taro leaves and the leaves folded around to form a bundle. This is then placed in a wrapper of banana leaves and steamed in the ground oven for a couple of hours. The outer leaves are removed and the ror is ready to eat and enjoy. The favorite drinks are coconut liquid, water, or *jerkara,* the fermented sap of the coconut blossom.

A MARQUESAN DINNER PER INDIVIDUAL

SARDINES (3½ ounces)
ROR, breadfruit with coconut cream, (1 cup)
TARO LEAVES (2 ounces)
MANGO (1 fruit)

A MARQUESAN DINNER FROM YOUR KITCHEN

CANNED SARDINES IN MUSTARD SAUCE, 4 cans,
    3¾ ounces per can
BAKED SWEET POTATOES, 4
TROPICAL FRUIT COCKTAIL
BAKED SWISS CHARD IN COCONUT CREAM

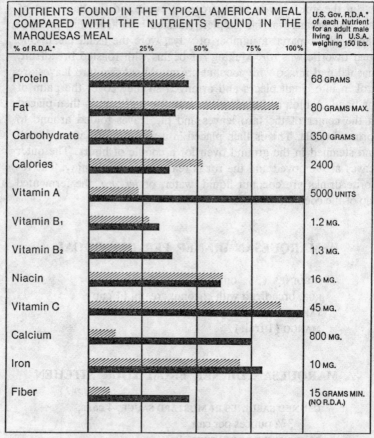

NUTRIENTS FOUND IN THE TYPICAL AMERICAN MEAL COMPARED WITH THE NUTRIENTS FOUND IN THE MARQUESAS MEAL	U.S. Gov. R.D.A.* of each Nutrient for an adult male living in U.S.A. weighing 150 lbs.
Protein	68 GRAMS
Fat	80 GRAMS MAX.
Carbohydrate	350 GRAMS
Calories	2400
Vitamin A	5000 UNITS
Vitamin B₁	1.2 MG.
Vitamin B₂	1.3 MG.
Niacin	16 MG.
Vitamin C	45 MG.
Calcium	800 MG.
Iron	10 MG.
Fiber	15 GRAMS MIN. (NO R.D.A.)

*R.D.A. is the recommended daily nutrient allowance intended to meet the needs of a *healthy* individual.

Diagonal lines represent the American meal.

The chief sources of nutrients in the Marquesan meal are:

PROTEIN	fish
FAT	coconut cream
CARBOHYDRATE	breadfruit
CALORIES	breadfruit and coconut cream
VITAMIN A	mango
VITAMIN B_1	breadfruit
VITAMIN B_2	fish
NIACIN	fish
VITAMIN C	mango
CALCIUM	fish bones
IRON	fish bones
FIBER	breadfruit

Sweet Potatoes

Wash potatoes, place on a flat pan, and bake in a 350° oven about 30 minutes, or until soft. When potatoes have baked 20 minutes, prick them with a fork or knife to allow steam to escape.

Serve them whole and hold in the hand to eat, skin and all. If you desire, you may dip them in melted butter as you eat them.

Tropical Fruit Cocktail

1 cup papaya, cubed
2 bananas, sliced
1 cup mango, cubed
1 cup fresh pineapple, sliced and cubed
3 tablespoons lime juice
1 tablespoon honey
½ cup toasted coconut (see below)

Combine lime juice, honey, and any juices from the fruit. Toss the fruit in the dressing, add toasted coconut, and serve. Fruit may be served in coconut shells, the pineapple shell, or seashells. Any combination of fruits may be used, or just substitute 4 sliced bananas.

Toasted Coconut

Spread grated coconut on a cookie sheet and toast in a 300° oven until slightly brown. It doesn't take long. Stir if it browns too fast on the edges. If you have a fresh coconut, you can remove the nut from the shell and make slivers with a vegetable peeler in place of grating it. These make good snacks.

Toasted Wheat Germ, Seeds, and Nuts

To preserve their protein quality, spread raw wheat germ, seeds, or nuts evenly on a shallow pan. Bake in a 200° to 225° oven for one hour or until browned and crisp. Stir occasionally to prevent burning. If you're in a hurry or you're planning to use them in baking, toast them at 300° to 350° for 15 to 20 minutes. Stir frequently to prevent burning.

Coconut Cream

  1½ cups shredded, unsweetened coconut. (Unsweetened shredded coconut is available at health food stores or you can buy a fresh coconut and grate its meat.)
  1 cup boiling water or hot milk

Combine coconut and hot liquid. Allow to stand 30 minutes. Drain cream into a bowl. Put coconut in a square of cheese cloth or other porous material and squeeze remaining coconut cream out with your hands. It is easier to squeeze about ⅓ of the coconut at a time. Discard coconut.

Baked Swiss Chard in Coconut Cream

  1½ pounds fresh chard chopped (reserve 4 large leaves) or 2 packages of frozen chopped chard
  ¾ cup coconut cream plus liquid left from cooking chard to make 1 cup (if more liquid remains, reduce it by boiling after the chard is removed). You may substitute half-and-half or milk for coconut cream.
  2 eggs, beaten
  1 teaspoon salt
  ¼ teaspoon nutmeg
  2 tablespoons grated unsweetened coconut
  Dash of white pepper

Cook chard until tender and add coconut cream. Combine eggs, salt, nutmeg, pepper. Add to slightly cooled coconut cream and chard mixture. Add coconut and mix well. Cut the four reserved leaves in half lengthwise and remove stems. Dip the leaves in warm water to soften, or lay them on top of chopped chard as it cooks. Place one leaf-half across the bottom of a lightly oiled individual casserole. Place the other leaf-half at right angles to it. Let the leaves extend up the sides of the container. If they are too wide, cut each into 4 strips. Fill with chard mixture and fold extended leaves over the filling. Bake at 300° for 15 minutes or only until set. The filled chard envelopes may be removed from the casseroles to serve. They can be served with fish and sweet potato on a large leaf or in abalone shells.

Fish with Coconut Cream

> *1 pound thin fish fillets*
> *¼ cup unsweetened, grated coconut*
> *⅓ cup chopped cooked shrimp or other shellfish*
> *1 tablespoon parsley, finely chopped*
> *4 medium mushrooms, chopped*
> *1 green onion, including green top, chopped*
> *¾ cup coconut cream (page 26); sour cream may be substituted*
> *1 pound cooked greens*
> *2 limes*
> *4 large leaves such as Swiss chard; dip in boiling water 3 minutes; drain well*
> *Salt to taste*

Divide fillets into 4 strips. Squeeze lime juice over them, then dip into coconut cream. Mix coconut, shrimp, onion, parsley, and mushrooms with 2 tablespoons coconut cream. Spread ¼ of the mixture on each fillet and roll them up jelly-roll fashion. Wrap each roll in a leaf and fasten closed with a toothpick or string. Set rolls close together in a greased baking dish. Heat remaining coconut cream and pour over the fish. Bake covered in a 300° oven just until the fish turns solid white, about 30 to 40 minutes.

To serve, remove fish from pan. Thicken remaining broth with arrowroot, if desired, and mix with cooked greens. Salt to taste. Place greens in individual dishes or coconut shells and set a fish roll on top. Serve lime wedges on the side so that each diner can squeeze some on his fish. A good addition to this meal would be sweet potatoes and fresh pineapple spears.

In later years the Marquesans used chopped pork in place of the shellfish. If you use pork, you must cook it first so that no red color remains.

Marinated Scallops

> *1 pound fresh scallops or any white-fleshed fish except cod or halibut*
> *¾ cup fresh lime juice*
> *1 small red onion, thinly sliced*
> *¼ cup unsweetened grated coconut*

Cut fish into scallop-size pieces. Place fish and onion slices in a heavy enamel dish; cover with lime juice and marinate 8 to 12 hours. Drain fish and onions; mix with grated coconut and salt to taste. The fish has actually cooked in the lime juice and is ready to eat.

The marinated fish is good served in a salad of raw vegetables. Make the salad dressing by mixing the lime juice left from marinating the fish with oil and a little dry mustard or garlic.

Fried Smelts

> *1 pound smelts or other small fish, cleaned but left whole. (Remove head if you wish.)*
> *¼ cup yellow cornmeal or dry whole grain bread crumbs*
> *½ teaspoon salt*
> *1 teaspoon grated lime rind*
> *¼ cup lime juice or coconut milk*
> *Coconut or vegetable oil*
> *1 lime, cut into wedges*

Heat oil in a frying pan to a depth of one-half the thickness of a smelt. Roll smelt in lime juice and dredge in a mixture of cornmeal, salt, and lime rind. Place fish in hot oil and turn when golden brown, 2 to 5 minutes; brown other side. Serve with lime wedges as soon as both sides are browned.

Banana "Poi"

> *2 cups mashed ripe bananas*
> *1 tablespoon fresh lime juice*
> *½ cup coconut cream (follow directions on page 26, but use 2 cups of coconut to 1 cup of hot water) (whipped cow's cream, sour cream, or yogurt may be substituted)*

Mash banana with hands or blender to make a smooth paste. Add lime juice. Gradually add the coconut cream, stirring constantly. Sweeten to taste with honey, if necessary. Banana poi is a good dip for pieces of raw fruit, sliced cooked sweet potatoes, or toasted coconut strips (see page 25).

Coconut Pudding, "Haupia"

> 2 cups coconut cream, page 26 (for a more nutritious pudding, use cow's milk or half-and-half, instead of water, to make coconut cream)
> 3 tablespoons honey
> 3 tablespoons arrowroot
> Dash of salt
> ¼ cup toasted coconut (page 25)

Heat honey and combine with arrowroot. Slowly stir coconut cream into honey mixture, stirring constantly. Heat until thickened but do not boil. Salt to taste. Mix in the toasted coconut and pour into a coconut shell or dish and set in refrigerator to chill.

Pineapple Rice Pudding

> 1 cup brown rice
> 4 cups pineapple juice
> ½ teaspoon salt
> 2 tablespoons butter
> Honey, to taste
> Cinnamon, to taste
> 1 cup toasted, shredded coconut (page 25)
> 1 cup fresh fruit, cut in small chunks
> Coconut cream (page 26)

Heat pineapple juice to boiling. Add rice and salt. Cover pan, reduce heat, and simmer 1 to 1½ hours or until the rice is very tender and the pineapple juice has been absorbed. Add butter, honey, cinnamon, and more salt to taste. Cool. When cool fold in toasted coconut and fresh fruit. Moisten with coconut cream, thick cow's cream, or yogurt.

Coconut Candy, "Amedama"

Mix grated, unsweetened coconut or coconut meal with honey (instead of honey, the Marquesans use a coconut syrup called jekemai), squeezing mixture with your hands very hard to make a stiff dough. Form dough into small balls the size of a marble and allow them to stand at room temperature for 2 hours. Refrigerate, covered, until ready to serve. They are very rich and should only be eaten as an accent food.

This mixture is also kneaded with mashed ripe bananas and a little lime juice or mashed steamed potatoes and formed into patties, which are wrapped in leaves and carried as a snack.

THE LIGHT BITE, MARQUESAN STYLE

A QUICK MEAL: Canned sardines, cold baked sweet potato, and a fresh fruit.

A SNACK: Mash cooked sweet potatoes. Season with coconut oil or butter and salt; form into small patties. Roll patties in warm honey, then toasted coconut. Eat cold or warm.

The Nomadic Tuareg
of the Sahara

It is said, "Allah removed all surplus human and animal life from the desert so there might be one place for Him to walk in peace . . . and so the Great Sahara is called the Garden of Allah."

Allah, however, shares His garden with a group of people unique in the world, the nomadic Tuareg.

The Sahara covers an area larger than the continental United States. Some of it is mountainous, much of it sand, and all of it arid. Annual rainfall is about two inches, and recently even this small amount has failed to materialize.

Geological evidence shows that as recently as the last Ice Age the Sahara was a dense jungle. Skeletal remains of South African animals have been found throughout much of the area. Centuries ago a cataclysmic earthquake drained what must have been lakes and a sea and created a vast desert. Into this barren, incredibly hostile wasteland, came the Tuareg. Related to the Berbers of the North African coastal areas, they are light-skinned, tall, handsome people. Being nomads, they have no use for civilization or farming and they look with contempt upon those who settled into agriculture. There is an ancient Tuareg saying: "Shame enters the family that tills the land."

Numbering about 300,000 (the figure is an educated guess because no accurate census has ever been taken), they are divided into two major groups, the northern Tuareg of Hoggar and the southerners of the Niger area. The northern Tuareg regard the southerners with a certain amount of disdain because they have intermarried with the local population and have discontinued, to some extent, the nomadic life.

Tuareg society has a rigid caste system; the nobles, who are strictly nomadic and consider any sort of work demeaning; their vassals, who travel with the tribe and do all the work including the cooking, herding, and general labor around the camp; and the slaves, who live permanently at the various oases that serve as Tuareg ports-of-call. The slaves, and they truly are, are well treated. They raise the food and make the goods used by the Tuareg nobles. Although they are allowed to keep a small portion of the food they raise, most of it goes to nobles of the tribes. There are subdivisions in this caste system, the Tuareg are a very complicated society, but by and large, everyone falls into one of these major castes.

Extremely religious, the Tuareg are Moslems although they have adapted many of the rules of Islam to life in their difficult environment. They are loyal to a fault, honorable and trustworthy with their friends, gracious with strangers, and devoted to their families. They are among the fiercest fighters in the world, neither asking nor giving quarter, hunters of superb skill and daring and, for many centuries, caravan hijackers of unquestioned success. When the French assumed control of North Africa, the Tuareg were the last to capitulate. Fierce pitched battles were fought across the desert sands and at fortified oases. When it all finally ended with the French clearly victorious, the Tuareg grudgingly treated them as equals. If the French had lost, they would have been treated as slaves. No one conquers a Tuareg, except of course, the Sahara.

Tuareg nomadic life is dictated by their huge herds of animals, said to outnumber the people forty to one. Their goats and sheep, camels and horses must be moved from grazing area to grazing area—the desert oases in winter, the mountains in summer. They rarely stay more than a month in one location as their huge herds quickly denude the land of all vegetation. These herds are absolutely vital to the Tuareg; they provide food, clothing, housing, a means of barter, and transportation. Because of the tribes' nomadic life, formal education is often overlooked, if not totally ignored. The French, knowing they could never change this pattern of living, sent teachers along with the tribes to try and educate the children and young men. Skill in simple arithmetic, reading, and writing was the most they could hope to achieve, but the Tuareg grudgingly admitted that their youngsters were better able to barter with traders if they knew a little about figures. They realized that for years they had been cheated by the shrewd and educated Arabs.

The Tuareg have one money crop, salt. They control most of the salt mines in the Sahara and they make yearly caravans to major North African cities, laden with salt to sell.

The horror of the salt mines can hardly be described. Tuareg slaves—men, women, and even children—dig and haul the salt slabs all year round. In summer the temperature soars to 150 degrees, but still they work. In winter, the nights are freezing and there is no protection from the fierce winds. Their only heat comes from burning camel dung. Men die of old age at forty, their skin tanned almost like leather from the dehydrating effects of heat and salt. Once or twice a year, the Tuareg caravans arrive at the mines. They buy the salt for a few pennies, load it on their camels and make the dangerous trip to Timbuktu or Hoggar, across the miles of trackless desert. With no maps or charts, somehow they know unerringly where they are. That these desert trips are dangerous indeed is borne out by the fact that caravans have disappeared entirely on several occasions. One recent disaster was the loss of a caravan of 1,200 camels and 200 men during a desert sand storm. They were buried by the raging storm and no trace of them was ever found. Comparable to the loss of a ship with all hands, such a catastrophe invites comparison between the Sahara and the sea.

Tuareg clothing is quite distinctive. Through the centuries, a certain type of dress has evolved that is well suited to the scorching heat and blowing sand of the desert. Many generations ago, the loose, smock-like garment all Tuareg wear was made of some kind of supple leather, deerskin or goatskin. This has been replaced by a lightweight cotton material. The smock is a single length of cloth, loosely tied at the sides, with a hole for the head. Wide-legged pantaloons are worn under the smock. Thong sandals, worn by everyone—men, women, and children—protect their feet from the searing sand, which, incidentally, can literally burn, making blistered feet a real danger on the desert.

The women wear a shawl around their shoulders, sometimes drawing it over their heads, but they are not veiled as so many Moslem women are. The men are veiled. Beginning about puberty, the men wear a veil that covers their entire face; only the eyes are visible. This veil is *never* removed in public and only rarely in the privacy of their families. The origin of the veil is lost in antiquity.

Undoubtedly it was first used as protection from the sun and sand, but no one can say when the custom of wearing it continuously began. The nobles wear veils dyed indigo blue, which rubs off and stains their skin; for years Tuareg noblemen have been called the Blue Men of the Desert. It is considered extremely offensive to see a man with his face exposed, a belief so rigid that very few pictures exist of Tuareg men, which is rather a pity as the Tuareg are extremely handsome. Some young and enlightened fellows who have just begun to wear the veil will allow their pictures to be taken, but this is rare. None of the older men would dream of removing their veils for a photographer.

Along with an array of beads and ornaments, every Tuareg noble wears a long, straight sword, the scabbard beautifully engraved, hanging from a wide belt. He also wears a dagger attached by a clip to his left arm. This is not a throwing knife—that is for savages; this is a close-quarter fighting knife. Gold is never used but the women are heavily laden with silver ornaments. They paint their fingers and toes with henna and darken their eyes with kohl. Tuareg women are noted for their beauty and arrogance.

The Tuareg are a matriarchal society; that is, they are ruled by a man but their lineage is traced through the women. From about fourteen or fifteen, the girls are carefully instructed by their mothers in the arts of love. Great emphasis is placed on sexual compatibility in marriage and the young women are encouraged to have as much sexual experience as possible before marriage. This is done with dignity and discretion and is not considered promiscuous. The woman usually chooses the man she wants to marry. He must of course be able to produce the bride price of seven female camels and he should be of the same caste. However, if a noblewoman marries a vassal, their children will be considered nobles. The Tuareg are generally in the middle twenties when they marry, rather old in comparison with many cultures.

Being a matriarchal society, the women have equal status with the men and unlike their sisters in most Moslem countries, they are not veiled. They may own property and are consulted in all tribal and family matters. The families are very close and display great affection for one another. The men respect all women, but they adore their wives.

That the Tuareg are extremely healthy and strong, with enormous endurance, comes as something of a surprise considering their diet and their environment. Their staple food is *couscous,* a coarse-ground grain stew of millet, wheat, and/or sorghum, steamed into a thick mush with vegetables and occasionally some meat. They eat this three times a day when in camp. The couscous is served with dates, goat cheese, yogurt, ghee (a form of butter), and several quarts of camel's milk. When they are traveling with their herds from oasis to oasis, their daily food is often restricted to camel's milk and dates. Occasionally, they will vary this with a bowl of steamed millet in the middle of the day.

A group of anthropologists who were traveling with the Tuareg decided that they'd had their fill of camel's milk and absolutely couldn't face another curdled cup. They drank water or tea instead. To their dismay, they quickly developed scurvy, a nutritional deficiency disease unknown among the Tuareg. The anthropologists decided the milk, fresh or sour, had better be included in their diet, no matter how sick of the taste they got. Camel's milk is comparable to goat's milk in nutritional quality. A daily intake of five quarts, not uncommon for an adult Tuareg, contains 50 units of Vitamin C, 7,800 units of Vitamin A, plus a good level of niacin. It has a better quality protein than cow's milk and is easier to digest. Milk and dates make an excellent nutritional combination. Milk, a near-perfect food, is low in iron and lacks fiber. Both of these are found in dates.

Although milk is liquid, it is a food. During digestion, it curdles and hardens into solid form so in addition to milk, the Tuareg have to drink huge quantities of water to maintain the body's fluid level in the blazing Sahara heat. They usually drink about three to five quarts a day in camp and sometimes twice that amount on the trail.

The milk, along with twelve or more cups of tea and several quarts of water, adds up to an incredible fluid intake. This, however, is the amount necessary to sustain life on the desert. The heat is so intense and searing, fluid loss is a constant hazard. A 5 percent loss of body fluid causes extreme fatigue and irrational behavior. The victim will follow a mirage and wander off into the desert to certain death. A 10 percent loss is usually fatal. Through the years, the Tuareg have developed a system of treating heat prostration that is pretty successful. They know a drink of water would be deadly so they tie a bunch of dates in a cloth, wet it, and squeeze drops into the victim's mouth. This method of revival has frequently worked.

Their custom of never removing the veil works something of a hardship on Tuareg men at mealtimes. Everyone sits in a circle on the floor with the common pot of couscous in the middle. Each dips his wooden spoon into the area directly in front of him to scoop out a bit. The men must lift their veils away from their faces and slip the spoonful of food into their mouths without showing their faces or disturbing their intricately wrapped drapery. It's not easy to get a meal down this way; foreigners who have tried declare it's impossible. As the bowl of couscous is being consumed, everyone is careful not to disturb the very center, as that untouched island of food is for Allah.

Tea is drunk constantly during festival seasons and four times a day the rest of the time: right after sunrise, at about two in the afternoon, late in the day, and immediately after sunset. There is a ritual in this tea drinking as stylized as the Japanese tea ceremony. Two pots are used, one to boil tea and one to boil water. Three two-ounce glasses are consumed each time—one for the host, one for the guest, and one for Allah. This never varies. The nobles regard their tea ceremony very seriously and stop whatever they are doing to observe the custom. Fortunately, they have little else to do in camp so these frequent tea breaks don't interfere with work to any extent. On the desert trails, custom is abandoned for convenience and tea is drunk when the opportunity arises, not at any special time.

Curiously, the Tuareg's limited diet is very well balanced. Camel's milk, dates, and grains are all high in nutritional quality. The grains used in the couscous provide satisfaction, energy, and bulk. Yogurt, a great favorite of the Tuareg, supplies essential enzymes and is an excellent source of protein and calcium. Another one of their basic foods, ghee, is made by melting goat's milk butter with salt and water. As it separates, the milky residue, much like the substance in clarified butter, is removed and mixed with their other foods. Ghee, which they rub on their bodies to protect them from the drying effects of the sun, is an important fat and Vitamin A source in their diet.

Camel's milk is consumed raw, fresh, or soured. It is never cooked. One of many Tuareg superstitions is that the camel will smell the boiling milk and refuse to produce any more. Fresh camel's milk is extremely sweet-tasting, but sours so quickly that cheese cannot be made from it. The Tuareg make their cheese and yogurt from goat's milk. In making cheese, this simple procedure is followed. They fill a goatskin bag with warm milk, tie it to their camel saddle and, during a day of travel, the cheese is produced. The cheese is dried rock-hard and grated as needed. Their yogurt starter is a piece of cloth that has been dipped into a batch of yogurt. This cloth can be dried, carried for days, dropped into a container of warm milk and, in a few hours, the yogurt is ready.

When the Tuareg eat meat, about once a week, it is usually game they have shot or a sickly sheep or goat culled from their herd. The animal is bled first according to Moslem custom, gutted, and immediately placed over the fire on a spit. The organs are cooked and eaten separately, as is the head, which usually serves as dessert. The Tuareg are very fond of spices, no doubt as a result of the many spice caravans they raided, and paprika, rich in bioflavonoids, is used generously. When food is scarce, as it frequently is, or when they are on a long caravan, the Tuareg often fast, more from necessity than choice. Even this imposed fasting, however, contributes to their well-being.

Studies have shown that animals that fast periodically live two-and-a-half to five times longer than animals that eat continuously. At a recent (1972) symposium on the relationship between nutrition and longevity, a group of experts in the field agreed that the restriction of food intake to the point that would be considered undernutrition by contemporary standards both lengthens the life and improves the health by reducing susceptibility to diseases of aging. A principal reason for disease and premature aging is disordered metabolism and the consequent retention of waste matter in the cells and tissues. Rational fasting, that is, a day or two of drinking juices and liquids with no intake of solid food, is a safe way of cleansing the body of accumulated toxins. This can help restore and normalize all the vital functions.

In spite of the Tuareg's harsh living conditions and uncertain food supply, they are extremely healthy people. Because of their high mineral diet of milk and millet, together with the Vitamin D they receive from the sun, their bones and teeth are sound and strong. Their life of strenuous exercise out in the open has given them great endurance, a source of wonder to Europeans who have had close contact with them. They can travel for days at a time and arrive at their destination showing no signs of fatigue. Infant mortality is quite high, due to their living conditions and the desert heat, but if a child survives to four or five, barring accidental death, he or she can expect to have a long and healthy life.

Few sights stir the imagination or evoke more admiration than that of a noble Tuareg, veiled in blue, sitting ramrod straight on a racing camel—a vision that must have struck terror in the hearts of caravan drivers in the past. The camels bred by the Tuareg are the finest in the world. Sought by traders all over North Africa, they are the Tuareg's most prized possession. They are pure white, fast, sturdy, and nearly indestructible. Camels can go three to five days without food or water with little or no ill effects. They can lose up to 22 percent of their body fluid and recover it in ten minutes at an oasis water hole. They can carry tremendous loads for days at a time; however, no domestic animal in the world has a worse disposition. With a malevolent look and screams of outrage, a camel that has been ridden for years will suddenly throw his rider and refuse to be mounted again. They are intractable, unmanageable, and absolutely vital to the Tuareg. No other animal—horse, donkey, or any beast of burden—can survive on the desert like the camel. Most Tuareg would rather starve than sacrifice one of their precious herd, but once in a while the choice must be made. To survive, the men will kill a camel. Like the cow, the camel is a ruminant with several stomachs. Once the decision has been made to kill the animal, it is opened up at the second stomach. This stomach contains a bloody, watery fluid that is nourishing and refreshing if somewhat repulsive to consume, and it can keep a human being alive. When a camel becomes old or sick, it is turned loose in the desert. It may or may not survive, *Insh Allah*. "It is the will of Allah."

Throughout the Sahara there is only one means of transportation that is more dependable than the camel and that is the truck. Slowly but inevitably, motor vehicles are replacing camels all across the desert wastes. Well-marked roads connect the various oases and newly created African countries have claimed large territories once part of the Tuareg's domain. When the land was being portioned out, the Tuareg were overlooked, so now there is no place they can call their own. To add to their problem, a severe drought has caused many of the desert oases to dry up and the huge grazing areas to disappear. The Tuareg, once masters of the

Sahara, are now its victims. Their enormous herds are dying from lack of food and water, and countless thousands of Tuareg are dying along with them. Unable to give up their nomadic ways, few of the haughty Tuareg have turned to farming, even though the various nations bordering the Sahara have urged them to do so, going so far as to offer them land and equipment.

Even if the rains come in time to save the remaining Tuareg, their way of life is virtually ended. After centuries of survival, there is no room, even in the vast Sahara, for their continued existence. Unlike many primitive cultures, it isn't altered diet that is the cause of their distress; the truck, the airplane, and the newly created African countries all are conspiring to defeat the proud, unconquered Tuareg. Their inflexibility in the face of encroaching civilization, their inability to adapt in order to survive, will eventually prove to be their downfall. The Tuareg camel caravans will disappear from the desert; their colorful encampments will no longer brighten an oasis; their riding contests, more like pitched battles than competitive sports, will be forgotten. The uncharted sweep of the Sahara will no longer be their domain. Allah will no longer share His garden with the Tuareg.

FOODS OF THE TUAREG

"Shame enters the family that tills the land." The Tuareg live, or perhaps die, by this ancient belief. Limited to what their herds produce or to food obtained at an oasis, the Tuareg diet is delicately balanced. If they cannot barter for food at a village, they must live on camel's milk, yogurt, and ghee. Still, they would rather starve than bring shame upon their families by farming.

Dates

The staple food of the Tuareg, dates, are as important to them as rice is to the Oriental. Because they are 78 percent natural sugar, dates are a fine energy source; they are called the bread of the desert. Dates add iron, potassium, niacin, and fiber to the basic milk diet and together they supply the Tuareg with nutrition of the highest quality. The very best dates are used for trade and barter, while those that are left may sometimes be stuffed into goatskins, pressed, and made into a sort of marmalade. Others are pitted and shaped into bricks, which keep for a long time and can be easily transported. Some dates are also dried and ground, pits and all, into meal, a form in which they are usually carried on a caravan. The meal is formed into a ball and, along with goat's milk, makes a nutritious snack or meal. When dates become sour, they are made into vinegar.

Grains

Millet is the most popular of the grains among the Tuareg, although wheat, barley, and sorghum are sometimes combined with it. Ground millet is the most frequent basis of couscous, the classic North African dish which is made from various grains. The grains are ground between ancient millstones that contribute bits of lime and roughage in the grinding process. The grain is broken up just enough to make it easy to eat, but all the nutrients are retained. Couscous is made by steaming the grain and setting it out to dry in the sun. When the couscous is needed, hot water is added and a thick, cereal-like food is formed. To this are added bits of meat, dried cheese, or vegetables. While on a caravan, the Tuareg often eat the couscous plain. As a convenience food it is unbeatable.

CHIEF SOURCES OF NUTRIENTS IN THE TUAREG DIET

PROTEIN	milk and milk products
FAT	cream
CARBOHYDRATE	millet
CALORIES	milk
VITAMIN A	cream
VITAMIN C	sprouts and milk in quantity
VITAMIN B_1	millet
VITAMIN B_2	milk
NIACIN	millet
CALCIUM	milk
IRON	millet
FIBER	millet

Flour made from ground millet is used in making noodles and bread. When on a caravan, the Tuareg make their bread by mixing flour and water, kneading it thoroughly on a saddle blanket that is spread on the ground, forming it into balls, and tossing them into the embers. When the bread is baked, the ashes are brushed off, the ball of dough is dipped into butter and eaten. Millet and camel milk and a few dates make up the usual meal while on the trail. Because the millet has an extremely high iron content, it makes a fine combination with milk. The easiest to digest of all the grains, millet has been shown to support life better than any of the other cereals. It contains three times more iron than any other grain and is one of the best sources of nitrilosides (B_{17}) available. When combined with milk, its protein quality is excellent.

Lentils and Garbanzos

These beans are commonly dried by the Tuareg. They are cooked in stews or ground into flour and used with millet in the making of noodles or porridge. Both of these beans are a fine source of incomplete protein, iron, B vitamins, and fiber. They are extremely rich in the essential amino acid, lysine, which makes up the deficiency of this amino acid in the millet. When combined with millet, they form a fine quality protein.*

Milk

The value of milk in human nutrition has been hotly disputed. Some authorities claim that milk is a perfect food for man—others insist that it is poison to man and causes allergies and respiratory problems. The answer seems to be quite simple: Milk is an excellent food for people whose ancestors herded dairy animals and traditionally lived on dairy products. Most white Americans of European ancestry fall into this group. Orientals do not; black Africans do not. After weaning, milk is not advisable in their diet and other substitutes should be found. Many who can't seem to tolerate whole fresh milk can take it in a soured form such as yogurt, cottage cheese, or buttermilk. Because fermented foods are partly predigested, they are easier to assimilate.

* Protein quality means the percent of protein in a given food that the body can actually use as protein.

The camel's and goat's milk used by the Tuareg is superior to cow's milk because it forms smaller curds in the stomach, which makes it easier to digest. These milks also contain slightly more minerals and vitamins. While this difference is insignificant in normal milk consumption, it becomes a factor when huge quantities are consumed, as in the case of the Tuareg. For instance, the Vitamin C in three quarts of raw camel's milk is enough to prevent scurvy, but even this quantity would be insufficient if it was pasteurized cow's milk. Whole raw milk is an excellent food. The protein quality is 82 percent, and is topped only by eggs, which boast a protein quality of 94 percent.* Milk is an excellent source of most vitamins and minerals and, in sufficient quantity, will support life and growth. When whole raw milk sours, it is still good food. A common dish of the Tuareg is the curd of camel's milk mixed with noodles and sprinkled with paprika. This quick meal can be eaten while on a caravan and is very nutritious.

Butter is made by churning milk in a goatskin bag tied to the camel's saddle. The butter churns during the course of a day's ride. Butter is not used in cooking, but the Tuareg dip their bread into it. Ghee is used in much the same manner. It is made by heating butter and adding salted water. The cooled mixture forms two layers; the milky lower layer is the ghee and the top layer is clarified butter. The ghee, which keeps better than butter, is eaten poured over noodles and grains. The cheese, yogurt, and ghee are made from goat's milk because camel's milk turns sour so quickly it is impossible to use. Camel's milk is for drinking or curds only. As indicated earlier, the Tuareg dry their cheese until it is rock hard, then grate it and mix it with their food.

Meat

The Tuareg are very fond of meat, but they do not like to slaughter animals, so meat isn't a major part of their diet. If it is sickly, a goat may be killed for a very special occasion. Gazelle, antelope, and wild desert sheep occasionally find their way to the table. Giraffe is considered the best of the game meats and ostrich is sometimes served, but the Blue Men don't like to kill for food. The men are skilled hunters and they enjoy the sport of the hunt, but

* Protein quality means the percent of protein in a given food that the body can actually use as protein.

often they will purposely miss their target. When in camp, they eat meat more frequently, once or even twice a week, but on caravans weeks may go by without the taste of meat. They even have a word in their language for "meat hunger"; and they will celebrate their arrival at an oasis with a huge gluttonous feast. The Tuareg are famous for the tender and delicious meat they serve, a result, probably, of the manner in which the animal is prepared. It is skinned, cleaned, and roasted before the flesh has had a chance to cool. The head is cooked separately and served as a dessert. It will be offered to an honored guest first. The Tuareg, understandably, do not eat fish, and the only eggs they eat are ostrich eggs.

Palm Oil

The solid yellowish or reddish oil obtained from the fruit of several species of palm is a real luxury food for these nomads. While it is never used in cooking, the Tuareg do make a sauce of palm oil, yogurt, and curry to pour over vegetables. Palm oil contains more saturated fat than most vegetable oils and is the only one that contains Vitamin A.

Spices

Spices are very important to the Tuareg. Like most people living in hot climates, Tuareg spice their foods heavily. Their favorites are red peppers, curry, and ginger, along with garlic, onion, and mint for their tea. Hot spicy foods are important for people in the desert climates, for they promote perspiration, which cools the body. Of course, additional salt must be taken to maintain the proper fluid balance. Probably their most important spice is paprika. It has been said that paprika was first used as a preservative for meats, and failing that, to conceal the fact that it had failed. It is an extremely good source of the bioflavonoids, the complex vitamins of the C family, and is important in the prevention of scurvy. The Tuareg sprinkle it heavily on their foods when on their caravans. Unlike our common black pepper, which can irritate the stomach lining, these spices stimulate digestive juices and aid the digestive process.

Mint and Peppermint

The Tuareg generally add mint leaves to green tea, or sometimes the tea is made entirely of mint. Mint and peppermint have long enjoyed a reputation as potent natural digestive aids. Peppermint has been used for a variety of ills since Egyptian times. It is a valuable herb for relieving the pain of gastrointestinal problems and it stimulates the digestive juices. Contradictory as it seems, hot beverages do cool a person down by stimulating perspiration. That this is well known to the Tuareg is evident from their custom of drinking hot tea four times a day.

Vegetables

The vegetables these desert people most frequently serve include squash, turnip, pumpkin, okra, carrots, artichoke, onions, peppers, tomatoes, garlic, and spinach. They are usually cooked as a stew to serve with couscous. Often the vegetables are steamed over the grain while it's being cooked, the vegetable juices seeping down and flavoring the grain so they are not wasted. Cooked carrots are an outstanding source of Vitamin A in the Tuareg stew. Because of the tough cellulose protecting their cells, much of the Vitamin A in raw carrots is unobtainable. Yellow squash, red peppers, and tomatoes, however, are other good sources of this vitamin. Sometimes the vegetables are air-dried and ground into flour to be made into a mush. A favorite meal is vegetable mush served with okra and spinach. The vegetable flour is also added to grain flour and made into noodles. When on caravan, sprouts of wild grasses may be gathered along the trail and added to the dinner. These sprouts are a source of Vitamin C for the traveling Tuareg.

Seeds

In summer the women and children gather seeds of wild grasses to dry for future use. These are crushed with a mortar and pestle and combined with other grains. Seeds add essential fat, Vitamins E and B, as well as protein and iron to the Tuareg diet. Melon seeds are a great favorite but hard to come by. They are saved for special occasions or honored guests.

Insects

Locusts are sometimes eaten by the Tuareg. They are usually roasted whole, the wings and legs being removed by the diner, who then dips the insect into salt. They are crunchy and taste something like pork. Locusts may also be dried and ground into meal to be used with grain flour. Dried locusts are an excellent source of protein; they contain up to 75 percent in contrast to fresh beef, whose protein content is about 25 to 36 percent. They are also a good source of B vitamins, iron, and Vitamin D. They are a fine food for hungry people.

DINING WITH A TUAREG FAMILY

Picture an encampment of brightly colored tents clustered among the palms of a desert oasis. Veiled men and unveiled women drift from tent to tent accompanied by the chink and jingle of bracelets and bejeweled necklaces. Camels, goats, and magnificent Arabian stallions are corraled a short distance away. A scene for a movie spectacular? A setting from the *Tales of the Arabian Nights?* Not at all! It's a Tuareg band at one of their regular stops. Resting, eating, repairing gear, and giving their animals a chance to graze before they push on to another oasis in their endless wandering about the Sahara.

An average Tuareg tent is made from about thirty or forty goatskins, while the head nobleman may have a huge tent formed from a hundred skins or more. The vibrant variety of shades and colors characteristic of a Tuareg encampment comes from the dyes rubbed on the goatskins during the curing process. The skins are cured by rubbing them with butter to which the dye is added. The seams are sewn together with thin strips of leather, while posts of tamarisk branches make up the frame over which the hides are stretched. The tent sides are open, but at night beautifully decorated reed mats are let down to form walls. The tent is always erected so the entrance faces east and the rising sun. Inside the tent the right side is for the men of the family and their possessions, and the left for the women. Exquisite and extremely valuable Persian rugs cover the dirt floors. Sometimes a great pile of rugs will be used as a couch. They must be shaken a couple of times a day as they are a favorite hiding place of the desert scorpion. For an adult the sting is wretchedly painful, but it can be fatal for a child.

Leather bags for storing grains and dates hang from the tamarisk tent frame. Drinking water is stored in skin sacks and butter in the horns of desert sheep. Clay pots are often used for cooking and simple wooden dishes, spoons, and bowls serve for tableware. The fire for cooking is always built away from the tent.

In camp everyone is busy. The women make butter, cheese, and yogurt and also grind the grains. The men repair saddles, see to their precious herds, or engage in a free-for-all on horseback that is euphemistically called a game. During the day everyone sort of snacks. The men like to take their frequent tea breaks with a group of friends, while the women and children content themselves with some milk and yogurt along with dates or a bowl of millet. But as evening approaches more dried dung is added to the fire. Wood is virtually unattainable on the desert so dung is the usual fuel. When the pot of couscous is ready, rugs or saddle blankets are placed in a circle and the family remove their sandals and gather to share their main meal. The common pot of couscous, with wooden spoons planted vertically in it, is placed in the center on a goatskin. At its side is the sauce and roasted meat, if any is to be served. As he eats, the man must hold his veil away with his left hand, which is quite a trick if he is trying to eat a piece of meat with his other hand. Everyone is careful not to encroach on his neighbor's share, nor on the little island that must be left in the center for Allah. From time to time a sauce is poured on the grain.

The Tuareg usually drink milk, water, or mint tea with their dinner. They like spices and use hot red peppers, ginger, and curry generously.

After dinner the fathers often recite poetry or sing to the family, accompanying themselves on a simple one-stringed instrument. The women always share in family events and at this time the mother may advise or instruct the children in these arts while the father often listens. As the fire dies and the sky becomes brilliant with the light from a million stars, the Tuareg must truly love their desert home.

A TUAREG DINNER PER INDIVIDUAL

MILLET, steamed, ½ cup uncooked
VEGETABLE STEW
  lentils, ⅓ cup uncooked
  onion, ½ medium size
  carrot, ½ large
  tomato, ½ medium size
  green pepper, ½ medium size
SAUCE, YOGURT, made from
  goat's milk, ½ cup
  palm oil, 1 tablespoon
  curry and powdered red pepper

A TUAREG DINNER FROM YOUR KITCHEN

VEGETABLE CURRY* ON MILLET WITH CURRY SAUCE

To serve vegetable curry place cooked millet on a large metal tray or platter. Place vegetables on top of the millet and pour some of the curry sauce over all. Sprinkle generously with paprika. Serve the extra curry sauce in a pitcher.

The condiments can be served in small dishes. Each diner can then sprinkle what he wants on his portion of food.

* For a special meal, roasted lamb shanks can be added.

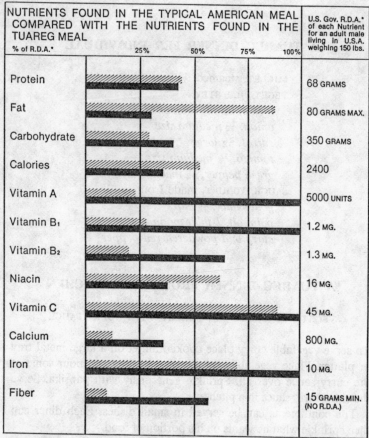

NUTRIENTS FOUND IN THE TYPICAL AMERICAN MEAL COMPARED WITH THE NUTRIENTS FOUND IN THE TUAREG MEAL					U.S. Gov. R.D.A.* of each Nutrient for an adult male living in U.S.A. weighing 150 lbs.
% of R.D.A.*	25%	50%	75%	100%	
Protein					68 GRAMS
Fat					80 GRAMS MAX.
Carbohydrate					350 GRAMS
Calories					2400
Vitamin A					5000 UNITS
Vitamin B$_1$					1.2 MG.
Vitamin B$_2$					1.3 MG.
Niacin					16 MG.
Vitamin C					45 MG.
Calcium					800 MG.
Iron					10 MG.
Fiber					15 GRAMS MIN. (NO R.D.A.)

*R.D.A. is the recommended daily nutrient allowance intended to meet the needs of a *healthy* individual.

Diagonal lines represent the American meal.

The chief sources of nutrients in the Tuareg meal are:

PROTEIN	lentils and millet
FAT	palm oil
CARBOHYDRATE	millet
CALORIES	millet
VITAMIN A	carrot
VITAMIN B_1	millet
VITAMIN B_2	millet
NIACIN	green pepper
VITAMIN C	green pepper
CALCIUM	yogurt
IRON	millet
FIBER	millet and lentils

Vegetable Curry

2 cups millet, raw
1⅓ cups lentils
14½-ounce can tomatoes
2 cloves garlic, minced
2 medium green peppers, cut in wedges
2 large carrots, cut in 1-inch pieces
2 medium onions, cut in wedges
1½ teaspoons curry powder, or to taste
½ tablespoon butter

Cook onions, curry, and garlic in butter until limp. Add juice from the tomatoes plus enough water to make 2¾ cup liquid. Bring to boil. Add lentils and tomatoes. Simmer, covered, 20 minutes or until lentils are almost tender. Add carrots and green peppers and simmer until carrots are just tender but still crisp, about 20 minutes. If much liquid remains, remove vegetables and reduce the liquid by boiling. Return vegetables to pan. Salt to taste and add more curry if you wish. (To add meat to the vegetable curry, see the Tuareg Lamb Shanks recipe on page 50.)

Millet

Bring 4 cups of water to boil; add 2 cups of millet. Simmer, covered, 30 minutes. Remove from heat but do not lift lid. Let millet stand 15 minutes. Add salt to taste. Place millet in large dish, put vegetable curry on top, and cover all with curry sauce (recipe follows).

Curry Sauce

2½ cups yogurt
3 tablespoons butter
Curry powder
Paprika

Melt butter; add yogurt and curry powder to taste. Heat sauce and blend carefully but do not cook or stir vigorously as this will thin the yogurt.

Condiments

Lentil or other sprouts; raw tomato, green onion (including tops), olives, dates, all chopped; walnuts or raisins.

For a celebration, lamb shanks would be a welcome addition to the vegetable curry. Reduce the millet and lentil portions by half and allow one small lamb shank per person. As an alternate, use heated marinade in place of curry sauce.

Tuareg Lamb Shanks

4 small lamb shanks (one per portion)
2 cups yogurt
1 cup chopped onion
2 cloves garlic, minced
1 teaspoon salt

Mix all ingredients together and marinate lamb shanks at least 24 hours, turning occasionally. Cook over a charcoal fire or broil until brown on the outside but still juicy within. Heat marinade, add curry powder to taste, and serve over the vegetables and millet. Chicken or turkey legs may be substituted for lamb shanks. Dry them and coat with oil before cooking. Turkey will require about 2 hours and chicken about 30 minutes to cook, as their internal temperature must reach 180 degrees. If they become too brown, place on a rack in a 300° oven to finish cooking. It is best to use a meat thermometer on turkey.

Couscous Dinner

> 2 cups couscous (semolina, available at specialty stores); you
> may substitute millet or other grain cooked in chicken broth
> for a more nutritious meal
> ¼ cup butter or sesame seed oil
> 1 pound lean stewing lamb or meat cut from a leg of lamb (1
> disjointed chicken may be substituted but reduce cooking time
> by about 45 minutes)
> 3 cups chicken broth plus 3 cups water including liquid from
> garbanzo beans
> 1 large onion, chopped
> 1 cup carrots, cut in ¾-inch pieces
> 1 cup parsnips, cut in 1-inch pieces
> 1 cup cooked garbanzo beans
> 1 cup green beans
> 1 cinnamon stick about 3 inches long
> 5 whole cloves
> 1 8-ounce package cream cheese
> 2 tablespoons lemon juice
> ½ cup pine nuts
> ½ cup green seedless grapes, or ¼ cup raisins

Cut meat into 1½-inch cubes and trim visible fat from it. In a frying
pan heat enough butter to brown the pine nuts lightly. Stir constantly
so they do not burn. Set nuts aside and add enough butter to the pan
to brown the lamb on all sides. Put browned lamb in a large kettle and
in the same pan used to brown the lamb, sauté the onions until they
are golden brown. Place onions, carrots, parsnips, 1 cup of chicken
broth, salt, cinnamon stick, and cloves in kettle with meat. Put prepared couscous (directions follow) or cooked grain on top of stew in
a steamer basket or colander. Cover pan and heat to boiling. Reduce
heat and simmer 1 hour. Add garbanzo beans, green beans, and
lemon juice and slowly blend the cream cheese mixed with 1 cup of
chicken broth into the stew. Simmer covered 30 minutes. Add grapes
and simmer 15 minutes or until meat and vegetables are tender.
Remove cinnamon stick. Mix the pine nuts into the stew.

Remove couscous to a large, shallow bowl and place meat and vegetables on top of it. Pour some of the broth over the couscous, keeping
the rest warm to add as you eat.

Couscous

Place the 2 cups of grain in a large kettle and pour 4 cups of boiling chicken broth over it. Cover pan and allow it to stand in a warm place 20 minutes. If it should become too dry, add more hot broth. Add 2 tablespoons of butter to the grain, and salt to taste.

Barbecued Heart

Cut heart into ½-inch slices. Brush with vegetable oil flavored with garlic. Cook on a grill over a charcoal fire, or broil only until the meat is light pink inside. Serve topped with warm sour cream or yogurt seasoned with chopped green onion and garlic powder to taste. Lentils are very good served with heart and sour cream.

Eggplant Stew

2 tablespoons olive oil
1 medium onion, chopped
1 clove garlic, minced
¾ pound eggplant, cut in 1-inch cubes
1 medium green pepper, cut in ¼-inch strips
1 medium zucchini, cut in ½-inch slices
1-pound can tomatoes, including juice
1 teaspoon dried basil leaves
1 teaspoon salt

Cook onion and garlic in oil until limp. Add remaining vegetables, cover and simmer, stirring occasionally until vegetables are tender, about 25 minutes. Remove vegetables and reduce remaining liquid by cooking over high heat uncovered. Pour concentrated liquid over vegetables. To serve sprinkle with dried and grated goat or romano cheese or cover with yogurt mixed with curry powder. This dish is very good eaten straight from the refrigerator as a snack.

Sesame Dip, "Humas"

2 cups garbanzo beans, cooked (other legumes may be used)
¾ cup sesame seeds, ground (other seeds or nuts may be used)
Sesame oil or other vegetable oil

Mash or whirl in a blender drained garbanzo beans and mix with ground sesame seed. Add enough oil to form a thick paste of the consistency of peanut butter. Chill. Serve as dip for vegetables or spread on whole grain bread or crackers. The Tuareg flavor the humas with garlic and lemon juice and pour a little olive oil over the top.

Lentil and Wheat Stew, "Imjudara"

½ cup lentils
3½ cups water
2 tablespoons vegetable oil
2 onions, chopped
1 to 2 cloves garlic, minced
¼ pound fresh mushrooms, sliced
1 cup bulgur (cracked wheat)
⅛ teaspoon oregano
⅛ teaspoon powdered cayenne
⅛ teaspoon paprika
6 green onions, including green tops, chopped
Salt to taste

Bring water to boil and add lentils. Cover, reduce heat, and simmer 30 minutes. Heat oil in a skillet and cook onion and garlic until onions are brown and just slightly burned. Add onions, garlic, bulgur, and spices to lentils. Cover and simmer until water is absorbed, about 15 to 20 minutes. Fold in the raw mushrooms, chopped green onions, and salt to taste. Serve imjudara topped with yogurt or sour cream flavored with curry powder.

Bulgur Salad, "Tabbouleh"

½ cup bulgur (parboiled cracked wheat)   ⅓ cup lemon juice
1 cup minced parsley   ½ teaspoon salt
⅓ cup green onion including tops, minced   ¼ teaspoon pepper
1 clove garlic, minced   ¼ cup pine nuts
¼ cup fresh mint, minced   ⅓ cup olive oil
2 cups tomatoes, peeled and
  coarsely chopped

Add bulgur to 1 cup hot water. Cover pan and allow it to stand in a warm spot 15 to 20 minutes, until the water is absorbed. Place bulgur in a bowl and allow it to cool. Add green onions, garlic, pine nuts, parsley, mint, and tomatoes. Stir in lemon juice, salt and pepper. Let stand ½ hour so that flavors can blend. Add oil and serve. Romaine lettuce leaves can be used for scooping up the salad.

Date Balls

4 ounces cream cheese
1½ cups dates, chopped (cut dates with shears dipped in cold water)
½ cup pine nuts or walnuts, coarsely broken

Work the mixture with your hands until well blended. If a stiffer mixture is desired, add ground sesame seeds or toasted whole grain bread crumbs. Form into small balls or patties. Cover and refrigerate until ready to serve. For a special treat they may be served with a dip of yogurt or sour cream flavored with vanilla extract, cinnamon, or brandy and a bit of honey.

Yogurt

To make thick yogurt, combine up to ½ cup of noninstant powdered milk or 1 cup of instant powdered milk with 1 quart of regular milk. Heat milk to 200° and then cool it to 100°. When milk reaches 100°, mix ¼ cup of commercial yogurt into it. Pour mixture into glass jars with lids or into coffee or custard cups. Cover each container with its lid or aluminum foil. Set cups in a pan of 100° water. Cover and place in a warm area, between 90° and 115°. Do not disturb for three to five hours.

The best method to maintain the correct temperature is to make the yogurt in your oven. If your oven light can remain on while the oven door is closed, place a 100-watt bulb in your oven light socket. Use an outdoor weather thermometer to check the temperature. If the oven gets too hot, try a lower wattage bulb. Sometimes the little appliance light bulb along with the pilot light of a gas oven is sufficient. Temperatures of above 120° will kill the yogurt culture, and those below 90° will produce sour milk. Be sure to replace the light bulb with your appliance bulb when you finish. When the yogurt has the consistency of heavy cream, it is ready to refrigerate. Homemade yogurt is not as thick or stable as commercial yogurt, which has stabilizers added. You can make yogurt without the addition of powdered milk, but your finished product will be thinner.

All containers and utensils used to make yogurt should be very clean. It is a good idea to dip them in boiling water before use. Do not disturb yogurt while it is incubating. If you wish to flavor it with honey, blackstrap molasses, vanilla, or crushed fruits, do so just before serving. Yogurt can be used in place of sour cream or buttermilk in most recipes but it must be handled more carefully. You should not stir or heat it any more than is necessary as it becomes watery and will not hold its shape.

THE LIGHT BITE, TUAREG STYLE

A QUICK MEAL: Cheese Curd Curry with Arabic pocket bread. (Corn tortillas or chapattis may be used instead of the Arab bread.)

To make cheese curd curry, mix dry-curd cottage cheese (ricotta) with pine nuts or other seeds or nuts, chopped dates or raisins, and chopped raw fruit or vegetables. Season to taste with curry powder, cinnamon, salt, garlic, or honey. Pour a curry sauce of yogurt mixed with curry and garlic or cinnamon and honey over the mixture. Good combinations are: dates, oranges, green onion, pecans, curry, and chopped sprouts; apples, celery, raisins, cinnamon, and walnuts; or tomatoes, cucumbers or summer squash, cooked green beans, onions, lentil sprouts, garlic, and sunflower seeds.

A SNACK: Pitted dates with cream cheese placed in the center. Cream cheese may be mixed with powdered cinnamon and chopped pine nuts.

Hunza in the Himalayas

All the elements necessary for the maintenance of life are found in the air we breathe, the water we drink, and the food we eat. Nowhere on earth are these elements found in greater perfection than Hunza, the isolated country high in the Himalayas.

The valley floor is 7,500 feet above sea level and the surrounding mountains rise to over 20,000 feet. With no industry and few cars, nothing pollutes the clear mountain air. Mineral water, in great abundance, rushes down from surrounding glaciers and irrigates the fields. Food grown in lovingly tended gardens is of superb quality, mineral rich, wholesome and delicious.

It comes as no surprise that the people of Hunza have outstanding health and tremendous vigor. Their life span exceeds the norm of industrialized society by twenty-five to forty years, and by all accounts their mental and emotional health is as enviable as their physical health.

Nothing, from reading the many books and articles about Hunza to experiencing the terrifying sixty-nine-mile ride from Gilgit in Pakistan, prepares the visitor for his first sight of the valley. Incredibly green and lush, the tiny villages are dwarfed by the snow-covered peaks of the towering mountains. From a distance the terraced fields that climb the steep hills from the valley floor present a multicolored mosaic of fantastic hues. The free-form shapes of the terraced fields contrast pleasingly with the closely grouped square homes of the Hunzakuts. The overwhelming verdance of the Hunza valley is nearly impossible to believe, it is so unlike dry, hot, dusty Pakistan to the south.

Legend has it, and there are many reasons to believe the story true, that about 2,300 years ago three Greek soldiers in the army of Alexander the Great deserted their troop in Persia and escaped with their Persian wives. Thinking that they would be pursued and punished, they fled into the most remote and impenetrable area of the Himalayas. The road, such as it is, did not exist at that time and it is believed that the three families made their way into the valley during winter while the Hunza River was frozen. The incredible difficulties of that trip can only be imagined.

Nevertheless, the three families founded Hunza. The physical appearance of the present residents is so unlike their neighbors in Pakistan or China that they surely must have come from an entirely different part of the world. Fair-skinned and dark-haired, the Hunzakuts have lean and muscular bodies. They are long-legged and fairly tall. The women bear a striking resemblance to the women in ancient Persian drawings.

No written history of Hunza exists, but it is fascinating to speculate about those early years. The deserters must have brought seeds with them because apricot, apple, and mulberry trees are not indigenous to that area of the world. As the population grew, there was not enough land bordering the river to raise all the food needed, so the terracing began. A stone wall would be painstakingly built and rich silt from the riverbed hand-carried and piled behind the wall. When the terrace was level with the top of the wall, it was ready for planting. Up and up the sides of the hills the terraces climb; some walls are twenty feet high and form a patch of garden only two or three feet wide and fifteen to twenty feet long.

Upstream, the Hunzakuts dug channels and developed an ingenious irrigation system. Huge slates hold back the water of the river; when they are removed, the water courses along ditches built next to the retaining walls. After a field is flooded, the slate is replaced and the next field down is flooded in the same manner. To prevent erosion, the terrace gardens are perfectly level. Modern engineers who have examined these terraces and the irrigation system swear that they were created by highly skilled people with an amazing knowledge of engineering and hydrodynamics.

When Marco Polo established a trade route to the Orient, it crossed the Hunza Valley and what amazing changes that must have brought. The Hunzakuts had lived in total isolation for many years and knew nothing of events in the rest of the world. The wild mountain sheep that are found in the area are named Marco

Polo sheep. He also introduced the Hunza national sport to the rest of the world and it is still called "polo."

Because of the valley's climate—dry, hot summers and cold, snowy winters—a particular manner of living emerged. The Hunzakuts built two-story homes, clustered tightly together to conserve land. They lived upstairs in summer and downstairs in winter, and they still do. In summer, food is eaten raw due to the shortage of firewood. Because everyone works in the fields from sunrise to dark during the summer, most holidays and feasts are held in the winter. In December, when the snows pile in drifts all across the valley, the communal wedding day is celebrated. All marriages in Hunza take place on the same day, early in December. Every family in the valley prepares a huge feast and it is one of the few occasions when some kind of meat is eaten, usually goat. A religious festival is held in February. Amid dancing and singing, another feast is enjoyed. During the rest of the year, the Hunzakuts eat very sparingly, rarely more than 2,000 calories a day.

Until recently, civilization has had little or no impact upon Hunza. The people lived as they had for hundreds of years. Other than the building of several schools, change has been imperceptible. Now, however, a new road into the country has been constructed, an airfield is being built, and a brand new Inter-Continental Hotel accommodates tourists who are eager to visit this mysterious and heretofore inaccessible land.

The Hunzakuts have not been uninformed about the rest of the world. The Mir (their ruler) and a few other families sent their children to England or the United States for higher education. Until now, their isolation has been a matter of choice. They love their homeland and prefer it the way it is, unsophisticated and serene.

The Hunzakuts are Moslems but with a few significant differences. Their women, by Moslem standards, are totally liberated. They work in the fields alongside the men. Dressed in pantaloons, they scramble up and down the terraces with amazing agility; they are not veiled and they can inherit property. They do not inherit fields because they are unable to tend them alone, but they do inherit homes and apricot trees. Unlike all other Moslems, the Hunzakuts make and consume an alcoholic beverage, a delightful wine made from grapes grown along the hillsides. This wine is extremely potent and at festivals is consumed in huge quantities with no apparent ill effect.

Hunzakuts are principally agrarian. They do raise a few cows, donkeys, and goats, but they feel that livestock eat more food than they produce so there are no large herds. They breed and take great pride in their wiry and spirited ponies. To criticize a man's horse is to insult him personally and he will immediately issue a challenge. This usually results in a horse race, at which a grand time is had by all.

Polo, unlike anything ever seen elsewhere, is the national pastime. There are no rules and no referees and the result is mayhem. There is also no age limit for the players and men in their nineties are out there tearing up and down the field. Things can get pretty rough and a gap-toothed grin is fairly common among the better players.

In a country full of amazing things, perhaps the most amazing of all is the physical and mental health of the inhabitants. There is no disease in Hunza. Imagine a country of 30,000 people with NO DISEASE. No vascular, muscular, organic, respiratory, or bone disease. No tooth decay, no dietary deficiency, nothing to cause illness or death. Men in their nineties or even early hundreds work in the fields daily. When they die, there is no known cause; everything has just worn out. Such longevity is an astounding phenomenon in itself, but there is no particular reason to strive for a long life if the quality of that life is not enjoyable. In Hunza, the oldest men are a viable part of the community. Honored and respected, they are greatly admired and their advice is frequently sought. They sit at the side of the Mir at his daily meetings and give their opinions on the affairs of the day. The men remain virile and productive into their nineties. It is not unusual for a twenty-year-old man to be the uncle of a forty-year-old man. The women go through menopause in their fifties, but the men continue to father children for many, many years.

Infant mortality is rare. Accidental death is the most common problem. The children occasionally fall from the terrace walls or tumble off a cliff. Injuries, usually broken bones, are treated by a villager skilled in bone setting. The Hunzakuts' remarkable recuperative powers enable them to remove the splint from a broken bone in about three weeks. The limb is mended and whole in that short length of time.

Because of the limitations in land and food, the Hunzakuts are extremely conscious of overpopulation. Families generally have two or three children at widely spaced intervals. A woman nurses her child up to three years and it is considered a grave problem if she becomes pregnant during that time. They feel the unborn child cannot get proper nourishment if the mother is feeding another child. The husband bears the brunt of his neighbors' disapproval; impregnating his nursing wife is a serious breach of custom.

If a man marries more than once, he may have two families, one grown and with children of their own, and several youngsters by the new wife.

Hunza children are curious, high-spirited, and friendly. They take to strangers quickly and show no signs of shyness or insecurity. Children are expected to help with the chores, carrying pails of fertilizer to the fields, helping the family at harvest, and tending the few animals. Because they have no pets (which eat too much and are unproductive), the children make pets of their farm animals. They may carry their chickens about or lead their goats or donkeys around on a leash and give them names. The children have perfect teeth and well-formed dental arches. They clean their teeth with small twigs and have no idea what toothpaste is for.

In the past few visitors from the outside world were permitted to enter Hunza. Those that were allowed in were usually doctors doing some specific research on geriatrics, ophthalmology, dentistry, or the cardiovascular system. Their reports are identical; the dentists say "no tooth decay," the ophthalmologists find "twenty-twenty vision in people up to 100 years of age." Dr. Paul Dudley White made the trip to Hunza in 1964 and after testing a group of men between ninety and 110 years of age, he found that not one of them showed a single sign of coronary disease, high blood pressure, or high cholesterol.

Along with their superb health, the Hunzakuts are extremely happy people. There is no crime in Hunza; there are no police, no jails, no army, no money, no hunger—and no stress.

The Mir and the elders sit in judgment on any subjects with a complaint. The most common cases involve water rights. Someone irrigated his fields at a time not allotted to him. The neighbor on the terrace below was deprived of his full measure. The guilty party is fined and must pay his neighbor a bushel of grain or a quantity of fruit.

Divorce exists but is fairly rare. If a wife cannot budget her food to stretch through the winter, the husband may get a divorce. No one starves, even if the mismanaging wife runs out of food, but the embarrassment is too much for the husband.

Because visitors are not permitted to stay in Hunza through the winter, little is known of their day-to-day life from October until the snows melt in May. Very likely the men hunt Marco Polo sheep in the mountains with aged rifles obtained from the Pakistani Army. The women probably use their time spinning and weaving cloth and knitting the traditional Hunza headgear, a long woolen cap that is rolled up to form a brim. In cold weather this brim is rolled down to keep neck and ears warm. The women are expert at needlework and embroider beautiful designs on their clothes. Some time is spent out-of-doors every day, winter and summer. In spite of their low-calorie and -fat diet, the Hunzakuts are remarkably resistant to cold. They enjoy swimming in their icy water all year round.

With the coming of spring, everything in Hunza shifts into high gear. The terraces must be examined carefully and repairs made, the tiny fields cleared of winter debris and prepared for planting. The all-important compost heap is turned over, and everyone in the family begins the task of carrying fertilizer to their fields. By early spring, most of their food is gone, and their diet is restricted to the few remaining dried fruits, chapattis, and what few potatoes are left. At a time when extra food is needed by the hardworking Hunzakuts, very little is available. They must wait for the new crops to grow.

The Hunzakuts revere their land with an almost religious fervor. They feel that only if they give to the soil will it provide for them. What is removed must be returned. Every scrap of food left from a meal goes into their compost heap, along with droppings from livestock, and stems and leaves left from the harvest. Even bones are ground to powder and returned to the soil. As a result, rich black topsoil, up to two feet deep, produces food of amazing quantity and quality. Trees so laden with fruit that their branches must be propped shade tiny fields of wheat, millet, and vegetables. Corn and peppers, tomatoes and carrots, spinach and radishes, onions and potatoes, all of outstanding flavor and texture grow in beautiful profusion up the mountainsides. Analysis of the soil has shown that it is extremely rich in minerals and is virtually germ-free.

Healthy, insect-resistant plants thrive without spraying and the vegetables are said to be the best-tasting in the world. In addition, they are about the most nutritious because of the constant renewal of minerals and trace elements through composted waste and mineral-rich water. By contrast, an alarming decrease in the nutritional quality of United States supermarket vegetables has many nutritionists very concerned.

At one time, the Pakistani government warned Hunza that a huge infestation of insects was expected and their crops were in danger. They offered to send pesticides to protect the Hunza food supply, but the Mir and his elders decided against this plan and instead made up a spray of fire ash and water that proved successful in repelling insects and didn't harm their soil or plants. One enterprising chemical fertilizer salesman convinced the Hunzakuts that they could increase harvests with his product, but after two years the farmers discovered that more water was needed to grow their crops and their corn was drying up too fast. They simply stored the rest of the chemical fertilizer and went back to their organic methods. Now chemical fertilizers are prohibited by law in Hunza.

Water for fields and home comes from melting glacial streams. It roars down the mountainside in a never-ending torrent, turning the mill wheels and irrigating the gardens. This water is a pearly grey color, extremely rich in minerals. When left in a glass overnight, it retains the milky color; the minerals remain in suspension and no sediment forms on the bottom. The Hunzakuts swear that their amazing health is due to their glacial water, a claim that would be hard to dispute. Recent studies that compare mineral-rich or "hard" water with mineral-free or "soft" water show that the high calcium and phosphorous content of hard water plays a significant role in preventing coronary problems. Striking evidence comes from Monroe County, Florida, where the water supply was suddenly changed from rainwater with a hardness of about 5 parts per million to deep-well water with a hardness almost 400 times greater. Within four years, the death rate from cardiovascular disease dropped from the 500–700 level to a 200–300 level.

The Hunza diet consists of fruits, vegetables and grains, and milk products, with a bit of meat from time to time. In summer, they usually eat their food raw and they especially like immature raw corn. No meal is complete without four or five chapattis per person. Chapattis are made from coarsely ground grain such as wheat, millet, or oats, and enough water to soften the dough. The dough is formed into round, flat patties and quickly cooked on a hot grill. When traveling, a Hunzakut will carry along a bag of grain and a hand mill to make chapattis for his meal. It is felt that freshly ground grain makes the best chapattis. Hunzakuts thresh their grain in a style that goes back to biblical times. They spread the sheaves of grain on a paved surface and tether several animals —some goats, a couple of donkeys—to a pole in the center. Around and around they go, their sharp hooves separating the grain from the chaff. Their droppings are immediately removed and added to the compost heap. The grain is then stored in earthen jugs and, when needed, is coarsely ground at community mills. These mills are built over the river and the rushing waters endlessly turn the wheels.

For breakfast, Hunzakuts generally have a grain porridge mixed with fresh or dried apricots; several chapattis; and tea made with herbs and mint, salted instead of sugared. Hunza has no sugar and imports none; they sweeten with honey.

Lunch in summer is fresh, raw vegetables or fruits and nuts and more chapattis. Dinner will be much the same with the addition of a curry stew, buttermilk, or whey.

Goat's milk is extremely rich and produces a fine heavy cream, which the Hunzakuts churn into butter, and then carefully wrap and store. For some reason, very old butter that has been stored for years is preferred to freshly churned butter. They also make cheese, yogurt, buttermilk, and whey from goat's milk. The cheese and butter are an important source of fat in the Hunza diet.

There is no other culture in the world that has apricots as the staple food. The Hunzakuts are certainly unique in this. Their trees are the staff of life. They represent the wealth of an individual. Young Hunza girls look with great favor on a man who has a couple of apricot trees. Their devotion to the tree and the fruit it bears is almost a religion. Much of the crop is dried for use in the winter. The apricots are cut in half and the seeds set aside. The fruit is then placed in huge, flat baskets with plenty of space around each piece, and left to dry on the roofs. Other fruits are dried in a similar fashion, pears, apples, peaches, and mulberries, but the apricot is clearly the favorite. The fruits are then stored in a dry, airy room. Hanging in great clusters, they are a beautiful and colorful sight. Sometimes the dried fruits are eaten plain, but when water is added, they swell almost to their original size. They are soaked overnight, mashed, and added to porridge; more water can be added to make the fruit into a soupy mixture, and in winter the children mix thick mashed apricots with snow to make a delicious ice cream.

To the Hunzakuts, apricot pits are almost as important as the fruit. When an apricot is eaten fresh, the pit is cracked and the kernel eaten also. It has an almond flavor and is a rich source of nutrients, especially the controversial Vitamin B_{17}. A tree that produces a bitter pit is destroyed rather than have the unpleasant flavor contaminate their oil (see below). The pit testing is done by a village elder whose main function in life is to sample various pits and decide whether they are of suitable quality. This is an important position and the taster is highly regarded.

Extracting oil from the apricot kernels is a long and tedious process. In order to lighten the task, this is done with an air of festivity. The whole family, dressed in their very finest clothes, gathers on the roof of their home. First the pit is cracked and the kernel removed. After it is pounded into a fine powder with a stone, a small amount is placed in a pot over low heat and sprinkled with a bit of water. As the mixture heats, the oil begins to seep out. The paste is kneaded by hand to extract the oil, which is then stored in jars. The Hunzakuts use this oil for everything. They pour it over greens as a salad dressing, and they use it in cooking. It is considered a fine cosmetic and is applied to skin and hair. Newborn babies are rubbed with it, and all children up to the age of five receive one teaspoonful per day. The oil has a delightful almond flavor, stores very well, and does not readily turn rancid.

Garbanzo beans and lentils grown on the terraced gardens are dried and used in stews. They are a fine source of incomplete protein, iron, and B vitamins and, when sprouted and eaten raw as the Hunzakuts frequently do, their enzymes, vitamin content, and protein quality are all enhanced.

Nuts, primarily walnuts, are found in abundance in Hunza. Nuts, fruits, and a glass of glacial water provide a fine and nutritious meal. Nuts are also added to stews or chopped and mixed with fruit.

When Hunzakuts do eat meat on holidays or celebrations, it is usually goat prepared as a stew or curry. They enjoy this highly spiced food but eat very small portions.

New studies into the value of walking have shown how vitally important this form of exercise is. It not only strengthens the heart and increases lung capacity, it actually increases bone density. The process of aging is slowed in people who are habitually active.

Since they have no cars or pack animals, the Hunzakuts walk everywhere. A twenty- or thirty-mile walk is nothing special; they don't even bother to rest after arriving at their destination. With a long, loping stride and a huge lung capacity, they can carry heavy loads across their mountainous country at amazing speeds. The energy and endurance of the Hunzakuts can be credited to what they *don't* eat as well as to what they do eat. The U.S. Department of Agriculture estimates the average American ingests about 3,300 calories per day, which includes 100 grams of protein, 157 grams of fat, and 380 grams of carbohydrates. The Hunzakuts consume about 1,900 calories a day, 50 grams of protein, 36 grams of fat, and 354 grams of carbohydrates. Studies show that while the American consumes almost twice the calories of the Hunzakut, his daily vitamin and mineral intake is much lower—thanks to the American diet of refined foods and flesh meat.

The high vitamin and mineral diet of the Hunzakuts enables them to wrest from a difficult environment the foods needed for their vitamin and mineral-rich diet. Without eating energy-producing food, they couldn't raise energy-producing food. They understand this cycle very well and live harmoniously with it. They return to the soil that which is needed by the soil. They grow in summer so they may eat in winter, neither asking too much nor taking too little.

It is hoped that this perfectly balanced existence can continue in spite of the country's changing circumstances. The recently deposed Mir has observed that "progress" is inevitable. His once remote and inaccessible country has now been fully annexed by Pakistan and the last vestiges of autonomy abolished.

What this will mean to the future of tiny Hunza one can only guess. Sadly the Mir remarked that it would be foolish to think Hunza could remain isolated in today's world. His only hope was that their tranquil way of life would not be too violently disrupted and that their basic resources, the pure air of the Karakoram peaks and their turbid but uncontaminated glacial water, would not become polluted.

THE FOODS OF HUNZA

Hunzakuts are lacto-vegetarians, that is, their diet is almost entirely grains and raw milk products, supplemented with vegetables and fruits. This isn't necessarily through choice; they have so little arable land, they simply can't afford to raise animals for meat. Their animals must supply milk in exchange for the grain they eat. They also supply something else of great value—the manure that helps to make Hunza soil the richest and most productive in the world.

Grains

Numerous grains are grown by the Hunzakuts, but wheat is the dominant one. The grains are coarsely ground and combined to make chapattis, the staple bread eaten at every meal. The chapatti is a pancake made of water and freshly ground grains, cooked about three minutes on a hot griddle. Freshly ground grains are added to stews and made into cereals. The protein quality of grain is improved 25 percent when it is eaten with a dairy product.

CHIEF SOURCES OF NUTRIENTS IN THE HUNZA DIET

PROTEIN	wheat and dairy products together
FAT	apricot seed oil and dairy products
CARBOHYDRATE	wheat
CALORIES	wheat
VITAMIN A	fruit and greens
VITAMIN C	fruit and greens
VITAMIN B_1	wheat
VITAMIN B_2	milk products
NIACIN	wheat
CALCIUM	milk products
IRON	wheat
FIBER	wheat

Next to oats, wheat contains the largest amount of usable protein of all grains. Its germ is the richest known source of Vitamin E, protein the quality of meat, and the B vitamin complex in good amounts. In its natural state, wheat will keep fresh for many years, but when it is ground into flour, its Vitamin E is quickly destroyed by oxygen and the product becomes rancid. In Hunza, the grain is ground fresh daily. In the United States, whole grain flour should be kept refrigerated in an airtight container and used within a short period of time.

The primary source of the C complex vitamin rutin is in buckwheat. Rutin has been found to strengthen capillaries. Buckwheat is the only grain to contain a large amount of calcium. It is also one of the few commercially grown grains in the United States that is so hardy it is seldom sprayed with insecticides.

A good source of the trace minerals, if they are present in the soil, barley is easier to digest than wheat. It is outstanding in soup, as it tends to create body heat, and is very filling. Barley stews are undoubtedly a frequent meal during the long Hunza winters, although too much barley tends to increase body weight more readily than other grains.

Animal tests have revealed that rye develops muscles whereas wheat promotes fat. Rye eaters are usually leaner than wheat eaters. Rye contains high levels of potassium, Vitamin E, magnesium, silicone, and unsaturated fatty acids, making it an important food in the prevention of heart diseases.

The Hunzakuts grow a little corn, but they don't usually save it for grain. They prefer to eat the immature ears raw, as soon as they appear on the stalk.

The only alkaline-forming grain, millet is also an excellent source of iron, Vitamin B_1, and so many minerals that they counteract acids. It contains Vitamin B_{17}, also found in apricot pits, and is considered to be one of the most easily digested of all grains.

Legumes

Soybeans, garbanzo beans, and lentils are the major legumes grown in Hunza. They are eaten fresh, dried and cooked, ground into flour, and sprouted. Beans are an excellent source of iron, B vitamins, potassium, cellulose, and incomplete protein. When

COMPARISON OF NUTRIENTS FOUND IN 100 GRAMS
OF WHOLE RAW GRAINS AND LEGUMES

	Iron (mg.)	Calcium (mg.)	Calories	Vitamin B_1 (mg.)	Vitamin B_2 (mg.)	Niacin (mg.)	Protein (grams)	Protein Quality (percent)
Wheat	3.1	36	330	.57	.12	4.3	14.0	60
Corn	2.4	20	355	.38	.11	2.0	9.2	51
Buckwheat	3.1	114	335	.60	.00	4.4	11.7	65
Barley	2.7	34	348	.21	.07	3.7	9.6	60
Millet	6.8	20	327	.73	.38	2.3	9.9	55
Rye	3.7	38	334	.43	.22	1.6	12.1	58
Oats	4.5	53	390	.60	.14	1.0	14.2	66
Rice*	1.6	32	360	.34	.05	4.7	7.5	70
Garbanzos	6.9	150	360	.31	.15	2.0	20.5	43
Lentils	6.8	79	340	.37	.22	2.0	24.7	30
Red beans	6.9	110	343	.51	.20	2.3	22.5	38
Soybeans	8.4	226	403	1.10	.31	2.2	34.1	61

* Rice is not grown in Hunza.

eaten with grains, seeds, or milk, they form a fine quality protein, and become a major source of this essential nutrient.

To sprout their beans, the Hunzakuts will soak them for a day or two, then spread them on wet cloths in the sun. The sprouts are usually eaten raw just as the tiny leaf turns green. Garbanzo sprouts are an unusual source of B_{12}, a vitamin usually associated only with animal products. Sprouts, of course, are one of the finest foods one can eat.

Vegetables

About 70 percent of the vegetables in the Hunza diet are eaten raw. (It is an unfortunate fact that only about 5 percent of the American diet is fresh vegetables, usually in the form of a salad made with iceberg lettuce.) Those vegetables that are cooked are usually steamed in a small amount of water, which is consumed with the food. The stews are not comparable to a typical Irish stew that simmers for hours; they are cooked only briefly, and contain various combinations of grains and vegetables. Because firewood is in such short supply, food is eaten raw whenever possible. In winter, fuel that is used to heat the house also cooks the food. Vegetables left over from the harvest will be dried and used in winter months, put in stews, or ground and added to chapattis or cereal. All the familiar vegetables are grown: potatoes, carrots, bell peppers, turnips, onions, radishes, and greens, including dandelions.

The potato is rare in that it is a complete food. However, to sustain life, the entire potato must be eaten because the major food value is found just under the skin, and at least some of them must be eaten raw. In Hunza, potatoes are baked in the coals of a small fire, steamed whole, or eaten raw directly from the field. The Hunzakuts' method of cooking potatoes preserves the Vitamin C. The protein quality of potatoes is quite good, but is improved with the addition of a little milk or cheese. The potato is probably the Hunzakuts' most important vegetable as it is stored for winter and eaten when little else is available.

Bell peppers are extremely nutritious. Their white membrane is an excellent source of bioflavonoids and pectin. Red peppers are mature green peppers and supply ten times more Vitamin A and twice the Vitamin C of the immature green pepper. One hundred grams of red pepper contains four times the Vitamin C found in 100 grams of orange. Bell peppers are sweet-tasting and should be eaten raw.

Karam is a vivid green leafy vegetable that resembles spinach. It is a great favorite in Hunza, eaten daily during its season and dried for winter use. It provides calcium, iron, and Vitamin A.

Fruits

More important than vegetables, milk products, or grains are the fruits grown in Hunza. A huge crop of apricots, apples, pears, and peaches is harvested each year. The Hunzakuts depend upon this one type of food for their day-to-day meals. If a Hunzakut ate nothing but fruit and its seeds, and drank his high-mineral water, he could maintain his health. The seeds are a source of protein, unsaturated fat, Vitamins B and E, magnesium, and other minerals. Fruit provides Vitamins A and C as well as fibers vital for proper digestion, while additional minerals, including calcium, are supplied by his water.

Virtually a staple food in Hunza, apricots are eaten fresh, along with their pits, and dried and stored for winter use; even the pits are pressed for oil. They are eaten in some form at most meals.

Apricots contain a fine quality carbohydrate and each one supplies an impressive 1,000 units of Vitamin A. The iron in apricots ranks with that of liver, kidneys, and eggs in ease of absorption. As mentioned earlier, oil pressed from the seeds is used in cooking, as a medicine, as a vitamin source for infants and children, and as a cosmetic. It is a very stable oil and can withstand high temperatures. A good source of Vitamin E and essential fatty acids, it also keeps very well without turning rancid.

While apples contain only traces of most vitamins, they are one of the best sources of pectin known. Pectin has been found to reduce high cholesterol, prevent atherosclerosis, and remove poisons from the body. Apples aid digestion and, when eaten before a meal, will help overcome constipation. Some dentists feel that eating a slice or two of raw apple after a meal not only removes particles of food from between the teeth but also stimulates the gum tissues and actually reduces tooth decay by causing a salivary flow.

Nuts

The most abundant nut in Hunza, the walnut resists spoiling when left in the shell, but becomes rancid more easily than other nuts when shelled. Hunzakuts usually eat them raw and sometimes add them to stews. Walnuts are light and easy to carry so they are frequently taken along on trips. They are cracked and eaten along the way with some dried fruit. Walnuts are the best source of the essential fatty acids.

The almond is the other nut grown in Hunza. It is the most stable of all nuts, providing more protein, calories, iron, calcium, potassium, B vitamins, and saturated fats than most other nuts. It also contains some Vitamin D.

Milk and Milk Products

In Hunza, milk is usually consumed as buttermilk, whey, yogurt, cottage cheese, or ghee. Because these mountain farmers have no way to keep their milk fresh, fermented forms are utilized. Milk is never cooked. Goat's milk is the most common variety consumed and it is preferable to cow's milk as it contains a better quality protein and more niacin and thiamine. Easier to digest and stronger tasting, it makes a fine cheese. These milk products, along with grains, are the chief protein source in Hunza.

Cultured milk products are true wonder foods. They contain high quality proteins, minerals, enzymes, and all the known vitamins, including B_{12} and D. Being predigested by bacterial action, they are utilized by the body faster and more easily than fresh milk. They are a natural antibiotic and help manufacture the B vitamins and Vitamin K in the intestines.

The best butter is made by churning yak milk in a goatskin bag. The yak is a large, long-haired type of ox found in central Asia. Its milk is very rich and makes huge quantities of butter. This butter is a great favorite of the Hunzakuts, but they follow an unusual procedure in making it. After it is churned, it is wrapped in paper made from thin slices of wood, and stored underground. They believe the older and stronger it is, the richer it is. Fresh butter is virtually never eaten, but old butter, like old wine, is savored and enjoyed.

Another form of butter is made by allowing raw milk to stand at room temperature until it thickens naturally. When it forms a thick, gleaming white curd, it is used like butter. It is said to be absolutely delicious, and contains the fat-soluble Vitamins A and D.

Whey, a watery residue, is the byproduct of ghee or cottage cheese. Hunzakuts drink it at meals. Whey contains half the calcium of milk and only one-fourth the protein; however, it is a good source of sodium and lactose (milk sugar). Lactose is not digested in the stomach, but travels into the large intestine where it serves as a food for beneficial intestinal flora, keeping the organ healthy so it can do its job of digesting foods properly. This helps in the retention of minerals in the system, especially calcium, phosphorus, and magnesium.

Scarce Foods

Even though meat is well liked, it is a rare treat. When it is prepared for a special occasion, it is never served separately but always as part of a stew or curry, providing bulk and flavor. Since most Hunza festive holidays take place in winter, this is when meat is usually featured. Occasionally a Marco Polo sheep will be killed, but the most common meats are yak and goat.

Since chickens peck seeds and seeds are more valuable than eggs, until recently no chickens were allowed in Hunza. Now there are a few, but their eggs are considered a great luxury.

Water

It hardly seems appropriate to list water as one of the foods of the Hunzakuts, but their healthful water is so unique it must be included. The water of Hunza is so mineral rich and nutritious that, if need be, it can be substituted for a meal. It comes from melting glaciers, and as it races down along its rocky stream bed, it picks up minerals and trace elements. These minerals are in such minute particles they remain in suspension in the water even if left standing for several days. The glacial water of Hunza has long been credited with contributing to the outstanding health of these people. No matter where a person is in Hunza, there is always an irrigation stream nearby where he can quench his thirst or get water to make his chapattis.

DINING WITH A HUNZAKUT FAMILY

Hunza and its people seem so remote and romantic. Surely it was Hunza James Hilton described when he wrote of Shangri-La, but in truth, the people are not mysterious, they are more often mischievous; they aren't mystic, they are extremely pragmatic. A perfect example is the typical Hunza home. It is four-square, solid, and two-storied. In summer the family lives on the second floor and the flat roof is used for drying fruit and pressing oil. In winter, they move to the first floor to be near the hearth. The Hunza house has no fireplace. In the center of the first floor room is a raised hearth where the food is cooked. Above this is a hole in the ceiling and directly over that, a smaller hole in the roof. Cooking is done on a metal tripod that holds the iron kettle and an iron griddle is used to cook the chapattis. A wooden spoon is used to stir the food. Potatoes, corn, and squash are cooked in the ashes. It is important that all the food that is to be cooked be prepared with only one fire. Wood is scarce and animal dung is saved for compost, so only small twigs and dry grass are burned.

There are a few pieces of simple, low, wooden furniture in the room and often an area where the floor is raised about one foot. It is covered with beautiful rugs and this is where the meals are eaten. A walnut bowl filled with curry, soup, or stew is placed in the center and each diner dips his food from it. There are no plates and silverware. The diners usually break a chapatti into small pieces with the right hand, shape it into a scoop, and pick up soft food with it. Occasionally, a wooden spoon is used for soup while the right hand is used to dip into grains from the common bowl.

Buttermilk whey or tea, the common beverages drunk with meals, are served in earthenware cups. Salt and milk are added to tea.

Since their food is so flavorful because of the minerals it contains, the Hunzakuts need little seasoning. Wild mint is the favorite and is often made into tea. Sometimes thyme, green pepper, ginger, and curry powder are used.

In spring, as the first vegetables begin to mature, most food is eaten raw. Only a small fire is made to cook the chapattis.

Every meal will feature five chapattis per person and apricots in some form—dried, soaked, mashed, made into jam, or mixed with snow.

A HUNZAKUT DINNER PER INDIVIDUAL

KARAM CURRY:
   karam, 5½ ounces (or spinach)
   yogurt, ¼ cup
   almonds, 2 tablespoons
   apricot oil, 1 tablespoon
   lentil sprouts, 2 tablespoons
CHAPATTIS, 75 grams of wheat,
   about five chapattis

CARROTS, 2 small
RADISHES, 4 small
GREEN ONIONS WITH TOPS, 2
BELL PEPPERS, ¼ medium
DANDELION GREENS, 4 leaves
APRICOT JAM, 4 dried halves
BUTTERMILK, 8 ounces

A HUNZAKUT DINNER FROM YOUR KITCHEN

SPINACH CURRY*
CHAPATTIS
APRICOT JAM, or fresh apricots (2 each)
RAW VEGETABLES
   Carrots
   Radishes
   Green Onions
   Sliced Tomatoes

* For a special meal, cubes of lamb can be added to the spinach curry.

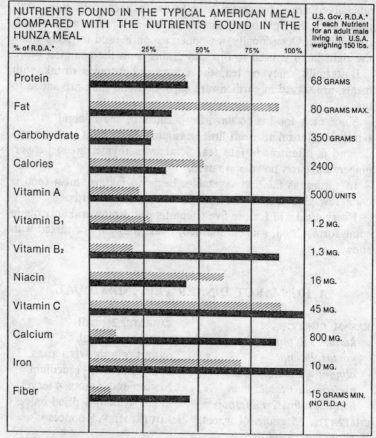

NUTRIENTS FOUND IN THE TYPICAL AMERICAN MEAL COMPARED WITH THE NUTRIENTS FOUND IN THE HUNZA MEAL	U.S. Gov. R.D.A.* of each Nutrient for an adult male living in U.S.A. weighing 150 lbs.
% of R.D.A.* 25% 50% 75% 100%	
Protein	68 GRAMS
Fat	80 GRAMS MAX.
Carbohydrate	350 GRAMS
Calories	2400
Vitamin A	5000 UNITS
Vitamin B₁	1.2 MG.
Vitamin B₂	1.3 MG.
Niacin	16 MG.
Vitamin C	45 MG.
Calcium	800 MG.
Iron	10 MG.
Fiber	15 GRAMS MIN. (NO R.D.A.)

*R.D.A. is the recommended daily nutrient allowance intended to meet the needs of a *healthy* individual.

Diagonal lines represent the American meal.

The chief sources of nutrients in the Hunza meal are:

PROTEIN	milk and wheat chapattis
FAT	apricot oil
CARBOHYDRATE	wheat chapattis
CALORIES	wheat chapattis
VITAMIN A	karam
VITAMIN B_1	wheat chapattis
VITAMIN B_2	buttermilk
NIACIN	wheat chapattis
VITAMIN C	karam
CALCIUM	buttermilk
IRON	karam
FIBER	wheat chapattis

Spinach Curry

1½ pounds spinach, chopped fine, or 2 packages frozen chopped spinach
a few young dandelion leaves, chopped fine
1 cup plain yogurt
1½ teaspoons curry powder, or to taste
½ cup ground almonds
1 tablespoon fine chopped onion
1 teaspoon salt or to taste
1 tablespoon butter

Cook onion in butter until limp; add spinach and dandelion leaves and cook, covered, just until tender. Add just as little water as possible. When spinach is cooked, add ground almonds, curry powder, and salt. Mix well. Fold in yogurt gently and only heat the curry. Do not cook or yogurt will become thin.

Serve spinach curry in a bowl. Top with the following:

1½ cups small-curd cottage cheese

Heat cottage cheese and add chopped green onions and curry powder to taste.

Serve the following condiments to sprinkle over your spinach curry if you desire: Chopped hard cooked eggs; chopped green onions, including their tops; raisins; cubed apples; lentil sprouts; chopped parsley.

Hunza Wheat Cakes, "Chapattis"

> 2½ cups whole wheat flour
> ½ cup toasted wheat germ
> ⅓ cup melted butter
> 1 teaspoon salt
> About 1 cup water or buttermilk

Blend flour, wheat germ, salt, and butter in a bowl. Gradually stir in the liquid until the dough holds together. On a lightly floured board, knead the dough until smooth, about 5 minutes. Cover dough and allow to stand 20 to 30 minutes. Divide dough into balls approximately 2 inches in diameter. Pat them into ⅛-inch thick circles between your hands or roll them on a floured board. Bake cakes on a medium hot, lightly oiled frying pan or griddle until light brown. In Hunza they continually flop them back and forth. Or you can make the chapattis ¼ inch thick and bake them in a 300° oven on an oiled cookie sheet. Wrap chapattis in a dish towel to keep them warm. They may be reheated in the broiler, but are best eaten when fresh.

Apricot Jam

> 16 dried apricots, cut fine with scissors or knife
> 1 tablespoon lemon juice
> 2 teaspoons honey
> ¼ teaspoon almond extract
> 3 tablespoons yogurt

Cover apricots with just enough warm water to cover. Allow them to stand overnight or up to 24 hours. Add lemon juice, honey, and almond extract and press into a thick paste with spoon, your hand, or in a blender. Fold in yogurt. Any dried fruit or combinations of dried fruits may be prepared in this manner. Spoonfuls of this jam can be frozen or mixed with chopped nuts and coconut and eaten as candy.

Hunza Lamb Curry

For a very special occasion, lamb is used.

> ¾ *pound lean, boneless lamb cut into 1½-inch cubes*
> *1 tablespoon butter*
> ¼ *cup chopped onion*
> *1½ teaspoons curry powder or to taste*
> *1½ teaspoons salt*
> *1 cup plain yogurt*

Mix yogurt, salt, onion, and curry. Marinate lamb cubes 24 hours, turning occasionally. Remove lamb from the marinade. Drain meat and dry it with a paper towel. Melt the butter in a frying pan and brown the meat until it loses its red color but is still light pink in the center. To serve lamb curry, cook 1½ cups of any grain such as cracked wheat or millet to use in place of chapattis. Use the marinade in which the meat was tenderized in place of yogurt, curry, onions, and salt in spinach curry. Serve spinach curry on grain and arrange lamb cubes around edge of dish. The cottage cheese can be omitted or served as an optional condiment.

Winter Stew

> ½ *cup lentils*
> *2 cups water*
> *1½ teaspoons salt*
> *1½ cups potatoes, cubed; scrub skins but do not peel*
> *1½ cups carrots, thinly sliced*
> ½ *cup light cream*
> ¾ *teaspoon powdered tarragon*
> ¼ *cup almonds, chopped*
> *2 tablespoons butter*

Bring water to a boil and add lentils. Cover pan, reduce heat, and simmer 30 minutes or until the lentils are almost tender. Add potatoes and carrots. Cover pan and simmer until vegetables are tender and water is absorbed. Add cream and simmer 5 minutes, stirring occasionally. Stir in tarragon, almonds, butter, and salt to taste. In Hunza crushed, dried mint leaves are often added to the stew.

Barley and Garbanzo Curry

1 cup whole barley
2 cups cooked garbanzo beans
2 tablespoons butter
3 cups chicken, beef, or vegetable broth (if using canned garbanzos, use the liquid from the can as part of the broth)
1 bay leaf
1 teaspoon dill seed
1 cup yogurt
½ cup green onions, chopped
Curry powder, to taste
Salt, to taste

Sauté barley in butter about 5 minutes, or until slightly brown. Bring broth to a boil, add bay leaf, dill seeds, and browned barley. Cover pan and reduce heat to simmer. Cook until barley is tender and broth absorbed, about 1 hour. Add more broth if needed. When barley is cooked, remove bay leaf and add garbanzo beans, onions, yogurt, curry powder, and salt. Mix well and bring just to a boil. Remove from heat and allow curry to stand covered for 15 minutes so that the barley will absorb the yogurt. Serve curry with a large vegetable salad flavored with dry mint, and chapattis. Top curry with chopped dried apricots if you desire.

Summer Soup

½ cup green onions including green tops, finely chopped
3 ears raw young corn; cut corn from cob and scrape milk from cob with knife
1 cup cucumber, diced finely; peel only if skin is tough
4 large mushrooms, chopped
1 cup peas; use frozen peas, defrosted but raw
1 large tomato, chopped
½ cup fresh asparagus tips, if available
½ sweet red pepper or green bell pepper, finely chopped
½ cup watercress, spinach, or ¼ cup parsley, finely chopped
2 teaspoons dry mint leaves, finely chopped (optional)
4 cups yogurt
¼ cup almonds, chopped
Salt to taste

Combine the vegetables and refrigerate, covered, until well chilled. Fold yogurt into chilled vegetables and salt to taste. Curry powder or garlic powder may be added to soup if you desire. Sprinkle with almonds. Soup may be served cold, at room temperature, or heated to body temperature. Served with chapattis, this soup makes a complete meal.

Hunza Breakfast

1 cup whole wheat, rice, rye, barley, oats, or millet, or a combination of these
4 cups boiling water (milk may be substituted but do not boil)
1 teaspoon salt
2 tablespoons butter or apricot oil
Dried apricots (or other dried fruit), diced and soaked overnight in yogurt, milk, pineapple juice, apple juice, or water to cover
½ cup almonds or walnuts, chopped

Grind grain in a grinder (a coffee grinder will work) or a blender. Bring water to a rolling boil. Add cereal, cover pan, reduce heat and simmer until cereal is tender, about 15 to 20 minutes. Stir cereal occasionally and add more liquid if necessary. When cooked, mix in dried fruit and the liquid in which it was soaked, nuts, butter, salt, and honey or blackstrap molasses to taste. Vanilla extract or cinnamon enhance its flavor. In Hunza chopped fresh mint is often added to the cereal. Add cream or yogurt to make the right consistency. Cereal may be eaten warm or at room temperature.

Raw Applesauce

3 apples
¼ cup honey, or to taste
1 tablespoon lemon juice
¼ teaspoon cinnamon

Core apples, quarter, and put through food grinder. Mix with lemon juice, honey and cinnamon. You may chop ingredients in the blender. If more liquid is needed to start blender chopping, use apple juice. Applesauce should be prepared shortly before it is to be served.

Fruit Leather

Make a purée of any fresh fruit or mixture of fresh fruits. Add pine-apple or apple juice if fruit is dry. The blender works best, especially for hard fruits like apples. Sweeten purée with honey and flavor with vanilla, almond extract, lemon juice, or any desired spice. Spread the purée thinly on a lightly oiled cookie sheet and set in the sun to dry, as they do in Hunza. It may also be dried by placing it in your oven. Prop the oven door open 2 or 3 inches to allow the moisture to escape. Keep the temperature in your oven between 125° and 150°. Usually a 100-watt light bulb placed in your oven light socket will maintain the proper temperature. You will have to experiment to see what wattage bulb you need. Be sure to remove the light bulb when you have finished drying the fruit. When the fruit is dry but still pliable, peel it off the pan and cut it in small strips with a pair of scissors. Store fruit leather in an airtight container in the refrigerator.

Fruit and Nut Snack

> 1 cup dried apricots
> 1 cup other dried fruit, or a combination of several
> 1 cup almonds, ground
> 1 cup walnuts, chopped

Put dried fruit through a food grinder. (If some of the dried fruit is very hard, before grinding it, soak it in a small amount of fruit juice until it becomes semisoft.) Mix almond meal, walnuts, and chopped fruit with your hands to form a firm mixture. If mixture is too dry, add a small amount of juice—apple, pineapple, or grape, or even brandy—so that small solid patties can be formed. If mixture should become too thin, add more ground nuts or some dried whole grain bread crumbs. In Hunza the patties are wrapped in birch leaves and known as "Traveler's Food."

Mint Tea

> 2½ tablespoons fresh mint leaves, chopped, or 2 tablespoons
>   dried mint leaves, crushed
> 1 quart water

Bring water to boil and pour it over the leaves. Let the tea steep for 5 to 10 minutes. Serve with salt or honey to taste.

Sprouts

All seeds can be sprouted. Mung beans, lentils, rye, and alfalfa are those used most frequently. Radish, pea, and garbanzo sprouts are good accent foods. You must be sure the seeds you sprout have not been chemically treated. It is safest to buy the seeds you use for sprouting at a health food store.

To sprout small seeds, including lentils, place about 1½ tablespoons of the seed in a quart jar and cover with water. Put a piece of cheese-cloth over the mouth of the bottle and fasten it in place with a rubber band. Place the jar in a cupboard or other dark place. Soak seeds 12 hours; then drain the water from the seeds through the cheesecloth and run fresh water into the jar to rinse the seeds. The water used to soak the seeds can be used to water your plants, mixed with your pet's food or used in a stew. Drain the water from the jar and return the seeds to the cupboard. After draining the rinse water from the seeds, you can store the jars in the cupboard, cheesecloth side down, on a cake rack placed over a pan to catch any water that drains out. Rinse and drain the seeds every 12 hours. They will be ready to eat in 3 to 4 days. When they have reached their desired length, set them in the sun for an hour or so to turn their leaves green.

To sprout large seeds like garbanzos, peas, and kidney beans, first soak them overnight in plenty of water; they will double in volume. In the morning rinse the seeds and spread them in a colander; cover them with several layers of damp paper toweling and set in a warm place, as on top of your refrigerator. Remove the towels twice a day and rinse the seeds. Dampen the towels and replace them on top of the seeds. Repeat until sprouts are ready to eat.

To remove the hulls from sprouted seeds, cover the sprouts with water, and the hulls will come to the top. Drain and repeat until most of the hulls are removed. It is safe to eat the hulls and there is no need to remove them if you prefer not to.

Raw sprouts are such a nutritious food, they should never be cooked. They are good used with lettuce in salads or as a lettuce sub-stitute in sandwiches or tacos. Sprouts can be mixed with other foods after the foods have been cooked. They can be folded into a cheese or Spanish omelet or scrambled into eggs on the very last scramble. They are good used in place of pasta with spaghetti sauce, peanut sauce, curry, stroganoff, or cream sauce, and are good condiments on various foods and soups.

THE LIGHT BITE, HUNZA STYLE

A QUICK MEAL: Hunza breakfast (page 79) made with milk instead of water, or ¼ cup cottage cheese per serving added after the cereal has cooked. A raw fresh fruit would complete the meal. The cereal may be kept hot in a thermos or eaten at room temperature.

A SNACK: A purée of any fresh fruit added to an equal amount of yogurt. Add honey, vanilla, almond extract or brandy to taste. In Hunza they use mint. This mixture may be partly frozen, then mixed to the mush stage and eaten as a "slush."

The Digueños
of Southern California

Of the tens of thousands of aboriginal Americans who made their homes in California before the arrival of the Europeans, pitifully few remain today. Living on reservations, eking out a substandard existence on tiny unproductive farms, or joining the ranks of unskilled urban workers, their tragic history is often ignored.

Estimated at more than 300,000 in 1800, by 1910 the California Indian population had been reduced to 16,000.

The Digueños of the San Diego area are typical of many California tribes. Although their contact with Europeans was earlier than most, they suffered much the same fate.

In an effort to consolidate their western territories, Spanish soldiers and missionaries were sent into California in the eighteenth century to establish a series of forts and missions. The San Diego Mission was built in 1769 and the mission fathers immediately set about gathering the local Indian population into the fold. The Spanish name *Digueño* was given to the Indian groups who made their home in the area, but the Indians actually had their own tribal names and each tribe had its well-defined territory. Linguistic differences and tribal customs kept the groups separate and distinct, but the Spanish chose to ignore the differences and lumped the entire population under one designation. This intermingling of tribes caused great distress among all the Indians.

The Digueños were a branch of Yuma Indians from the southern Colorado River area. They lived and traveled around San Diego Bay; Mission, or False, Bay just to the north; La Jolla on the coast; inland to the mountains and deserts; and south into Baja California. Mission Valley, the valley of the San Diego River, was their favorite spot for permanent homes.

It is hard to imagine what the area must have looked like then. There were immense groves of oak everywhere. Pine trees grew in abundance along the coast; the morning fogs provided enough moisture for them to thrive in the semiarid climate. Streams of fresh, clear water ran down the sides of surrounding hills and the San Diego River tumbled toward the sea over a series of falls. Wild game abounded in the hills, fish and shellfish were plentiful along the shore, and countless varieties of edible plants were available for the picking. It is not surprising that the people who lived in this lovely and bountiful area were as benign as the climate—serene, happy, and peaceful.

The women were the food-gatherers. They knew every bush and shrub, every plant and flower. This knowledge they passed on to their daughters, teaching them how to select mushrooms, when to pick certain berries, where to find the best reeds for basket-making, and how to pick the spiny cactus. Their diet was incredibly varied. They ate more than one hundred types of plants along with their fish and game. The staple food was acorn mush, served hot or cold.

When gathering the acorns, the women slung a net holding a large flat basket across their backs. The net hung from their foreheads and to protect their heads, they wore a beautifully patterned woven cap. Laughing and chattering, groups of women and their daughters would move about in the groves of oak trees, filling their baskets to the brim. Then, singing songs of their harvest and thanking their gods for the abundance of food, they would return to the village to begin the tedious job of preparing the acorns.

The predominant sound in any Digueño village was the tap-tap-tap of mortar on pestle, the sound of acorn flour being made. The acorns were first cracked and allowed to dry for a few days. Then the nuts were removed and pounded with a rock into flour. Only a few nuts at a time were pounded, so the job went on all day. Sometimes a stone bowl or pestle was used but often the acorns were hammered in natural depressions found in huge boulders near the river. There might be several of these depressions on each rock so the women could gossip or sing together while working. When one hole got too deep, another would be started. Many of these pitted rocks can still be seen along the banks of the San Diego River up near Adobe Falls.

The acorn flour had to be leached of its tannic acid after it was pounded to remove the poison and the bitter taste. A small amount of flour was put into a basket and water poured through it dozens of times, hot water speeding up the process. Frequently the women would dig a hole in the sandy river bed and leach the flour in that manner. A lot of sand and stone got mixed in with the flour, a fact that accounts for the worn teeth found in many Digueño skeletal remains. The teeth were sound and showed little sign of decay, but some were worn away nearly to the gums.

After leaching, the flour was dried and stored in huge narrow-necked clay jugs. The women cooked up a large batch of acorn mush every morning. This pinkish, bland dish, rather like oatmeal, was a great favorite of the Digueños. Indeed, it was served at nearly every meal. When the village moved on to a new hunting or gathering area, the jugs filled with acorn flour, grains, or dried berries, would be buried near their permanent homes.

The Digueños led a seminomadic life, moving from area to area as the seasons progressed. The geography of San Diego County varies dramatically from the shoreline beaches and tide pools to the valley of the San Diego River on into the mountains and further east to the searing desert, all within a few days' walk for an Indian group. They took full advantage of this geographic variety. Spring would find them in the desert gathering yucca, ocotillo, and other cactus plants. Early summer was spent along the coast, fishing and gathering piñon nuts; winter found them in their permanent homes in the valley. The men hunted game in the mountains and hills nearly all year round.

Desert plants provided a variety of foods for the knowledgeable Indians. Nothing was overlooked. The yucca blossoms were cooked and eaten fresh, or dried for later use. The stalk of the yucca plant made a fine soap treasured by the Digueños. The tuna cactus has a juicy red fruit they found delicious and refreshing, while its leaves were steamed and eaten. Learning how to remove the spines without getting stuck was quite a trick. Ocotillo grew in abundance and the desert in spring was alive with this cactus' brilliant red flowers. The blossoms of the ocotillo were cooked and eaten and its long stalks were used as fences in the villages.

The century plant, or agave, was another food the desert provided. In early spring, when the agave begin to bud, the women gathered basketfuls while the men prepared the fire pit. After they put a layer of leaves over the hot coals, they placed the agave buds in the pit. The buds were covered with more leaves, and sand was piled over the pit. The next day, when the pit was uncovered, the agave buds, now cooked to a sweet, juicy mass, were enjoyed by the tribe.

Chia seeds, from a mustard-like plant that grows all over San Diego County, were great favorites of the Diegueños. The women filled their baskets with chia seeds by beating the dry plant head over a tightly woven basket. Dried chia seeds, rich in oil, were ground into flour and mixed with other seeds, tangy mustard, wild rye or oats, and made into *pinole,* another mush-like staple food. They also toasted the chia seeds by tossing them in a basket containing hot rocks. Toasted chia seeds were always carried along by the Diegueños when they traveled. The seeds, along with dried berries, made a filling snack.

By late spring, the desert had lost its brilliance. The tiny wild flowers wilted in the heat and blossoming cactus gave way to brown, dried tumbleweed and sage. It was time to move on.

From spring through summer, grunion, a beautiful silvery fish, engage in a mating practice unique in the marine world. During the high tides, they rush onto the beaches of California to lay their eggs in the sand. By the thousands—the millions—in the light of the full moon, grunion surge ashore, each wave carrying more fish toward land. Using their tails to dig a hole in the sand, they drop their eggs and wriggle back across the beach toward the receding waves.

Attuned as they were to nature and their environment, the Diegueños always knew when the grunion would run and they looked forward to these evenings. They would gather on the beaches and light fires to attract the grunion to their particular spot. While singing and laughing, joking and gossiping, they would keep a sharp eye for the first wave that carried the fish toward shore. When the run began in earnest, everyone, young and old, would scamper up and down the beaches, grabbing the flashing fish, getting soaked by waves, and having the time of their lives. The grunion, which run every full moon from March until about August, were an important part of the Diegueño diet. These small fish, a type of silversides, were cooked and eaten whole, or dried and used later in fish stew. The Diegueños were sharp traders and used the dried fish for barter with other tribes.

Abalone, all but extinct in California tide pools today, were gathered in huge quantities by the Digueños. They pried these delectable mollusks off the rocks, pounded the meat to make it tender, and then lightly cooked it in clay dishes. What they didn't eat right away was dried and stored. The lovely abalone shells, with their subtle mother-of-pearl colors, were used as utensils or cut into small discs and used as money.

The men caught other fish, using hooks, spears, or nets. During the height of summer, groups of Digueños would camp along the marshes of south San Diego Bay to gather salt for their tribe. It was also a brisk trade item.

The Digueños used more seasoning than most primitive groups. They had wild sage and mustard, salt, wild onions, and for sweetening, honey along with a good many types of berries.

Their diet sounds almost ideal. Greens, seeds, nuts and berries, fish and game, wild fowl and their eggs made up the menu. The rich variety of their foods ensured a long and healthy life. Skeletal remains have shown no evidence of physical deformity and little tooth decay. Because their diet was so complete, with elements lacking in one food found in another, illness must have been rare. They did have a variety of medicinal herbs to be used in case of sickness and, of course, the medicine man, or shaman, was expected to perform miracles. But, basically, the body's remarkable recuperative powers performed the miracle.

According to Dr. Henry Bieler, "80–85 percent of all types of human ailments are self-limited. Given a good diet and a reasonably healthy system, illnesses run their course and the individual recovers." This certainly must have been the case with the Digueños. They were healthy, happy, and long-lived. Good food, fresh air, and exercise were their best preventive medicines.

The Digueño culture was beautiful in its simplicity. Their educational, moral, and ethical system was completely integrated into their religious ceremonies. During these events, the history of the tribe was learned, the lessons for the future taught, and the standards of behavior reinforced. The most important ceremony in the life of a Digueño was the initiation rites of puberty. Frequently these rites were held for a number of young people who reached the appropriate age together.

The boys' initiation ceremonies began with the drinking of a Jimson weed potion. This narcotic is very strong, sometimes fatal, and it took several days for its effects to wear off. During this time the boys had weird hallucinations and dreams that were to play an important part in their lives. If they dreamed about a particular animal, they must never kill that animal for the rest of their lives; to do so would bring death. Other taboos resulted from their dreams—when they should hunt or fish, where they should live. After the effects of the drug wore off, the instruction in tribal life began. Ground paintings showing the universe as a circle were drawn by the chief, with all the major forces of life portrayed as abstract designs. Evil was depicted in the form of a spider or snake. Each symbol was pointed out to the initiates, along with exhortations to do the proper things so life would be long and happy. There were no words for "right" or "wrong" in their language; their concept of morality was based upon a belief in a system of cause and effect. If certain things were done, good would result. The boys' initiation ceremony ended with a tribal dance and feasts. Gifts were given to the young men, who were now considered adults and expected to take their places in tribal society.

The initiation for the girls was more bizarre. A deep hole was dug in the sand and filled with hot rocks. After the sand had been thoroughly heated, the rocks were removed and the girl was buried in the hole with only her head and arms free. For up to a week she had to remain buried and during that time she was not permitted to eat or speak or touch her head. Twigs were used if the need to scratch arose.

Meanwhile, dances were performed all around the initiate. Songs and chants telling of the woman's role in tribal life were sung. When the girl was removed from the hole, the ground paintings were done for her. The universe, the moon, the stars, and symbolic animals were drawn and explained. At this time, the taboos were described. She was told about birth and the delivery of children, how she must live apart from her family prior to childbirth and during her menstrual cycle.

These religious ceremonies were a vital part of the education of Digueño children. When the mission priests halted this practice, they didn't realize they were eliminating an important aspect of Digueño life. The young men and women grew up with no knowledge of their past, their traditions, or their expected role in tribal life. The girls suffered especially. Without any information about menstruation, childbearing, or child care, infant mortality rose alarmingly.

After the initiation ceremonies, the young men joined their older brothers and fathers in hunting and fishing. The most frequently caught game was rabbit which, along with fish, was their major source of protein. The DiguEños used a rabbit stick, rather like a boomerang, to kill the animals. They were very adept with this stick and could even hit birds on the wing. In hunting deer, the DiguEños stalked their prey wearing a deer skull, complete with antlers, on their heads. If they stayed upwind of the deer, they could get close enough to use the bow and arrow effectively. Deer were hard to catch, however; the animals could escape into rugged hills and arroyos where tracking them was all but impossible, so these Indians really depended on the ubiquitous rabbit for most of their meat. Rabbit has the lowest fat content of any North American animal and there is little fat in fish so the DiguEños might have suffered from fat starvation. Fortunately, the pine nut and chia have a high fat content. They ate enough of these foods along with acorns so that their fat intake was sufficient.

The DiguEños were pretty casual about clothes. They had to be functional, sturdy, and as brief as possible. The children went naked except during the coldest weather. The men wore a sort of deerskin loincloth and the women wore a skirt vaguely reminiscent of a hula skirt. It was made from the supple inner bark of trees or strips of tule reeds. It consisted of a woven belt with strips of bark or reeds attached to the front, which was quite short, and to the back, which came to the calf. These split skirts afforded great mobility and were often decorated with a bit of shell at the end of each strip. Sometimes they were dyed bright colors.

Blankets were made by cutting rabbit skins into very narrow strips and weaving them together. These soft, warm, and beautiful creations were the pride of the DiguEño family and some can still be seen in museums. However, the DiguEños had a practice of burning all the possessions of a person who had died. They felt this prevented the spirit from returning to earth. Unhappily, much was lost in this manner, so few artifacts were left for anthropologists to investigate.

The healthy, carefree, happy life of the DiguEño ended with the establishment of the missions. By force and guile the Indians were herded into the mission compounds, where they subsequently died by the thousands. In 1818, the Spanish governor reported that 64,000 Indians had been baptized—and 41,000 of them were dead.

Those that didn't succumb to mistreatment, poor diet, or disease, died of psychological depression. It was the practice of the mission fathers to separate the males and females with absolutely no regard for family ties. From age seven, males were housed in one compound and females in another. This unnatural arrangement led to serious emotional problems and many of the Diguñeos, unable to understand or accommodate, simply died for no apparent reason. Their way of life destroyed, their religion forbidden, they had nothing left to live for.

Disease swept through the mission Indian population, unused to crowding and close confinement and debilitated by strange, unhealthy foods. Tuberculosis, the scourge of Indians everywhere, accounted for nearly half the mission Indian deaths. Nearly all of the Indians developed diseases of the eyes and many of them became blind. The children suffered misshapen bodies, while tooth decay was rampant among all of them. Forced to work harder for the missionaries than they ever had in their lives of wandering, the Diguñeos frequently tried to escape and sometimes were successful. Family ties were so strong, however, they would not try to escape unless they could all leave together, so many remained and died.

After secularization of the mission lands following Mexican independence, the surviving Diguñeos tried to renew their tribal ways, but a new and formidable obstacle now faced them. Increasing numbers of whites were moving into their traditional hunting and gathering areas. The Indians would establish a village only to be told that the land belonged to a white man. "Move on." Slowly, inexorably, they were pushed into the hills, the deserts, into lands that could not support them. They had never been cultivators. Food had always been plentiful and the semiarid climate couldn't produce crops without irrigation. Now they weren't able to stay in one place long enough to raise a crop, even if they wanted to plant. The tribes splintered and disappeared. In their place, small family groups wandered here and there, working at a rancho, picking crops, anything to stay alive. Many of the families headed south across the border into Baja California. There they had the freedom to move about with no encroaching civilization to interfere. They recognized no borders and Baja had long been part of their hunting territory.

The tragic and beautiful autobiography of Delfina Cuero, a Digueño living in Baja, describes her life of wandering. From the viewpoint of one family, the process of acculturation, what anthropologists call the absorption of one culture into another, is told in touching detail. With no way to prove she is indeed an American in the truest sense, Delfina is not allowed to live in the United States.

These people have managed to maintain their independence during the years when many Indians were forced into dependency upon the federal government. Now they ask: "Can our grandchildren go to your schools? There is no longer room for hunters or gatherers. We can no longer teach them to survive. They must learn new skills from you. Is there room for us in America?"

FOODS OF THE DIGUEÑOS

"With all their hardships the California Indians were seldom sick. They were in general strong, hardy and much healthier than the many thousands who lived daily in abundance and on choicest fare that the skill of Parisian cooks can prepare. Gout, apoplexy, dropsy and colds were said to be almost unknown among them and they attained general freedom from such diseases as tuberculosis, smallpox, measles, trachoma and syphilis. Cancer was very rare, even in old age, and other degenerative processes were not often met."

Begert, an early anthropologist, wrote this in 1869 in his report to the Smithsonian Institute, "An Account of the Aboriginal Inhabitants of the California Peninsula." His wonder at the health and stamina of the Indians was understandable. Compared to his diet, their food was strange indeed.

Their two staple forms of food were *atole* and *pinole*. Atole was the thick, soup-like food made from ground nuts and seeds, usually acorns. Pinole was the fine flour made by grinding seeds of grasses and flowering annuals. It was sometimes made into mush, but frequently eaten dry. Bulbs, roots, stalks, and other parts of plants were cooked in the "earth oven," a pit dug in the ground and lined with heated rocks, filled with the food to be cooked, covered and left to steam, sometimes for up to twenty-four hours. Cooking vessels were watertight baskets lined with pitch. When the baskets were filled with water and the food to be prepared, very hot rocks were placed in them, which caused the water to boil. Or, food was sometimes placed in a clay pot and buried in hot ashes.

Nuts and Seeds

Acorns. Atole was the chief food, making up over half the Digueños' daily diet. After the acorns were gathered, they would be stored in their shells until needed. At that time they would be shelled and the nut inside, dry by this time, would be pounded with mortar and pestle, often just a rock and a hollow stone. The acorn flour had to be leached of its poisonous tannic acid and this was done in one of two ways: putting the flour into a large shallow basket and running water through it, or digging a hole in the sandy river bank and pouring water over the flour. Either way, a lot of abrasive material found its way into the atole. Most of the acorn flour was made into the mush mentioned earlier. Some of it was set aside for bread-making, which was done by building a hard-wood fire on a flat stone and letting it burn for about half an hour. Then the embers were brushed aside and the bread dough placed on the rock. They covered the loaf entirely with the embers and the hot coals were replaced. A sharp stick would be stuck into the bread from time to time, and when it emerged clean the bread was done. All the coals and ashes were brushed away and the loaf was ready to eat.

The bread, which was quite sweet, hardened as it cooled. It could be kept for weeks. When needed, it was softened by soaking it in water. The men carried acorn bread on their trips and found it was the most compact and nourishing food they could take along. The Digueños flavored their atole with bone meal, fire ash, and occasionally clay. They received calcium from the bone meal and fire ash, and iron from the clay.

CHIEF SOURCES OF NUTRIENTS
IN THE DIGUEÑO DIET

PROTEIN	rabbit and shellfish
FAT	nuts
CARBOHYDRATE	acorns
CALORIES	acorns
VITAMIN A	fresh greens
VITAMIN C	fresh greens, flowers, and fruits
VITAMIN B_1	acorns
VITAMIN B_2	acorns
NIACIN	rabbit and shellfish
CALCIUM	ground bones
IRON	nuts and acorns
FIBER	acorns, wild greens

It has been estimated that over 500 pounds of acorns were gathered by each Indian family every year. Through the centuries, more humans have eaten acorns as a staple food than any of the grains. Acorns are a member of the nut family and contain Vitamins A and the B complex, and unsaturated fatty acids. The nutrients found in acorns more closely resemble those in grains than in nuts. Compared with wheat they contain about half the protein, twice the fat, and about the same amount of calories. Ecologists believe that acorns are a neglected source of nutritious food, but in preparing most types of acorns, it is essential to remove the poisonous tannic acid.

Piñon nuts. Pine nuts, or piñon, are found in the mountains of Southern California at altitudes of 3,500 to 9,000 feet. They were an important food item for the Digueños who traveled many miles to harvest the crop. Using long poles, the men would knock the pine cones from the tree. Gathered by the women and children, the cones would be piled up in great heaps and set on fire. It was a simple task to remove the nuts from the charred cones. Next they would be shelled by rolling a stone pestle lightly over them, and the hulls would be winnowed out. The small white seed was then ready to be eaten raw or roasted.

Piñon nuts are an extremely concentrated food. They contain a large amount of incomplete protein, Vitamin B_1, niacin, and iron. They are an excellent source of oil, containing about 50 percent; they do not become rancid quickly so they can be stored for long periods. Pine nuts were the chief source of the essential fatty acids in the Digueños' otherwise low-fat diet.

Chia and Wild Mustard.   Chia is a type of wild sage that grows over large areas of Southern California. Its tiny gray-brown seeds are harvested by shaking the heads of the plant over flat, tightly woven baskets. Generally, the Indians ground the dried or roasted seed into a flour, which was eaten raw or made into a thin gruel. Whole chia seeds were a favorite snack and were carried in leather pouches by the men and boys. Chia seeds have a high food value, as they are rich in proteins and easily digested fat. They become jelly-like when soaked in water. One teaspoonful of chia seed was said to be enough to keep an Indian nourished for up to twenty-four hours on a forced march.

Wild mustard seed was gathered from the hills and the seeds were sprinkled over other foods to add flavor. Sometimes the seeds would be pounded into a fine powder and mixed with water to produce mustard.

Wild Plants

Mescal.   Mescal, agave, and century plant are different names for a large cactus-like plant that grows in great abundance in the rocky hills of the Southwest and Southern California. Spring, when the plant sent up its flowers, was one of the most enjoyable times of year for the Digueños. Large groups would gather to prepare an earth oven, and as the preparations were underway, it was a wonderful opportunity to tell ancient legends, meet old friends, and sing songs. The camp would last for weeks. The groups would return to the same location year after year so the pit was used repeatedly.

The flower of the agave is a huge stalk covered with tiny golden blossoms that emerges from the center of the plant, and the thick stem is fibrous and moist. The Digueños would cut the stem and remove the blossoms. These latter would be boiled and dried to be kept for winter use; they could be stored for years without losing their sweet, delicate flavor. The very young and tender leaves of the agave would be eaten raw and the seeds collected and added to the family's supply. The huge center stem, now stripped of its blossoms, was placed in the earth oven and steamed for up to twenty-four hours. When it was removed, it had cooked into a brown juicy mass, very sweet and nutritious. The Diguenos happily stuffed themselves with all they could eat of this delicious treat, then dried the rest for use in winter.

Mesquite. Mesquite, a common shrub found in low areas and washes throughout the Southwest, has a long yellow bean that was collected and stored in great quantities. While gathering the beans, the Diguenos consumed many of them fresh-picked and raw. The rest were dried and ground for later use. In preparing the mesquite gruel, a quantity of water would be added to the ground beans and allowed to ferment slightly. This improved the flavor. Cakes were made from the bean flour and were sometimes the only food carried on a long journey. As they were 25 percent sugar, they provided a quick energy lift and their high protein content sustained this effect. Mesquite wood was considered the most desirable because its fire is slow-burning and hot. The tree produces a clear gum when cut and the Diguenos gathered this gum and used it in a number of ways. Dissolved in water, it was an effective treatment for sore throats, and also soothed sore eyes. It was used as a glue and, when boiled, it made a black dye for painting pottery. This black dye, mixed with mud, was plastered on the hair for a day or two and, when it was removed, it had covered any gray hairs, restored the deep black sheen, and even killed any lice.

Screwbean. This is a shrub closely related to the mesquite, but not quite as common. The beans are similar to the mesquite, but a bit smaller and more bitter. In a rather complicated treatment, the Diguenos reduced this bitterness to produce a bean that was extremely sweet. The procedure involved placing the beans in a large pit lined with arrowhead leaves. The beans were layered alternately with the leaves until the pit was full. They were sprinkled with water to keep them moist and after about a month they were removed and dried for storage. Sometimes the beans became wormy in this process, but the worms were ground up along with the beans, thus increasing the protein content. Pods of the screwbean were boiled down to make a thick, very sweet syrup similar to molasses that was a favorite sweetener.

Yucca. This, found all over the Southwest, was by far the most important plant to the Digueños because of its many uses. The fiber was used in clothing, and the stem has a soap-like quality. When left to ripen on the yucca, the fruit turns very sweet, and was a favorite treat for the Digueños. Deer, birds, and insects also value this fruit, so it was usually picked green and left to ripen in the sun. Much of the yucca fruit was dried for future use. When water was added to the dried fruit, a delicious drink resulted.

Holly, Islay, Manzanita. Toyon, or California holly, is a small bushy tree or shrub that grows in the hills and canyons of California. It has bright scarlet berries that were gathered and roasted by the Digueños. The early Spanish settlers crushed the berries and made a pleasant cider from the juice. From the bark and tender leaves a soothing tea was brewed which the Indians used as a cure for stomachache.

Islay, or holly-leaved cherry, produces seeds that were dried and ground into powder. After leaching the flour, the Digueños added it to acorn meal. The fruit was not eaten.

Manzanita is a common bush of the Southwest. The Indians collected the ripe berries by shaking the branches of the bush over baskets. They ate the berries fresh, but also dried and stored large quantities for winter use. The pulp of the manzanita berries is sweet and, when dried and pounded into powder, it can be added to water to make a delicious drink. The Digueños collected the seeds, from which they made a fine flour which they used to make cookies.

Wild Onion. One of the most abundant and widespread of the wild foods, it is found all over the United States. It is easy to recognize from its smell. The Indians ate onions in large quantities, not as a seasoning or flavoring, but as a vegetable. They ate the entire plant, bulb and shoots, raw or cooked. When the tops are also used, the strong odor is reduced because the tops contain chlorophyll that may clear the breath. Not only that, the tops are extremely nutritious. Following is a comparison of 100 grams of onion bulb and onion tops:

	Vitamin A (units)	Vitamin C (mg.)	Vitamin B_1 (mg.)	Vitamin B_2 (mg.)	Iron (mg.)	Calcium (mg.)	Niacin (mg.)	Carbo-hydrate (grams)
Bulbs	trace	25	.05	.04	.6	40	.4	10.5
Tops	4,000	51	.07	.10	2.2	56	.6	5.5

Cacti. Tuna, or Indian fig, is a large cactus that was introduced into California from Mexico. The Indians made much use of the fruit, which they broke off the plant with a stick. Fine spines on the fruit had to be brushed off, after which they were peeled. The orange, juicy fruit is sweet, soft, and contains soft seeds. Containing a good quantity of Vitamin C, they were eaten raw. The young pods were gathered before the spines hardened and were roasted in the earth oven to be eaten as a vegetable.

Beavertail cactus is similar to the tuna and is eaten in the same manner.

Cattail. Cattail, a versatile favorite of the Indians, grows in marshy areas. It provided a complete and nutritious meal from its many edible parts. The thick creeping roots were roasted, made into soup, or dried and ground into meal. The pollen was used in making bread, the young shoots were eaten raw, and the bulb was baked like a potato. The food value of the roots is similar to that of corn or rice. The large bulb-like sprout, located where the stem joins the root, was baked inside leaves. It has a sweetish taste like a water chestnut. The core or marrow of the young plant was eaten raw or cooked. The flower spikes that appear before the pollen forms, were also eaten raw or made into a soup. The pollen was gathered and, when cooked with water, became a porridge; or it was formed into loaves and baked like bread. Truly, the cattail is a valuable plant, overlooked by modern people but highly regarded by the Digueños.

The young spikes can be boiled in salted water, husked just like corn, and eaten like an ear of corn—right off the cob. They have a delicate, sweet flavor that most people like. When the young plants are about two feet high, it is time to gather "cossack asparagus." Peeled down to the tender center, these shoots are white, delicate, and delicious. The pollen of cattail is an incredibly rich nutritional food source. It is virtually a complete food and a little over an ounce, thirty-five grams, contains all the nutritional requirements of the average person. As little as twenty grams a day would constitute a survival diet. The tails contain all the enzymes known to be necessary for good health; the pollen has seven times more protein than eggs. It also has natural antibiotical properties that have been said to cure anemia, constipation, prostate problems, and maladies of old age. It is also rich in nucleic acids. All of these amazing facts were revealed in a study by Alen Caillas, a French agriculturist who analyzed cattail pollen. When this pollen is added to other foods, it adds a buttery color and a corn-like taste.

Fungus. Fungi gave additional variety to the Digueño diet. Small mushrooms were occasionally gathered from the trunks of dead trees, and larger mushrooms were found in the meadows. A real delicacy was a white fungus found on the trunk of cottonwood trees. None of these was an important item in the diet because the Indians were aware of the danger in making a mistake and gathering the wrong species. It is safest for modern cooks to stick to commercially grown varieties, although wild mushrooms have a marvelous flavor. As a food, mushrooms are excellent. Ounce for ounce, they are richer in protein than any other vegetable, and they are a source of Vitamin B_{12}, iodine, and Vitamin D. They are also low in calories and carbohydrates. Mushrooms are a fungus and have no seeds or roots. The spores creep through the soil like cobwebs and lie dormant until the right conditions exist, then spring up overnight. Researchers at Duke University report that the spores of some mushrooms may be a promising source of antibiotics.

Tule, or arrowhead. Tule is a reed-like plant that grows at the edges of ponds and streams. The Digueños harvested the roots of this attractive water plant in late summer and baked them in the embers of the fire. They ate them skinned and whole, or mashed and mixed with screwbean syrup. The tubers, which are about the size of an egg, are pure white inside and have a sweetish taste and starchy texture. Surplus was dried and eaten later.

Peppergrass. Peppergrass is a weedy annual widespread throughout California. Its small red seed was gathered by the Digueños. It was usually toasted by tossing it in a basket with hot stones, then ground and added to pinole. Because of its peppery taste, it was often used to season other foods. The leaves were eaten raw or boiled. The leaves are spicier in taste the higher they grow on the peppergrass plant.

Wild greens.   Wild cabbage, prince's plume, and many other wild greens were added to boiling water and cooked until tender. They were then removed and rinsed several times in cold water. This was done to remove the slightly bitter taste. It also removed many vitamins and minerals. The leached greens were often laid out on rocks to dry for winter use. Large quantities of wild greens were consumed raw. Greens collected along the shore line have a desirable salty taste.

Lamb's quarters (also called wild spinach), shepherd's purse, dock, and dandelions are all weeds that the Diguenos frequently cooked and ate in the spring. The crown of the dandelion, found between the leaves and the root, was steamed and eaten like a potato.

The Diguenos gathered and dried kelp, which they used as a seasoning. Dried kelp keeps well and is important for good health. It contains over forty-one trace minerals, calcium, protein, Vitamin C, and is the best-known source of iodine.

Eggs

Diguenos gathered the eggs of wild birds and ate them raw right on the spot. If the eggs were to be cooked and eaten later, they would first be tested by putting them in water. If the egg sank, it was good to eat, but if it floated, incubation was well advanced so it was gently replaced in the nest. The Diguenos cooked eggs by pushing a small green twig through the egg and placing it over a bed of coals. After they turned the egg for about ten minutes, it was ready to eat or carry along on the trail. Eggs were a great favorite of the Diguenos, a fact which contributed to their good health, as eggs are a near-perfect food.

Meat

The favorite day-to-day meat of the Diguenos was rabbit. Other game they caught fairly regularly was deer, wild birds, squirrels, snakes, mice, and lizards. Large game was usually roasted over a fire or cooked in the earth oven. Smaller game was pounded on rocks to break up the bones, and added to the atole. Dried bones of larger animals were ground into a powder and also added to atole. This bone meal was the chief source of calcium for the Indians. Dried bone meal contains up to 800 milligrams of calcium, 375 milligrams of phosphorus and 1.7 milligrams of iron per one-half teaspoon.

Rabbit is a fine-textured lean meat with very little fat. The wild rabbit is the leanest animal in North America, and Indians who depended upon this meat often suffered fat hunger. Luckily, the oil in pine nuts, chia, and other seeds balanced the Diegueños' low-fat diet. Boys were encouraged to eat the eyes of the rabbit, as this was supposed to make them sharp-eyed, and it really did. The fat around the eye and the retina is the richest of all animal sources of Vitamin A, which is essential for good eyesight.

Seafood

The abalone, a large single-shelled mollusk that lives in tide pools, was gathered in huge quantities all along the beaches. The meat, which is tough, was pounded on the rocks before cooking. It was often dried and saved for later use or for bartering. Other seafood enjoyed was octopus, crab, grunion, scallops, starfish, and smaller fish found in the bays and inlets. The fish were usually roasted over a bed of hot coals or baked in the earth oven. All of the fish was consumed; the tail, fins, and head were added to the soups and the bones ground into meal to be used as a flavoring for other foods. Much of the catch was sun-dried. Fillets of fish would be threaded on sharpened sticks and stuck into the ground so the air circulated freely. This dried fish kept very well and was carried inland to be used for barter with desert tribes.

Insects

Many insects were gathered by the Diegueños in the larval as well as the adult stages. Roasted grasshoppers, with legs and wings removed, were very popular and were said to resemble pork in taste. Another popular treat was roasted bee larvae, which was said to taste like oily peanuts. In a comparison of 100 grams of insect and beefsteak there are:

	Protein (grams)	Iron (mg.)	Vitamin B_1 (mg.)	Vitamin B_2 (mg.)	Niacin (mg.)	Fat (grams)	Calories
100 grams larvae	16.3	1.7	.23	.46	3.3	4.6	130
100 grams adult	15.5	1.0	.23	.54	2.8	6.4	139
100 grams beefsteak	14.7	2.2	.06	.13	3.5	37.1	397

DINING WITH A DIGUEÑO FAMILY

The serene and harmonious life of the Digueños was reflected in their living habits. Their house, or wickiup, an easily dismantled assortment of branches and bush fronds, could be transported and reerected quickly and easily. The frame of the wickiup was sturdy branches that had been bent to form a conical shaped dwelling, usually about twelve feet in diameter. It was covered with palm fronds or brush and lined with some sort of fabric or pelt. The Digueños rarely did more than sleep in the wickiup, however, for all the chores of the day took place outside. The family usually ate cold atole mush and some fruit and seeds for breakfast. The day's activities kept them from sharing a midday meal, usually some sort of snack. The women would be gathering acorns or pounding the kernels, fetching water from the river, curing pelts or hides, busy at any one of a dozen tasks. The men and boys would be off hunting rabbit or deer, climbing around the tide pools, gathering clams and abalone, or sitting in tribal discussions.

At dinner the family gathered in front of their wickiup to enjoy the evening meal together. Sitting in a circle on a fur blanket or woven rug with the bowl or basket of atole in the middle, they would eat and chat about the day's events. They would dip their hands into the common pot, using all their fingers to form a cup.

For centuries the Digueños used gourds, shells, or tightly woven baskets for cooking and eating utensils. In later years they traded for pottery vessels made by the desert tribes. The Digueño baskets were woven so tightly and were so well covered with pitch that they were watertight and food could be cooked in them. This was done by using wooden tongs to drop hot stones into the water-filled baskets.

In addition to the atole, the Diegueños would usually have roasted rabbit or some seafood. A basket of fruits, berries, and seeds accompanied every meal. Fresh raw greens in summer or dried greens soaked in water during the winter were zestily spiced with onion, mustard, sage, or kelp. Bone meal and occasionally even clay were used to flavor the atole.

After dinner, the family listened with rapt attention while the father recounted his day's adventures. Later the mother brought out the ever-present basket of acorns and, as they sang the tribal songs, the whole family joined in the endless task of removing the shells by cracking them with their teeth. Later, around the fire, the men carved their rabbit sticks, and the boys fashioned arrows by running thin branches through deeply grooved stones that had been heated to temper the wood. The women and girls wove narrow strips of rabbit fur into beautiful and softly luxurious robes.

It evokes a tranquil scene: the cluster of thatched dwellings, the glowing fires, and the sounds of singing and laughter as the families performed their evening chores or visited with one another.

That these hunters and gatherers were doomed becomes apparent when one considers the enormous amount of land needed to sustain each family. Geographic limitations and encroaching civilizations prevented the Diegueños from obtaining their food in their accustomed way, so it was only a matter of time until they either disappeared or became acculturated.

A DIGUEÑO DINNER PER INDIVIDUAL

RABBIT, 4 ounces
ACORN MUSH, 3½ ounces dry acorn
BONE MEAL, ½ teaspoon
PINE NUTS, 2 tablespoons
WILD GREENS, 2½-ounce mixture of
    dandelion, mustard, and sorrel
MUSHROOMS, 2 medium
WILD ONIONS, 4 young onions, including their tops
PUMPKIN, ½ cup
HONEY, 1½ teaspoons

A DIGUEÑO DINNER FROM YOUR KITCHEN

SALAD (assorted greens and onions)
OIL AND VINEGAR DRESSING
BARBECUED RABBIT (chicken may be substituted)
BUCKWHEAT GROATS WITH PUMPKIN SEEDS
PUMPKIN SQUARES

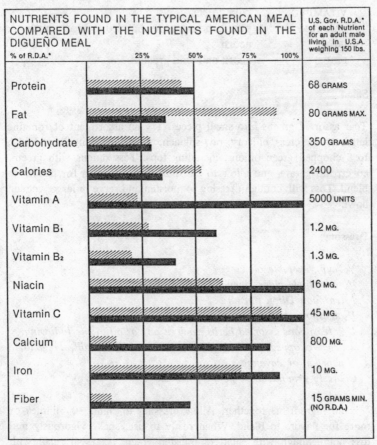

NUTRIENTS FOUND IN THE TYPICAL AMERICAN MEAL COMPARED WITH THE NUTRIENTS FOUND IN THE DIGUEÑO MEAL						U.S. Gov. R.D.A.* of each Nutrient for an adult male living in U.S.A. weighing 150 lbs.
% of R.D.A.*		25%	50%	75%	100%	
Protein						68 GRAMS
Fat						80 GRAMS MAX.
Carbohydrate						350 GRAMS
Calories						2400
Vitamin A						5000 UNITS
Vitamin B₁						1.2 MG.
Vitamin B₂						1.3 MG.
Niacin						16 MG.
Vitamin C						45 MG.
Calcium						800 MG.
Iron						10 MG.
Fiber						15 GRAMS MIN. (NO R.D.A.)

*R.D.A. is the recommended daily nutrient allowance intended to meet the needs of a *healthy* individual.
   Diagonal lines represent the American meal.

The chief sources of nutrients in the Digueño meal are:

PROTEIN	rabbit
FAT	pine nuts
CARBOHYDRATE	acorn
CALORIES	acorn
VITAMIN A	wild greens
VITAMIN B$_1$	acorn
VITAMIN B$_2$	wild greens
NIACIN	rabbit
VITAMIN C	wild greens
CALCIUM	powdered bone meal added to acorn mush
IRON	acorn
FIBER	acorn and wild greens

Salad

Tear assorted greens into small pieces. Try an assortment of romaine lettuce, watercress, chicory, raw spinach, and young dandelion. Add 6 to 8 chopped green onions, including tops. Toss onions with greens, cover, refrigerate, and allow to stand 20 minutes or so for flavors to blend. Toss with enough dressing to moisten and serve in large wooden bowl.

Dressing

¼ cup vegetable oil
¼ cup apple cider vinegar or lemon juice
1 teaspoon Dijon mustard
½ teaspoon salt
1½ teaspoons assorted herbs, such as any or all of the following:
    dried chopped parsley, chives, basil, tarragon, dill, oregano,
    paprika, or cayenne
Coarsely ground black pepper, to taste

Mix all ingredients together. Allow dressing to stand 30 minutes or more for flavors to blend. When ready to use, shake vigorously and toss only enough with salad to moisten greens. Garnish salad with canned beavertail pods if you wish. They are sold in the Mexican food section of many grocery stores and are called *napalitos*.

Rabbit

1 young frying rabbit cut in quarters

Coat rabbit with melted unsalted butter or vegetable oil. Barbecue over a charcoal fire or in your broiler. Turn rabbit several times during cooking. Baste with more butter or pan drippings when you turn it. Cook until tender, about 45 minutes. Cut up chicken may be substituted for rabbit and cooked the same way.

Buckwheat Groats

¼ pound (1¼ cups) buckwheat groats (or kasha)
2 teaspoons butter
1 medium onion, chopped
3 cups chicken broth
8 medium-size fresh mushrooms, quartered
¼ cup shelled pumpkin seeds or sunflower seeds
1 teaspoon bone meal powder

Melt butter in a saucepan. Add bone meal and chopped onions and cook until onions are soft. Add chicken broth and bring to boil. Add buckwheat groats; cover, and simmer until tender, about 20 minutes. Fold in raw mushrooms and pumpkin seeds. Add salt or soy sauce to taste.

Pumpkin Squares

1 pound pumpkin or yellow winter squash

Poke shell with a knife in several places to allow steam to escape. Bake pumpkin on a cookie sheet in a 350° oven until just tender, about 45 minutes. When cooked, cut into wedges, remove seeds, and cut flesh into 1-inch cubes, down to shell but not through it. Pour warm dressing over pumpkin squares and serve in shell.

Dressing

> 2 tablespoons butter
> 2 tablespoons honey
> 2 tablespoons prepared mustard
> ¼ teaspoon salt

Combine ingredients in a small pan and heat, but do not cook or boil.

Pumpkin Pudding

> 1 cup young corn kernels or 1 cup cream-style corn
> 1 cup pumpkin or acorn squash, finely chopped (or 1 cup canned pumpkin)
> ½ cup water (omit if using canned pumpkin)
> ½ teaspoon salt (omit if using canned pumpkin)
> 1 cup raw sunflower seeds, ground

Put corn kernels through a food grinder, retaining all the juice. Combine corn and chopped pumpkin and simmer, covered, stirring occasionally, until pumpkin is very tender. If using canned pumpkin, heat mixture to simmer and allow it to cook, stirring occasionally, about 10 minutes. Remove from heat and mash the pumpkin. Add sunflower seed meal to thicken. The pudding should be thick and gelatinous. If it is too thick, add a little hot water; if too thin, add more sunflower seed meal. Blackstrap molasses, maple syrup, or honey may be added; or canned chopped and seeded green chiles and salt may be added to taste. This pudding is good eaten hot or cold.

Piñon Nut–Sunflower Seed Cakes

> ½ cup sunflower seeds, ground
> ½ cup piñon nuts (also called pine nuts) or ½ cup pecans, ground
> Dash of salt

Add salt to ground nuts. Press 2 tablespoons of meal together with your hand to form a cookie-shaped cake. (If it just won't hold together, add a small amount of peanut butter.) Wrap the cakes individually in parchment paper, corn husks, or aluminum foil. Bake in a 300° oven until they are delicately brown, about 40 to 60 minutes.

The Indians wrapped the cakes in leaves and baked them in the ashes.

Cornmeal or Acorn Mush

> *1 cup acorn meal or cornmeal*
> *5 cups water (you may use milk to increase food value but don't let it boil)*
> *¾ teaspoon salt*
> *½ cup or more ground seeds or nuts, plus ¼ cup water (optional)*

Bring 4 cups water to boil. Gradually add the cornmeal, thinned with 1 cup of cold water. Reduce heat to simmer and cook, stirring constantly until it is smooth and thick (about 5 minutes). Reduce the heat to the lowest possible, or place mixture in the top of a double boiler and cook about 30 minutes, stirring occasionally. Mix in ground seeds or nuts with additional water, if needed. Turn mixture into an oiled loaf pan and cool. While the Indians enjoyed their mush in this form, many people find it more tasty if it is browned. Remove cold mush from pan. Slice into ¾-inch slices and sauté in hot butter or vegetable oil until golden brown on both sides. Serve with butter and honey or maple syrup.

Marrow Paste

> *Beef shank bones, cut in ½-inch pieces*
> *Sunflower or pumpkin seeds, ground*

Broil marrow bones, or simmer them in a small amount of water, until marrow is soft and easily removed from the bone. Remove marrow, place in a bowl, and mash. Add enough sunflower seed meal to make a mixture with a good spreading consistency. Add salt and garlic powder or chopped green onions to taste. Marrow paste makes a nice spread for whole grain bread or a dip for raw vegetables.

Jerky

> *2 pounds lean meat (beef flank or brisket are usually used). If using pork or wild meat, you must heat the meat slices to boiling just long enough to remove the red color*
> *½ cup soy sauce*
> *¼ teaspoon garlic salt*
> *¼ teaspoon coarsely ground black pepper*

Trim all visible fat from the meat and cut it lengthwise with the grain into long strips no more than ¼ inch thick. Combine soy sauce, garlic salt, and pepper. Pour over the meat and coat it well. Place meat on a wire rack placed on a baking sheet. The strips may touch but must not overlap. Place in the sun or bake at 150° in your oven for 10 to 12 hours. If drying the beef in the sun, you must protect it from insects and cover it at night to keep it dry. Often your gas pilot will give enough heat to oven-dry the meat. If not, you may place a light bulb in the oven light socket. Probably a 150-watt bulb will be adequate. Leave oven door open about 1 or 2 inches so that moisture can escape. Jerky is done when it is black on the outside and if, when bent, it will crack but not break. Store in airtight jars.

Pemmican

4 ounces jerky
4 ounces dried berries or fruit, chopped
1 teaspoon honey
4 ounces nuts or seeds, ground
2 tablespoons warm melted butter or rendered animal fat

Grind jerky in a blender or pound it until a powder is formed. Mix powder with warm butter, honey, and nuts. Knead mixture until it has the consistency of raw hamburger. More butter or nuts may be added to thicken or thin the mixture. Add dried fruit to pemmican and pack in a crock, rawhide, sausage casing, or plastic bag. Seal airtight. If kept in a cool, dry place, pemmican will keep indefinitely.

Granola, "Pinole"

4 cups rolled oats
½ cup almonds,
    coarsely chopped
¼ cup sunflower seeds
¼ cup sesame seeds
½ cup crude bran
½ cup wheat germ
½ cup unsweetened coconut

2 tablespoons brown sugar
2 tablespoons blackstrap molasses
¼ cup vegetable oil
1 tablespoon vanilla
½ cup raisins
½ teaspoon salt

Mix molasses, oil, and vanilla in a small bowl. Combine oats, seeds, nuts, bran, coconut, wheat germ, brown sugar, and salt in a large bowl. Pour molasses and oil mixture over it and mix thoroughly with your hand to an even consistency. Spread it out on a shallow baking pan. Bake in a 225° oven until fairly dry and golden brown, about 1½ to 2 hours. Stir occasionally to prevent burning. Remove from oven and add raisins. After granola has cooled, it will become crisper.

Eat either hot or cold as a cereal, with milk or other liquid. Chopped dried fruit soaked overnight in milk, fruit juice, or water is good poured on cereal in the morning.

Granola may be varied by adding other grains, nuts, or dried fruit. It should be stored in an airtight container in the refrigerator.

The Digueño often toasted the seeds of wild plants on hot rocks placed near the fire and ate them as a cereal. Later, grains were also toasted, then ground and mixed with seeds to form an early version of granola.

Dandelion Coffee

Collect dandelion roots; wash and scrape them well. Dice into small pieces, place on a flat pan, and dry in the sun or in your oven. (See drying directions for jerky on page 107.) When the roots are almost black, very dry and easily crumbled, remove them from the oven and allow to cool. Grind cooled roots in a blender or with a rolling pin.

For each cup of "coffee," place 1 teaspoon of dandelion root powder and 1 cup of water in a saucepan. Simmer, covered, 5 minutes. Add an ice cube to settle grounds. Serve with honey and cream if desired.

Cattail Pollen Flour

To gather pollen, place the pollen-laden cattail spikes in a plastic bag or a paper sack (you do not have to cut the spike from the plant). Close the bag around the stem and shake very hard. This pollen gives foods a butter color and a corn flavor. You may substitute equal amounts of pollen for flour up to one-half of the flour in many recipes. Cattail muffins are really good!

THE LIGHT BITE, DIGUEÑO STYLE

A QUICK MEAL: Cleaned, raw mushrooms marinated 24 hours in an oil and vinegar salad dressing, jerky or hard cooked eggs (you can mash the yolks with mustard, chopped onion, and a little marinade from the mushrooms), whole grain bread or sunflower cakes, and a fresh tomato or other fruit.

A SNACK: A mixture of seeds, nuts, and dried fruit. Try raw sunflower seeds, dry roasted peanuts, broken almonds, and raisins mixed in equal amounts.

The Gandans
of Lake Victoria

The equatorial sun beats down on a cluster of conical thatched huts. Beyond the huts a large field of banana trees lends vibrant color to the landscape. Their black trunks, shining green leaves, and brilliant white blossoms contrast vividly with the tawny huts and provide a stunning background for the village. Out past the carefully tilled fields, the rolling hills begin, home of python and puff adder, lynx and lion, elephant and hippo. Countless species of jungle birds and insects live here, some harmless, many fearfully dangerous. In the midst of this beauty and danger live the Gandans of Uganda.

Uganda lies astride the equator in central Africa. It is so remote that no explorer had ever seen the country before John Speke made his famous journey in search of the headwaters of the Nile and discovered Lake Victoria and the country bordering it, Uganda. His stories of the people and their customs were so bizarre no one took him seriously until Stanley confirmed his discoveries several years later. All this was in the 1860s, centuries after the coast of Africa had been thoroughly explored and mapped. Because of its nearly impassable terrain and the constant threat of death from fever, accident, or hostile natives, central Africa had remained an unknown mystery.

The Gandans lived undisturbed by the encroachment of civilization. No slavers made their way into the country, dragging off entire villages to die in the holds of slave ships or to spend their lives toiling in the fields of the New World. The Gandans and their complex society remained intact through the centuries and they retain their unique identity to this day.

They are members of the Bantu branch of Africans, and their

language is essentially Bantu. The root word *Ganda*—brother—has various prefixes. *Baganda* means the tribe; *Buganda* the country; *Luganda* the language. When Speke first encountered the Gandans, they had no writing, but messages were sent throughout the length and breadth of the country by means of drums. There were several hundred distinctive drum beats that transmitted signals to the population in a very efficient manner. All the news of the country was communicated in this way, the death of a king, a call to war, a gathering of the hunters, or simply local gossip.

The Bantus first inhabited Uganda about 3,000 years ago. Later, the country was invaded by a group of Hamitic people who established the villages that now make up Uganda. It was an ideal combination. The Bantus, a disorganized agricultural group, and the Hamites, a structured pastoral society, merged to form a successful nation.

The Gandan hierarchy consisted of the chief; one of his sisters, who acted as consort; and ten subchiefs representing each of the major sectors of Uganda. Every village had a petty chief and governmental jobs were passed out endlessly among the men—Keeper of the Drums, Guardian of the Fetishes, and on and on. There was hardly an adult male in Uganda who didn't hold some official title.

Polygamy was widely practiced and it was a poor man indeed who didn't have at least three wives. This arrangement was extremely successful and was actually necessary to ensure the food supply. The women tended the fields and one wife could hardly be expected to care for the banana grove, the yam patch, and the millet field while bearing the children and maintaining the home. Also, the women outnumbered the men about three to one. Because of warfare and the custom of human sacrifice, men were always in short supply. Too many unmarried women in the villages would be a source of trouble.

The climate is delightful. At an altitude of 4,300 feet, Uganda is on the high plateau of Africa. The temperature varies little throughout the year, it rarely gets over 85 degrees and the evenings are cool. There are two rainy seasons, April–May and September–October, and the Gandans sensibly established a six-month calendar, each with its planting and harvesting time. Being on the equator, the region experiences little seasonal variation.

Extremely handsome people, the Gandans are well proportioned and sturdy. They do not scarify, tattoo, or circumcise, and consider any marring of the human body disgusting. Their sexual habits were, and probably still are, very rigid, bordering on prudish. The body must be completely covered at all times. Adultery is punished harshly, although intrigues are carried on continuously more for excitement and fun than because of any serious dissatisfaction with the spouse. But it doesn't pay to get caught.

Extremely clean and sanitary, the Gandans bathe each morning and wash before and after meals. In their homes, the dirt floors are built up to about a foot above the ground; then the dirt is tamped down firmly and covered with woven mats. Fresh-cut banana leaves are placed on the mats daily. All household utensils are carefully wrapped in banana leaves and neatly stored. Each household consists of several buildings: the main house for sleeping, eating and visiting; a cookhouse; a privy; and a separate structure for the gods and fetishes worshipped daily.

The Gandan routine sounds almost ideal. They rise at sunrise, pay homage to their gods, and eat a small meal. Then everyone starts the daily chores, the men to fishing or cloth-making, the women to tending their fields or preparing the food. At noon they gather for lunch and spend the rest of the day visiting or amusing themselves. No one works after lunch. The Gandans are very sociable people and much of their day is spent seeing other members of the tribe or stopping by the home of a relative. Dinner is a time for story-telling, singing, and the repeating of ancient legends of the tribe. Each full moon, everyone takes a week off.

With a schedule like this, how does anything get done?

The Gandans are healthy, strong people, hard-working and vigorous. They possess more stamina than the people of other agricultural nations of Africa due, it is believed, to the abundance of freshwater fish available to them. Lake Victoria provides enough perch and tilapia, bass and trout to supply the whole country. Much of the catch is dried and carried inland for barter with other villages.

Years ago the Gandans established an intricate and well-maintained system of roads. Each small village built a road to the main village in that sector; the main villages then cared for the road to the capital. These roads crossed rivers and ravines, penetrated the densest forests, and climbed the steepest hills. There is no doubt that the Gandans' highly evolved road system contributed to the integrity of their society. Trips into the remotest areas of Uganda were easily undertaken and trade was brisk among the various settlements.

The men were superb hunters and seemed absolutely fearless as, armed with nothing but spears, they attacked an elephant or hippo. They also dug pitfalls along animal trails and caught an unwary buffalo or two in this manner. Wild game, however, was not their major source of protein; the animals were usually pretty lean and rangy with little fat on them. The fat of the land was a species of huge rat, highly prized by the Gandans. They caught this animal frequently and considered it a real delicacy.

The men fished Lake Victoria from boats, seined along the shore, or dropped long lines armed with dozens of barbless hooks into the lake. While waiting to haul in their lines, the men had no intercourse with their wives. This was just one of several sexual taboos and the result was a fairly effective method of population control.

Typical of most unsophisticated cultures, children are a source of pride and pleasure to the Gandan household. The women are devoted mothers, and the children reflect the care they receive. They are breast-fed until about three years old and the mothers are very careful about the food they eat during lactation, knowing it affects their babies. During the nursing period the mothers eat a special cereal made with red millet and quinoa. Red millet is rich in Vitamin A and has a calcium content five to ten times that of other grains. The quinoa is not only an important mineral source but it also has the remarkable ability to stimulate the flow of milk. The children are weaned abruptly at about three years and from then on they eat what the rest of the family eats. They rarely drink milk after weaning. This causes a drop in the body's production of lactase, an enzyme necessary in the digestion of milk, and may account for the fact that about 70 percent of adults of African extraction cannot tolerate milk.

The mainstay of the Gandans is their extensive banana groves. Every part of every tree is utilized in some manner. After the second year, the tree bears one hand of bananas and dies. The roots of the old trees are separated and planted, and leaves are placed around the base of the shoot as a mulch as well as a protection against insects and weeds. Banana leaves provide wrapping material; floor-covering; and, as food is wrapped in leaves and steamed, cooking utensils. The leaves are also used as cleaning cloths. In addition, they are fashioned into hats and, in the home, are piled on the floor to make a comfortable bed. The pithy stalk of the tree is used just like a sponge. Cut into small, easily handled pieces, it serves as napkins during the meal. Bananas are their staple food, and it is little wonder the Gandans feel it is the only crop worth planting.

In preparing the bananas for cooking, the fruit is picked green, then peeled, and usually steamed. In the cookhouse, a great pot hangs from a tripod of sticks over a fire pit. Into this pot the women place shredded banana leaves and the peeled bananas wrapped in fresh leaves. After steaming for several hours, the fruit is mashed. If it is properly done, a blob tossed up to the ceiling will stick. The steamed banana mash is rolled into small balls by each diner and dipped into the common pot containing a stew made from any sort of edible thing—fish, goat's meat, rats, caterpillars, leaves of wild or cultivated plants, vegetables, legumes, peanuts—the whole thing thickened with peanut or cassava flour. This stew, called *matoke,* is extremely nourishing and is served as lunch and dinner; in fact, many Gandans eat little else. The variations are endless so the meal is never the same twice.

The national beverage is *mwenge,* or banana beer. It is made by mashing overripe bananas in a large trough, adding millet flour and water, and waiting for the whole mess to ferment. This takes about three days. It is then strained into a gourd and considered ready to drink. Mwenge is served at all ceremonial occasions, during meetings of chiefs, after meals, and just about any time that seems appropriate.

Although the versatile banana is surely their most important plant, the Gandans do raise other foods—yams and millet, peanuts and cassava, tomatoes and sorghum. They collect a wide variety of wild greens that go into the gravy pot and, as a result, their diet is fairly extensive. Their main protein source is fish, and this they eat in huge quantities. Sometimes the fish is steamed whole, but usually it is cut up and cooked along with vegetables and served in the stew.

Along with the fish they catch and the crops they grow, the Gandans have a few other menu items that they esteem highly. Termites in Africa build huge hills, up to twenty feet high. After a rain they will leave their hills to mate and start new colonies. The

Gandans regard termite as a very tasty food indeed and, to scare up a termite feast, they cover the hill with banana leaves and pound on it to simulate the sound of rain. When the termites take wing, the Gandans are ready with nets. The insects are roasted or fried, or dried and ground into flour for future use.

Another seasonal favorite of the Gandans is gnats. These tiny insects swarm along the shore of Lake Victoria by the billions, and the children are sent out to gather up gourds full. The gnats are dried and made into a pie. Missionaries who have tried gnat pie declare it delicious and it is a favorite dish to serve visitors to Uganda. After the first shock, they invariably enjoy this strange food.

From time to time locusts invade the area, but pesticides aren't needed to control the hordes. The Gandans catch them for food. Very few escape to ravage the carefully tended gardens. The locusts are steamed and, after the wings and legs are removed, they are fried. The flavor is considered quite good and the protein content of locust, like most insects, is about equal to that of beef.

The Gandan diet also includes *manioc* (cassava), eaten in a variety of ways. Certain species of cassava contain a considerable amount of prussic acid and this highly toxic element is removed by an elaborate system of soaking and boiling. Other types of cassava are edible right out of the ground. It is imperative to know the difference.

Cassava is a secondary staple food of the Gandans and, depending on the variety, is roasted and eaten like a potato or, after proper treatment to remove the poison, ground into flour and added to the stew.

Cassava has the ability to thrive in impoverished soil, and as a result, is often planted in fields that have lost their productivity. In areas subject to occasional famines, cassava ranks high as a famine fighter. It grows rapidly and provides a good source of carbohydrates. The leaves contain a high level of Vitamins A and C as well as calcium.

After the cassava is harvested, the field lies fallow for up to ten years, when the planting cycle begins again with millet and sorghum, sweet potatoes and yams. Frequently a hedge of cassava surrounds the garden, and Henry Stanley's description of the well-tended Uganda garden makes it sound like a charming place.

It is laid out in several plats, with curving paths between. In it grow large sweet potatoes, yams, green peas, kidney beans, field beans, and tomatoes. The garden is bordered by manioc, coffee, and tobacco plants. On either side are small patches of millet, sesame, and sugar cane. Behind the house and courts and enfolding them, are the more extensive banana and plantain plantations and grain crops. . . .

Sorghum is another important item in the Gandan diet. This indigenous African grain grows in abundance throughout the continent. Similar to corn, it is prepared in much the same manner. The grains are pounded into a rough meal and mixed with steamed yams or cassava. The resulting thick paste is occasionally served along with stew in place of bananas in Gandan homes. The nutrients in sorghum are similar to those in corn.

This then was the society that Speke and Stanley found. Healthy, successful people, living at peace with their environment, if not with their tribal neighbors. Diseases that took such a dreadful toll of Europeans and Americans who lived in Africa seemed barely to touch the Gandans. In the 1890s, Uganda became a British protectorate and with the influx of foreigners determined to follow their own life style and eating habits, massive changes in the Gandan diet should have been expected. Curiously, this was not the case.

In the two major cities of Uganda, Entebbe and Kampala, new skyscrapers have risen, schools have been built, and technological progress can be observed everywhere; but just beyond the limits of these European-style cities, the conical, thatched homes of the Gandans still dot the countryside, each with its banana grove and patch of garden. The only significant change in the Gandans' diet has been an increase in the amount of meat they consume.

The menu of the major hotel in Kampala features *matoke,* the Gandan national dish. The only other item offered is a typically British meal of roast beef, Yorkshire pudding, and sherry trifle. Stores in villages all over the country have canned goods and flour for sale, but the Gandans prefer their traditional foods. They still catch huge perch out of Lake Victoria; they still make their mwenge beer, which they store in tall gourds and sell along the road; they still favor their gnat pie to the supersweet desserts enjoyed by the British; and best of all, they have retained their health and vigor to an amazing degree. Gandans have marvelous teeth and Dr. Price failed to find a single case of malformation of the dental arch among the rural population. In a survey of dental caries in a group of ten urban Gandans, Dr. Price did find twenty decayed teeth. They were all in the mouth of the hotel cook, who ate his meals at work and seemed to prefer European food. The rest of the survey group, all hotel employees, ate their meals at home.

In contrast to the Europeans who live in Africa and suffer the ravages of strange and exotic diseases endemic there, native Africans rarely get these diseases. They also seem immune to many civilized malfunctions such as appendicitis, diabetes, obesity, heart disease, and cancer. Dr. Denis P. Burkitt, a famous British physician who spent twenty years as a surgeon in a teaching hospital in Uganda, feels that the superior health of the natives is due mainly to their high-fiber diet. He found their fiber intake to be about 25 grams a day as compared with the American intake of less than 5 grams a day. The longer food remains in the intestines, the more chance there is of intestinal tissue being exposed to disease-causing elements. The high fiber content of a native African meal results in elimination in thirty-five hours. The typical meal of a European may remain in the intestinal tract for up to 100 hours. The whole or coarsely ground grains in the Gandan diet provide the fiber need for proper elimination. As a result, intestinal problems such as polyps, appendicitis, and cancer of the colon are virtually unknown. Doctors are now convinced that cancer of the intestines, rectum, or colon can be prevented by proper diet.

That Africans are generally immune to malaria has long puzzled scientists until investigations into sickle cell anemia provided the answer. Many thousands of years ago, a mutation or genetic change in blood cells occurred in Africans. This mutated blood cell, known as a sickle cell, provided resistance to malaria. Through natural selection, it spread all over the continent and those who carried this trait survived and passed it on to millions of their descendants.

In the United States, approximately 10 percent of the 22 million Afro-Americans carry the sickle cell trait. Of these over 50,000 have sickle cell anemia, a debilitating and fatal disease. It is caused by the sickle cell's inability to provide sufficient oxygen, which eventually results in reduced circulation and, finally, death.

However, in Africa, 25 percent of the population carry the sickle cells, but a medical survey covering a period of twenty-five years, 1925 to 1950, found less than 100 cases of sickle cell anemia. Researchers puzzled over this discrepancy, the strange fact that Africans who "ought" to have sickle cell anemia don't.

Meanwhile, work progressed on a treatment to inhibit the sickling factor in blood, and after considerable research, a drug called cyanate proved to be the most effective control. To do the job, however, cyanate must be taken continuously because new blood cells are constantly being manufactured. Some investigators felt that the absence of sickle cell anemia in Africa might indicate there was an alternate to constant medication, or as Robert Houston stated in the *American Journal of Clinical Nutrition:* "The evidence suggests the existence in Africa of an inhibiting environmental factor on the clinical manifestations of the disease." In other words, they've got something we haven't.

The logical reaction was to study the native African diet for clues to their apparent immunity. Are Africans protected through the foods they eat with some substance that Afro-Americans must take as a drug? The two richest natural sources of thiocyanate (from which cyanate is broken off by enzyme action in the red blood cell) are yams and cassava, both eaten in great quantities by native Africans. The cassava is made into a flour and yams are eaten daily throughout most of the continent. In addition, two other African foods, sorghum and millet, were found to be quite high in thiocyanates. Africans, on their native diet, consumed enough cyanate daily, roughly 1,000 milligrams, to protect them from sickle cell anemia. The average diet of the Afro-American rarely exceeds 25 milligrams per day. In truth, sickle cell anemia should be classified as a nutritional deficiency disease, just as scurvy is a Vitamin C deficiency and pellagra a niacin deficiency disease. More and more evidence supports the theory that the ethnic foods eaten by a particular group through generations are of prime health importance to that group. These foods possess a special survival value and altering the diet leads to the physical degeneration of the group. This certainly appears to be the case here. The native African diet provided protection; the Afro-American diet, conforming to American tastes, doesn't.

In many areas of Africa, local agriculture has been drastically changed. A European innovation was the large-scale production of cash crops for export: cacao, coffee, sugar, and tea. In Gambia, for instance, the culture of local food crops has been completely abandoned in favor of the production of peanuts. As a result, staple foods must be imported at high cost and the nutritional deficiency of the Gambians is causing considerable alarm. But in Uganda little is altered, every home has a garden sufficient to feed the family. Termites and locusts are still considered a delicacy and are gathered in much the same manner as before. The swarming gnats are caught by young and old, and it isn't uncommon in the cities to see a well-dressed lady stop her car by a street light that has attracted the gnats to fill a bucket with these insects. She will take them home to make a crunchy snack.

Strong and graceful, polite and independent, the Gandans have taken in stride the many changes in their society. Political upheavals have beset Uganda since the British departed in the 1960s, but along the shores of Lake Victoria the men still fish for perch, the women tend their gardens, and healthy, attractive children play about the homes.

A feeling persists that this will go on forever.

FOODS OF THE GANDANS

While the Gandans cultivate many common foods, the staple food crop and almost the only one they consider worth growing is the banana. Banana gruel is one of the first foods fed to babies. Thousands of natives eat little else but bananas all of their lives. Luckily, bananas are one of the few foods that can support life if eaten in quantities large enough to satisfy caloric needs.

CHIEF SOURCES OF NUTRIENTS
IN THE GANDAN DIET

PROTEIN	fish
FAT	peanuts
CARBOHYDRATE	bananas
CALORIES	bananas
VITAMIN A	greens
VITAMIN C	greens
VITAMIN B_1	bananas
VITAMIN B_2	bananas
NIACIN	fish
CALCIUM	greens
IRON	bananas and greens
FIBER	peanuts and greens

Of the dozens of varieties of bananas grown in Africa, the favorite of the Gandans is the short, fat, green matoke banana. It is eaten daily. When steamed it tastes more like wheat than banana. Few foods furnish as complete nutrition as the banana. It is easily digested, contains a fine quality protein, is safe for allergy sufferers, and is a storehouse of vitamins and minerals. As described earlier, the Gandans steam their bananas after wrapping the peeled fruit in leaves. They then mash the steamed fruit and form it into small balls. Using their fingers, they dip the balls into the common pot of stew. Dried bananas are made into flour, which makes a nutritious thickener for the Gandan stews, and first food for infants. Occasionally, banana tree roots are also dried and ground into flour to be added to stew.

Greens

The Gandans eat more than fifty-two varieties of greens, a combination of wild plants and some that are cultivated. Among their favorites are the leaves of cassava, pumpkin, and sweet potato. They grow spinach and chard. These greens are a major source of Vitamins A and C and calcium. When they are cooked in the stew along with tomatoes, the acid in the tomatoes helps retain the Vitamin C in the greens.

Melons

Watermelon is an indigenous plant of Africa, and a favorite of the Gandans. Most often they will mash the pulp to make a refreshing drink. Watermelon is a good source of liquid, and a fine source of most minerals and cellulose. It is also a mild stimulant for the kidneys. Its seeds contain a substance called cucurbocitrin which is said to have the ability to dilate small blood vessels and thus reduce blood pressure.

Cassava

This large, bushy plant is an important food source for much of Africa. It grows well all over the continent. It is a starchy, high-calorie food but one with few nutrients, only about half as much protein as corn. It does contain B_{17} and thiocyanate, an inhibitor of sickle cell anemia. The roots of the cassava are roasted or dried and pounded into flour known as tapioca. As indicated above, the poisonous variety must be pounded and leached of its poison (prussic acid) before being used. The Gandans use the powder to thicken their stews.

Salt

Sea salts are unavailable to the Gandans, but they have found an excellent substitute in the ashes of water hyacinth. The plant grows in abundance along the shores of Lake Victoria and is an excellent source of essential iodine. The women gather the hyacinth and char the stalks in a fire. It is then powdered and used just like salt. Inland Gandans will walk for days to barter for bags of this plant salt, which they use to protect their families from "big neck," their name for goiter.

Seeds

Sesame seeds are an excellent calcium source. The Gandans press the seeds for their high quality oil, which is extremely stable and resistant to spoiling. Sometimes the seeds are made into cakes for a treat or ground into powder and used to thicken a stew.

Vegetables

The favorite vegetables of the Gandans are sweet potatoes, yams, onions, tomatoes, and okra, along with a wide variety of greens. Most vegetables are never cooked separately, but are added to the stew pot. Generally, vegetables are cooked only a short time, just until tender.

Occasionally the sweet potato or yam is roasted in the fire or prepared like the banana and used in its place to eat with the stew. Sweet potatoes contain an easily assimilated carbohydrate, and are an excellent source of Vitamin A.

No stew is complete without a few tomatoes. The acid from the tomatoes helps the stew retain its Vitamin C and leaches calcium from the bones of fish or animals into the stew. Tomatoes are also a good Vitamin C source in themselves.

Okra is a great favorite of the Gandans because of its mucilaginous texture. It gives a slippery consistency to their stews. A therapeutic vegetable, okra has been used for aiding digestion and helping to overcome inflammation of the stomach and intestines. While it is low in calories, it is high in nutrients, including Vitamins A and C, calcium, and potassium.

Onions are another therapeutic vegetable. Their fumes contain a chemical that enters the blood and can kill germs and viruses. Onions are a source of calcium and Vitamin C. They add a spicy flavor to the stews.

Sorghum

Another indigenous African plant, sorghum grows on a tall stalk with a large cluster of seeds on the end. To some extent it resembles corn and has about the same food value. It is higher in protein and lower in fat than corn, however. The Gandans are about the only people who do not make a syrup from sorghum. They cook it fresh or dry it and pound it into flour to add to their stews.

Millet

One of the basic grains in the Gandan diet is millet. A high quality food, it is boiled and fed to small children and nursing mothers. Millet contains a good quality of B_1, iron, and potassium; it is rich in B_{17} and is the only alkaline-forming grain. The Gandans add millet to their stews or grind it to make a bread-like patty. Millet is very bland, easily digested, and has a soothing quality that aids in healing gastrointestinal inflammation. In the United States, millet is found most often in bird seed.

Fish

The major supplement to the Gandan's banana diet is fish. Because of the high level of protein and nutrients found in fish, Gandans are physically and mentally superior to those Africans whose diet consists mainly of grains and vegetables. The Gandans steam their fish after first wrapping them in banana leaves. Fish is also dried and added to the stew pot or used for barter with inland tribes. It is eaten daily in Uganda and the head is the favorite part.

Meat

Although the area abounds with wild animals, meat is generally eaten no more than once a week. The rat is the most highly prized of all meats. This is probably because the rat is the fattest of all range animals, and most likely makes a flavorful stew. When animals are slaughtered, their livers belong to the children. Women eat the ribs and the oldest male receives the eyes. Gandans raise few goats and chickens but usually use them to pay an occasional fine, or slaughter them only for a celebration. Meat for a feast is customarily wrapped in banana leaves and steamed with the bananas. It is cooked only long enough to make it chewable. Since the cooking temperature is always low, the protein quality and certain B vitamins are not destroyed. When meat is wrapped in leaves, nutrients that would be lost through exposure to air, light, or liquid are preserved.

Peanuts

The peanut was introduced into Africa by early explorers. It grows extremely well throughout the continent and is an important food item for many Africans. For the Gandans, whose diet is low in fat, the peanut is an important source of the unsaturated fatty acids. The peanut contains a good amount of incomplete protein and B vitamins. The brown papery skin has a considerable amount of thiamine, which is lost when the skin is removed. Fried and salted peanuts are a favorite snack of the Gandans. They frequently add a couple of handfuls of peanuts to their stews. Often the nuts are dried and ground into flour. Peanut flour can be used in place of wheat or grain flour. The resulting product will have four times the protein, twice the iron, and four times the niacin of wheat flour. Peanut flour is often added to the stew. In baking, only part of the wheat flour should be replaced with peanut flour as it has a stronger flavor and contains no gluten.

Insects

Nutritional analysis of insects provides some surprising information. Not only do insects contain as good a quality protein as meat, but they are low in calories. Also, they are a good source of the B vitamins and also contain Vitamin D.

The locust is a popular item in the Gandan diet. The insect is first steamed, and wings and legs removed. The body is then fried and lightly salted. Locusts can also be dried and ground into flour and stored for later use. One ounce of dried locust contains the calories, protein, and fat found in two cups of nonfat milk.

Termites are much fatter than locusts. They are usually fried in their own fat and served as a snack or as a supplement to the daily stew. Two ounces of fresh termites have the same calorie, protein, and fat content as two and three-quarter ounces of cheese.

Gnats are made into cakes by grinding them and adding water to make a sticky paste. They are then baked and served as a dessert.

DINING WITH A GANDAN FAMILY

The Gandans usually eat a light meal in the morning. The other two meals are pretty much alike: matoke (steamed banana mash) and dipping gravy made from vegetables and peanuts, and maybe a little fish or meat. A whole, steamed fish caught in Lake Victoria and a side dish of vegetables may also be served. The family usually eats together. At meals the people sit cross-legged on the floor around a neatly arranged cover of banana leaves. Each person has a wooden bowl, and a wicker basket of steaming food is placed in the center. Everyone is served a little mound of banana mash and some meat or fish if there is any. A few common receptacles contain gravy and extra vegetables. Each person rolls his *stodge* of banana mash into little pellets, and using his fingers, dips them into the gravy bowl, then transfers them daintily to his mouth. With a flat sponge made from the pith of banana, he carefully wipes his fingers. The sap in the stem removes the grease. A guest compliments his host by eating lustily and belching loudly.

Following each meal a little rest is allowed. Often the men chew on roasted coffee beans or drink mwenge, banana beer, while the children sit together and tell stories.

Ugandan food is usually rather bland. Various peppers and spices are sometimes used, but they are generally passed separately, to be added to the food as the diner wishes. They are not considered good for children. The various vegetables, meat and greens that go into the stew pot are cooked just soft enough to chew. Most of the other foods are steamed; often many different foods are steamed together in the same pot, each item being first wrapped in banana leaves.

Serving dishes are carved wooden bowls and gourds which are used for drinking vessels. The cookhouse is usually a separate building. Here a special iron pot is supported over a woodfire. The women, who do the cooking, put a little water and some shredded banana leaf fibers in the bottom of the pot, fill the pot with foods wrapped in green banana leaves, and allow the food to steam for two or three hours.

A UGANDAN DINNER PER INDIVIDUAL

BANANAS, 3
FISH, 3½ ounces, steamed
DIPPING GRAVY

    peanut meal, ¼ cup   *okra, ½ cup*
    tomato, ½ medium   *cassava leaves, 3½ ounces*
    onion, ¼ medium   *sesame oil, ½ tablespoon*

A GANDAN DINNER FROM YOUR KITCHEN

    STEAMED FISH
    STEAMED BEET TOPS AND COLLARD GREENS
    MASHED STEAMED BANANAS
    GROUND NUT SAUCE
    SLICED TOMATOES AND RED ONIONS

To serve, place fish, greens, bananas, sliced tomatoes, and sliced onions on a plate. Cover everything with a ground nut sauce. Extra sauce can be served in a wooden salad bowl or a gourd. Optional condiments can be placed in small bowls so that each diner can sprinkle what he wants over his food. Some ideas for condiments are chopped green onions including tops, chopped raw tomatoes, alfalfa sprouts, lentil sprouts, banana hunks, chile peppers chopped and with seeds removed, chopped hard-boiled egg, raisins, or hot whole peanuts.

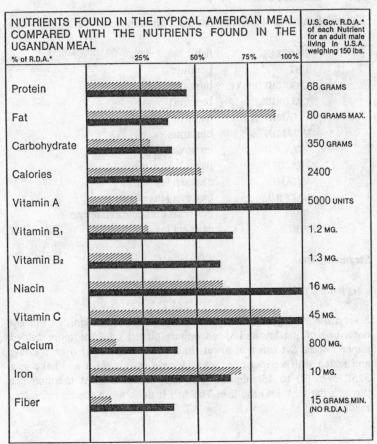

NUTRIENTS FOUND IN THE TYPICAL AMERICAN MEAL COMPARED WITH THE NUTRIENTS FOUND IN THE UGANDAN MEAL					U.S. Gov. R.D.A.* of each Nutrient for an adult male living in U.S.A. weighing 150 lbs.
% of R.D.A.*	25%	50%	75%	100%	
Protein					68 GRAMS
Fat					80 GRAMS MAX.
Carbohydrate					350 GRAMS
Calories					2400
Vitamin A					5000 UNITS
Vitamin B₁					1.2 MG.
Vitamin B₂					1.3 MG.
Niacin					16 MG.
Vitamin C					45 MG.
Calcium					800 MG.
Iron					10 MG.
Fiber					15 GRAMS MIN. (NO R.D.A.)

*R.D.A. is the recommended daily nutrient allowance intended to meet the needs of a *healthy* individual.

Diagonal lines represent the American meal.

The chief sources of nutrients in the Ugandan meal are:

PROTEIN	fish
FAT	peanuts
CARBOHYDRATE	bananas
CALORIES	bananas
VITAMIN A	cassava leaves
VITAMIN B_1	bananas
VITAMIN B_2	cassava leaves
NIACIN	fish
VITAMIN C	cassava leaves
CALCIUM	cassava leaves
IRON	bananas and cassava leaves
FIBER	cassava leaves

Steamed Fish

1 pound fish steak or whole dressed fish

Season fish with garlic, dill, parsley, and powdered onion. Set upright on a bed of parsley and sliced onions placed on 2 or more folded paper towels. Set fish and towels in a paper sack. Fold over opening and fasten with a paper clip. Set sack on a cookie sheet and bake in a 325° oven 30 to 45 minutes. You may insert a meat thermometer through the sack into the fish. The fish is done when the thermometer reads 140°.

Steamed Bananas

6 large or 9 small firm green bananas
2 tablespoons butter
2 tablespoons lemon juice, or to taste

Wash banana skins and place whole bananas in their skins in a covered baking pan. Add just enough water to cover the bottom of the pan. Cover and bake 20 to 45 minutes in a 325° oven. Bananas are done when their skins begin to burst and they are soft inside. Remove skins. Mash bananas well. Add salt, butter, and lemon juice to taste.

Ground Nut Sauce

1 onion, finely diced
2 large tomatoes, peeled and finely sliced
1 cup diced okra (optional)
1 cup unsalted peanuts, finely ground
¼ cup sesame seeds, finely ground
1 teaspoon curry powder
4 cups water
Salt to taste

Sauté onion, okra, tomatoes, and curry powder in a small amount of oil until onions are limp. Add nuts, seeds, and water. Bring to boil, then reduce heat to simmer. Stir constantly as the sauce boils until the simmering stage is reached. Continue cooking, uncovered, until nuts and okra are well cooked and the sauce is slightly thickened. Season to taste with salt.

Steamed Greens

1 package frozen or ¾ pound fresh chopped collard greens
1 bunch beet greens

Wash fresh greens and slice leaves in half along the stem, removing the stem. Stack leaves and shred across veins. Simmer greens in a very small amount of water or chicken broth until just tender. The chopped stems may be added to the ground nut sauce.

Festival Thick-Curried Chicken with Steamed Bananas, "Matoke"

2- to 3-pound frying chicken, disjointed
1 cup chicken broth
1½ cups okra or green beans, washed and with ends removed
2 large onions, sliced
3 tomatoes, peeled and sliced
½ cup unsalted peanuts, ground
1 clove garlic, minced
2 teaspoons curry powder, or to taste
1 large sweet potato, scrubbed and diced
Small can hot chiles or chile powder

Brown chicken in peanut or vegetable oil in open frying pan that has a lid. Place browned chicken in a kettle with chicken broth, cover, and simmer 30 minutes or until chicken is almost tender. Sauté onions in the pan used to brown the chicken, adding more oil if necessary. Cook onions until soft but not brown. When chicken has cooked 30 minutes, add tomatoes, garlic, curry powder, okra or beans, and sweet potatoes to the pan with the cooked onions. Mix 1 cup of chicken broth from the cooking chicken with the ground peanuts. Add mixture to pan with vegetables and mix to blend. Put drained chicken in the pan and coat with sauce. Simmer slowly, covered, stirring occasionally, until vegetables and chicken are tender and sauce is very thick. Add more chicken broth if mixture becomes too dry and more peanut meal or toasted bread crumbs if it is too thin. Add salt and more curry to taste. Serve curry with steamed bananas (page 129) and pass a bowl of finely chopped hot red peppers or chile powder so that each diner can season his portion to taste.

Ugandan Fish Soup

*1 pound any fish cut in 1-inch chunks (leave very small fish
    whole)*
3 cans tomatoes, 14½ ounces each
1 cup fish stock or clam juice (recipe for fish stock follows)
½ teaspoon salt
½ teaspoon whole thyme
1 bay leaf
Dash red pepper
Dash powdered saffron or turmeric
*2 cups unpeeled sweet potatoes, scrubbed and cut into ¾-inch
    cubes*
1½ cups okra or green beans, cut into ¾-inch lengths
1 medium onion, cut in 1-inch chunks
*¾ pound spinach, stems removed and finely chopped, leaves left
    in big pieces*

Combine tomatoes, fish stock, salt, thyme, bay leaf, and pepper in a
kettle. Bring to a boil, reduce heat, cover, and simmer for 20 minutes.
Discard bay leaf and press soup mixture through a strainer. Return to
the kettle and bring to a boil. Add sweet potatoes, okra, and onions.
Simmer, covered, until vegetables are tender. Add fish, spinach, and
saffron; simmer gently—do not boil—3 to 5 minutes, just until fish is
cooked and spinach has wilted.

Fish Stock

1 pound fish skin, backbones,   1 parsley sprig
*   heads, and collars   ½ bay leaf*
2½ cups water   ½ tablespoon each chopped carrot,
1 peppercorn   celery, and onion
1 small clove

Put all ingredients into a sauce pan, bring to boil, cover, and simmer
1½ hours. Strain stock.

Fried Brains in Ground Nut Sauce

1 pound fresh brains
1 egg, beaten
1 tablespoon water
1 teaspoon salt
Dry bread crumbs
Sesame or vegetable oil

Rinse brains under running cold water. Remove all membrane. Dry on a paper towel and cut into ¾-inch pieces. Dip each piece into a batter of egg, water, and salt. Roll in bread crumbs and allow to dry 15 to 20 minutes. Heat sesame or other vegetable oil in a frying pan. Sauté brains until golden brown and firm (about 20 minutes). Serve with ground nut sauce (page 129).

In Uganda, some okra would be sliced into ¾-inch pieces, dipped in the batter, rolled in the crumbs, and fried with the brains. While protein foods should never be cooked at high temperatures or to a well-done state because such treatment toughens the proteins, brains are an exception to this rule. Because of their soft texture, when they are cooked to a well-done state and their protein toughened, their texture is improved.

STODGES

(Stodges are eaten in place of a grain with a gravy or stew. Add liquid drained from cooking the following stodges to the stew.)

Banana and Vegetable Stodge

8 green bananas, peeled and sliced
2 medium tomatoes, peeled and finely diced
2 medium onions, minced
¼ cup water

Combine bananas, tomatoes, onions, and water. Cover pan and bring to a boil, then simmer until all ingredients are soft, about 20 minutes. Drain and mash. Add butter and salt to taste.

Sweet Potato Stodge

Cook sweet potatoes until tender. Cool slightly and remove skins. Mash well, add salt and butter to taste. Put mashed sweet potatoes into a deep mixing bowl and beat until they become stiff and very smooth.

Peanut and Bean Stodge

>   1 pound kidney or pinto beans, cooked
>   1 onion, finely chopped
>   2 tomatoes, skinned and chopped
>   1 tablespoon vegetable oil
>   ¼ cup peanut butter

Cook onion in oil until soft and slightly browned. Add tomatoes, and ¼ cup liquid from beans or water. Cover and simmer 5 minutes. Mash beans with a fork. Add to cooked vegetables with peanut butter and salt to taste. Cook over medium heat, stirring constantly until mixture is thick.

Sesame Cakes

>   1 cup sesame seeds, ground
>   ⅓ cup water
>   ¼ teaspoon salt

Mix sesame meal, salt, and enough water to make a very stiff batter. Press into 2-inch circles using 1 tablespoon of batter for each cake. Allow cakes to stand at room temperature 1 hour. Cook on a lightly oiled griddle over low heat until cakes are golden brown on both sides. Eat as bread or a cracker, warm or cooled. They are good eaten with raw honey or frosted with a mixture of equal parts of peanut butter and honey.

Peanut Butter Candy

Mix equal parts of peanut butter and honey together. Work with hands, adding enough ground sesame seeds to make a stiff dough. Form into small balls or patties. Store covered in the refrigerator. (Powdered milk, toasted wheat germ, carob powder, or ground nuts may be substituted for sesame seed meal and chopped nuts, chopped dried fruit, or coconut may be added.)

THE LIGHT BITE, UGANDAN STYLE

A QUICK MEAL: Cook cold fish, liver, kidney, or heart, dipped in ground nut sauce (page 129). For a different sauce, combine equal parts of catsup and peanut butter, then add a little chopped onion, garlic, and curry powder or chile powder. Whole grain bread or a sweet potato, a banana, and some peanuts in their shells could complete the meal.

A SNACK: Bananas cut in 1-inch chunks and rolled first in a mixture of peanut butter and honey and then in chopped nuts. These banana chunks may be frozen and eaten like popsicles.

The Eskimos
of the Pacific Coast

The Arctic regions of the world are so bleak and formidable, it comes almost as a surprise to find that anything can survive there for any length of time. But this area does sustain life—human, plant, and animal. Not in any great numbers, but enough to prove it can be done. Across the desolate Alaskan tundra are scattered tiny villages where Eskimos have lived successfully for many generations, wresting a livelihood from an uncompromising land.

The Algonquin Indians gave the name Eskimo to the people of the Arctic. It means "eaters of raw flesh" and the Indians found this practice incredible. The Eskimos, however, call themselves a name that translates into "the real people." Their ancient legends, passed on by word of mouth, are beautiful and poetic. The world was created by the raven. Man was formed from a pea pod and woman from clay. Their stories always involve animals—the bear, caribou, great whales, and other creatures—and demonstrate how closely their lives were linked to the environment.

Recent discoveries have confirmed what anthropologists have long suspected: that the area was first settled by nomadic people from Siberia crossing a land bridge into what is now Alaska. Physically, the Eskimos closely resemble the Mongols, with broad, flat faces and short, stocky bodies. Their hair is straight and black and rather sparse.

Beginning with Russian fur traders in the nineteenth century, contact with outsiders drastically altered Eskimo life. Typical of isolated people everywhere, the Eskimo developed a taste for the traders' food. His altered diet lowered his body's resistance to the traders' illnesses. Since he had no natural immunity to the diseases of civilization, tuberculosis, smallpox, and measles took a dreadful toll.

In Alaska today, Eskimos in the major cities such as Nome or Fairbanks have adopted American foods and customs and have completely abandoned their old ways. However, in the more isolated areas, Eskimos still live as they have for many years. There have been a few changes. Instead of handmade kayaks, they have boats with outboard motors. They have pretty much given up their nomadic life and stay in one area where the men may work at a nearby cannery instead of hunting bear and caribou; but the Eskimo men still trap mink, catch fish, and depend upon sea mammals for much of their families' food.

South of the Yukon, along the Kuskokwim River, are several small settlements. Typical of these villages is Napaskiak. With about 200 residents, it is considered a town of reasonable size for the area. Downstream is the town of Bethel, with about 800 people. Steamers can navigate up the river as far as Bethel, but from there goods must be loaded onto a stern-wheeler that can negotiate the shallow river with its shifting mudbanks. This means that the upstream towns have access to, and can get goods from, the outside world, but only during about two months of summer and at great expense. By and large, the men of Napaskiak use money earned from selling pelts for the purchase of outboard motors for their boats or a piece of equipment like a generator or a sewing machine. Little is left over for the purchase of commercial foods from the local merchants. Of necessity, they stick to their ethnic diet. A case of misplaced affection, however, is their habit of buying candy and bubble gum for their children.

Eskimo children are probably the most indulged in the world. As infants they are petted and played with constantly. A baby goes everywhere with its mother, riding in a sling attached to her shoulders. The woman's parka is made larger than the man's, big enough to accommodate the child before and after birth. Children are breast-fed for about three years. In the old days, the women avoided becoming pregnant during lactation; now, however, they are turning more and more to bottled formula and they frequently become pregnant every year. This recent development has had unfortunate side effects. The bottle-fed children are much more prone to rickets and their growth is slower than that of the breast-fed infants. This changing attitude about breast-feeding is generally confined to the cities, where bottled formula is available. In the remote villages, the women still breast-feed. At about three months, solid food is introduced into the infant diet. The first food is usually fish livers that the mother has chewed into a paste.

Another food supplement is fish roe gently simmered and mixed with seal oil. This is fed to the children daily. The mothers also cook tom cod livers and spoon off the oil to give their babies. Of all primitive cultures, the Eskimo baby probably had the healthiest start in life due to his cod liver oil and liver supplements. Because of difficult living conditions and lack of sanitation today, the infant mortality rate is quite high, 138 per 1,000 compared with 7.2 per 1,000 in the rest of the United States. The most frequent cause of infant death is amoebic dysentery or acute infectious diarrhea. In the past, Eskimos were nomadic people. They would travel in groups of several families, going from winter camp to spring camp, and then on to the summer hunting areas, never staying in one place more than a few months. Sanitation was never a serious problem until they began to remain in one area for a period of years. It was then that their rather casual attitude about sanitary facilities began to cause health problems and their babies started to die. Since statehood, tremendous efforts have been made to correct this situation through education and improved sewage disposal.

The Eskimos' stoic attitude about death borders on indifference. They live with danger—flood, fire, and famine—and regard these things as an inevitable part of life. The rate of accidental death for Eskimos is nearly four times that of the contiguous forty-eight states, 59.3 per 1,000 for the United States versus 206.7 for the Alaskan Eskimos. Barring accidental death, the Eskimos following their old customs and diet live long, healthy lives. Cheerful, gregarious, sturdy old men enchant the children with long elaborate stories illustrated with drawings made with a special ivory drawing stick. The pictures are drawn in mud or dirt and tell tales of travels across the frozen tundra, great whale hunts, and seasons of famine when they ate their dogs.

The Eskimo's high regard for his dogs is second only to his affection for his children. Dogs are killed for food only in the most desperate situations. Because the sled dogs are the sole means of transportation most of the year, their breeding and general health is of constant concern. Any man who neglects his dog is looked upon with scorn by his neighbors. The dogs fare very well by sophisticated standards. In times of plenty the most common dog food is the meaty flesh of the caribou. The head, the organs, and the neck and ribs are eaten by the family; the roasts and hindquarters are fed to the dogs. Eskimos feel this meat is the least desirable part of the animal. Of course, these portions don't contain the excellent nutrients and vitamins found in the head and organs, but the dogs do all right on their raw steak and roast diet.

Yearly trips to remote camps are made every fall when the snow is deep enough for the sleds. The Eskimo's amazing stamina and strength allow him to travel in subzero weather for days without succumbing to frostbite or exhaustion. At camp, the men set out their mink traps and hunt caribou. The sale of mink skins is still their major source of income. Skins are sold by the bundle and a bundle consists of thirty-two pelts, the number needed to make a parka. This standard measure exists throughout the fur industry.

In the past, the whole family went along to the winter camp. There was plenty to do and having the women along to cook and help with the skinning, tanning, and drying of the pelts meant the men could spend more time on the trail. However, the schoolmistress in Napaskiak announced that any family who took their children out of school to go to winter camp would be prosecuted. The men reluctantly go alone now. They always return in December to celebrate the Christian and Russian Orthodox holidays at that time, and they greatly enjoy both.

The traditional food of the Eskimo is fish—raw, frozen, cooked, or dried. Salmon is the fish most frequently eaten but they also eat blackfish, halibut, needlefish, whitefish, and stickleback. Huge runs of salmon surge up the Kuskokwim River from spring to midsummer, and the Eskimos catch them by the thousands. The women are experts and fillet the fish with great speed and agility. They sit on the ground by a huge pile of salmon and, after removing the heads, they gut the fish. The heads are thrown in one container, the guts in another, and any roe is tossed into another can. The fish are skillfully boned and placed on drying racks. The heads may be cooked and eaten that day or buried and allowed to ferment. When fermented, they have the flavor of strong cheese. Roe, one of the finest natural foods, is also dried and is used as a food supplement for the small children and expectant mothers. After the salmon is dried, it is smoked and stored for future use.

Arctic weather is so harsh that extra fat is essential in the Eskimo diet. Just as the seal and walrus need a thick layer of body fat to serve as insulation against the cold and as a source of energy, so does the Eskimo. After only a few weeks of abstaining from eating fat, he will become weak and violently ill. If his diet is not supplemented with large quantities of fat, death will soon follow. The chief cause of death among inland hunting parties is fat starvation.

Since fish contains little or no fat, blubber is the Eskimos' main fat source, and they eat enormous amounts of it, raw or fermented. Producing fermented seal oil from blubber is quite an undertaking. In early spring the men go seal hunting. In catching the animal, great care is taken not to damage its skin. In a very risky maneuver, the seal is clubbed to death instead of being harpooned or shot. The innards of the seal are removed through the mouth and the skin is peeled off very carefully so that it ends up inside out. All meat clinging to the skin is removed. The blubber is cut into small strips and stuffed into the skin with the fur inside and the opening is sewn tightly shut. The stuffed seal, weighing up to 250 pounds, is then placed on a high rack to protect it from dogs or other animals and allowed to ferment in the warm summer sun. Sometimes a black cloth will be placed above the racks of seal pokes. This raises the temperature several degrees and speeds up fermentation.

After a couple of months, the blubber is ready to eat. It has melted and fermented into a syrupy, amber fluid with a slightly vinegary taste. Vilhjalmur Stefansson, the anthropologist who spent many years with the Eskimos, found the flavor delicious and became fond of it. Fermented blubber is used in great quantities daily by the Eskimos. Every piece of fish they eat is first dipped into the oil. When it is poured over berries, it is called "agutuk," or Eskimo ice cream. It is fed to babies and mixed with nearly every food they eat, from greens to fruits. Greens and berries are stored in seal oil for winter use.

In spite of the enormous cholesterol intake they receive from the blubber, heart disease among Eskimos is quite rare. Today, it accounts for 65.6 deaths per 100,000 as opposed to 370 per 100,000 for all ethnic groups in the United States. Evidence is mounting that the body's ability to metabolize fat is the crucial factor in preventing cardiovascular disorders rather than the amount of saturated fat in the diet.

Dr. Price, who visited the Eskimos in the early 1930s to examine their health and tooth development, had seal oil analyzed and found it richer in Vitamin A than nearly any food he had ever found. Although the Eskimos eat the fatty layers of many sea mammals, seal oil provides the major portion of fat in their diet.

During the summer, the Eskimo meal includes berries, greens, sorrel grass, kelp, migrating birds and their eggs, and groundnuts. These last aren't really nuts in the accepted sense; they are really a tuberous growth, rather like a potato.

Caribou is an important food source for many inland Eskimos and, in a roundabout way, the cause of a growing problem. Recently, scientists from the Hanford Laboratory of the Atomic Energy Commission examined over 100 Eskimos and found alarmingly high levels of cesium-137 in their bodies. The reason for this unusually high concentration arises from the unique food chain of the Arctic. Lichen acts as a "blotting paper" and picks up radioactive fallout. Lichen is the main food of the caribou and the Eskimos in turn eat the caribou. Cesium-137, similar to potassium, accumulates in the muscles and, in sufficient quantity, could present a genetic hazard.

The native Eskimo diet may prove to be essential in preventing dangerous accumulations of radioactive material in the body. Tests conducted on laboratory animals have shown that they have resistance to high-level radiation when fed a diet rich in calcium and bone marrow, liver, iodine, protein, and kelp. Most of these essential foods are part of the Eskimo's daily diet so they do have some protection from radiation hazards with their native foods.

Limited as the Eskimo diet is, it supplies all the elements required for good health and regeneration of cells. Fish livers are extremely rich in most of the vitamins and minerals. The stomach contents of sea mammals provide elements often missing in the daily diet. Sorrel grass mixed with seal oil is an excellent source of vitamins. Heads of fish, highly nutritious and desirable, have huge concentrations of Vitamin A and iron. They are usually given to the children. Heads of seal and walrus are not too popular, so they are fed to the dogs, but the flippers are a great favorite. An excellent source of calcium, they are often fermented and saved for a treat.

The stomachs of sea mammals are sometimes eaten as well as the intestines, after a careful cleaning. The lungs are inflated and all the air forced out. They are then cut in strips and dried, to be added to fish stews. Clams from the stomach of freshly caught walrus are considered a great delicacy and are eaten on the spot.

Dr. Price found that the native Eskimo diet provides five times the calcium and more than ten times the Vitamins A and D found in the average American diet. Their iron intake is well above the recommended levels and comes mainly from blackfish, needlefish, and the flesh of sea mammals. Seal tissue contains 19.6 grams of iron in four ounces of flesh, twice the amount in beef liver. The Eskimo intake of Vitamin B_1 is apt to be low since this vitamin is found mainly in grains and seeds, items noticeably missing in their diet. The B_1 is essential in metabolizing sugars and carbohydrates, but as the native Eskimo diet contains virtually no sugars or starches, their requirements for B_1 are proportionately lower.

Other B vitamins that would tend to be low in an all-fish diet are to some extent manufactured in the human intestines if the intestinal flora is healthy. The intake of fermented seal oil provides the lactic acid needed to maintain a high level of healthy flora.

There is scientific evidence that the Eskimos' health was among the finest in the world before they succumbed to the diet of the white man. Explorer Vilhjalmur Stefansson's experiments on diet in the Arctic proved that the good health of the Eskimo depended upon a diet of raw meat, including blood, liver, and bone marrow mainly from seal, walrus, and fish.

Truly few diets in the world are as delicately balanced as the native Eskimo diet. One element missing or one element added can disrupt this perfect balance irreparably. Unfortunately, this has happened in areas where local markets sell manufactured and refined foods. As soon as the Eskimos start eating these manufactured foods, their carefully balanced diet is disrupted and disease begins. The amount of tooth decay among Eskimos is in direct proportion to the amount of manufactured foods they eat. On their native diet, little or no decay is present. The teeth of old people are ground down nearly to the gums from chewing on hide, but the teeth are sound and no pulp is exposed. When they increase their intake of sugars and starches in the form of refined and manufactured foods, decay increases as much as 150 percent. Urban Eskimos now have about the worst teeth in the world. In addition, cancer, arthritis, and other degenerative diseases are seen where none existed before. The Eskimo loses the natural immunity that heretofore protected him. Tuberculosis, one of the most serious health problems among Eskimos, accounts for many deaths. In one village recently, of 180 people tested, forty-five were found to be actively tubercular. The old people, with the wisdom of their years, say that tuberculosis started when the *gussuk* (white man) came to the area and only began to be a serious problem when the Eskimos started to eat gussuk food, which they consider to be of very poor quality. The increase in tuberculosis relates directly to the increase in eating refined and manufactured foods.

When the diet is nutritionally adequate, the body has an amazing ability to resist infectious diseases, from tuberculosis to measles, and live in harmony even with intestinal parasites. If the least deficiency in any nutrient develops from famine or diet change and the body, because of previous isolation, has built up no resistance to a disease, the effects are disastrous.

In the past the usual Eskimo breakfast consisted of fish, smoked or frozen. Frozen fish was eaten raw and slightly thawed. It was cut into strips and, with one end of the strip in the mouth, a bite was cut off near the lips with a sharp knife. Lunch would be about the same as breakfast, depending on the season. If berries or greens were available, they would be part of the menu. The common pot of seal oil was always present. This oil was never used for cooking, only as an addition to their other foods. Dinner may have consisted of live blackfish, gently simmered until barely cooked. These were eaten whole and the liquid was also consumed. In spring and summer, the eggs of migrating wild fowl were also part of the menu. Animal blood, either fresh or frozen, was added to a broth of boiled fish and stirred rapidly. It thickened into a heavy sauce and made a filling and nourishing meal. The menu described was more varied than usual. It was quite common for the Eskimos to eat salmon three times a day until the supply was exhausted; then, if caribou was available, they ate that for every meal. In early spring, they would eat wild bird eggs morning, noon, and night until the nesting season was over. Not much thought was given to variety; they would eat what was available as long as it was available. They ate the entire animal, usually raw, and thus obtained all the essential nutrients.

Many Eskimos still cling to their old social customs. Every rural Eskimo village has at least one bathhouse and Napaskiak has several. It is here that the men gather daily to gossip, joke, and enjoy themselves. The bathhouse is a square, planked structure with a tunnel entrance and a firepit in the center. The men sit on benches around the wall and after visiting for a while, they build a roaring fire. When it stops smoking and turns to embers, the vent in the roof is closed and the contest begins. As the heat rises, sometimes up to 200 degrees, the losers begin to crawl, weak and gasping, out of the bathhouse. The last man remaining, if he is still conscious, is regarded as the winner and enjoys hero status for his show of stamina. The women frequently complain about the amount of time the men spend in the baths, neglecting their children and their work. Usually a trip to the movies in Bethel will quiet the situation.

The custom of the *kashgee,* or bathhouse, goes back far into the past and was part of the Eskimo culture long before the gussuks arrived. In those days the men practically lived in the large bathhouses; their wives would even bring their food to them at mealtimes. The hot room, or sauna, has therapeutic and rejuvenating properties, according to the famous nutritionist Dr. Paavo Airola. "Overheating stimulates and speeds up the metabolic processes and inhibits the growth of pathogenic bacteria. The vital organs and glands are stimulated and the body's own healing restorative capacity is increased. Accumulated toxins are eliminated through perspiration. Skin is the largest eliminative organ and about 30 percent of body waste is in the form of sweat. The chemical analysis of sweat shows that it contains nearly the same constituents as urine." So what may appear to be a social indulgence of the Eskimos is really a vital element in their staying healthy. In areas where the kashgee has been forgotten, the well-being of the Eskimo has suffered greatly.

Eskimos are probably the most gregarious and sociable people in the world. They love parties and celebrations and if one village has a particularly good run of salmon or a very successful caribou hunt, they invite everyone from other villages for miles around to a party. This party involves the exchanging of gifts, singing, dancing, and feasting and often goes on for days. It usually ends when the host village runs out of food. The idea of saving their food for the long winter before the salmon run again in the spring just never occurs to them. The food is to eat; more will come along.

Sometimes, however, it doesn't. Salmon are unpredictable and occasionally the runs are alarmingly small. When this happens, the village is in desperate trouble. The old men and women fish through the ice for what they can catch, some blackfish, a stickle-back or two; the young boys go hunting rabbit or ptarmigan. The men risk their lives to hunt polar bear for food. One starving group of Eskimos found a grounded whale and thought they had been saved. Unfortunately, the whale had been grounded too long and the entire group died of botulism. Such events are rare today with the local markets selling processed foods, but the Eskimo is simply exchanging one problem for another.

Eskimo family life reflects their cheerful dispositions. Their children are adored and indulged. They are never punished. Ridicule or verbal disapproval is sufficient to induce approved behavior. There are no puberty rites and young people are encouraged to have frequent sexual experiences before settling down with one mate. There is no such thing as an illegitimate child; in fact, marriage ceremonies are rare. A new baby is always welcomed into the family. Women are highly esteemed and are consulted about all decisions regarding home or family.

The charming image of a domed house artfully made from blocks of ice is, unfortunately, a myth. Eskimos did build temporary shelters of snow or ice while hunting, but their homes were quite different. According to Stefansson, they were positively tropical. Made of wood salvaged during the spring floods, the houses were large, square, and windowless. Entry was through an underground tunnel that also provided ventilation. A typical house got very warm during the winter with the snow on the roof providing insulation and the whale oil fire providing heat. As soon as they entered, the family stripped off all outdoor garments as fast as possible to prevent their getting wet with perspiration. Everyone inside the house wore little or no clothing during the day and used only a light blanket at night.

In May, when the snow began to melt, the family moved into tents to avoid the prodigious leaking. By then it was time to move on to their seal-hunting grounds.

Eskimo utensils of old were truly pieces of art. Lovingly carved from whale bone or wood during the long winters, they were handed down through the families for generations. The art of carving has largely disappeared, and wooden bowls and bone spoons have been replaced by plastics and stainless steel. But one item is in use as much today as it was hundreds of years ago. That is the women's knife, or *ulu*. It is more like a cleaver with a hand grip in the center than a proper knife. Skillfully employed, these knives are used for butchering sea mammals, cutting meat, cutting pelts for parkas, and even cutting grass for inner soles in *mukluks,* the Eskimo boots. It is an impressive sight to watch an Eskimo woman deftly wielding this rather cumbersome blade.

Acculturation has changed the more urban Eskimo's life considerably; however, the inhospitable climate has limited their exposure to outside influences. In the tiny villages like Napaskiak, the old ways prevail. Eskimo is the language, not English; the boys are taught to hunt and fish; the women and girls dry the catch; and the bathhouse is still the center of social life.

FOODS OF THE ESKIMOS

The fragile diet of the Eskimos varies greatly from season to season, but to many people it would hardly be considered well balanced or even adequate. With about 90 percent of their food intake consisting of fish and sea mammals, the Eskimos still manage to get all the nutrients they need for good health. Balance in this limited menu is maintained by eating the entire amimal. They survive quite well in their hostile environment when they stick to their traditional foods.

Fish

Salmon, the major fish consumed by the Eskimos of the southwest Yukon-Kuskokwim area, run during the summer. In their season, the various subspecies of salmon—dog, chinook, coho, sockeye, and pink—are caught in great numbers. During the warm months, the all-salmon diet is a bit more varied because greens and berries are available, but salmon is still the main food. A large portion of the catch will be filleted and sun-dried. The heads and innards will be buried in grass-lined pits and fermented. All the roe is detached and what is left over from the daily meal will also be sun-dried. Roe, the first food supplement for children, is usually saved for the youngsters and pregnant women. Roe is extremely nutritious. Dr. Price found it to be one of the best foods in the world. Besides its amino acids, vitamins, and minerals, it contains special growth factors when eaten raw. Roe can be delicious when cooked properly.

It has a tender consistency and the flavor of chicken breast. The milt of the male salmon is saved for the fathers, as it is supposed to reinforce their reproductive efficiency.

CHIEF SOURCES OF NUTRIENTS IN THE ESKIMO DIET

PROTEIN	fish and mammals
FAT	seal oil
CARBOHYDRATE	berries
CALORIES	seal oil
VITAMIN A	seal oil, organ meats, fish oils, flesh of salmon, eyes and fatty pads behind eyes, roe, bone marrow, stomach contents
VITAMIN C	fresh raw flesh, raw organ meats, adrenal glands, stomach contents, greens, berries, and kelp
VITAMIN B_1	whole fish and mammals, including their organs
VITAMIN B_2	whole fish and mammals, and their organs
NIACIN	whole fish and mammals, and their organs
CALCIUM	bones, blood, stomach contents, kelp
IRON	organ meats, bones, bone marrow, stomach contents, roe, muscular tissue of diving sea mammals
FIBER	undigested parts of the fish or mammal
VITAMIN D	fish liver oils, bone marrow, oily fish flesh, bird feathers, roe

Other fish caught in season are blackfish, tom cod and ling cod, flounder, grayling, herring, stickleback, pike, smelt, sculpin, trout, and whitefish. These are occasionally cooked for the evening meal by placing them in a bit of water and just barely simmering them, but much of the catch is eaten raw while half-frozen. Again, the entire fish is eaten, the head with its fat-rich pads behind the eye being the most popular. Calcium is obtained when the small bones of the fish are eaten. Blackfish and needlefish are rich in this nutrient. By eating the entire fish—the head, the organs, and the roe—the Eskimos get all the nutrients needed for good health and they thrive on this diet. Excess small fish are strung on willow shoots to dry in the sun.

Sea Mammals

A great favorite of the Eskimos is the various sea mammals of the area. An entire upriver village will move to the shore to catch a supply of walrus, seal, baleen whale, and beluga whale. Some of the meat will be eaten fresh, usually raw, and the rest will be frozen or dried. All the animal will be consumed in the following ways:

The liver, a special treat, will be eaten raw and half-frozen, with seal oil or fermented until it has the flavor of strong cheese.

The stomach is occasionally eaten, after careful cleaning. Sometimes a walrus stomach will be filled with blubber and boiled.

The kidneys are eaten fresh, raw, half-frozen, or chopped and cooked. They are a special treat for the children.

The head will be boiled and eaten completely. The young boys consider this the choicest part.

The intestines will be thoroughly cleaned, then dried or cooked by boiling or frying. They are often finely chopped and mixed with berries and seal oil.

Embryo seals are skinned, boiled whole, and eaten completely.

Seal and walrus flippers are considered a great delicacy. They are buried and allowed to ferment. When removed from the pit, they are rather musty and taste like a strong cheese. A bit of fermented flipper will be served after dinner in much the same manner that we serve cheese after a meal.

Seal Oil

The major source of much-needed oil in the Eskimo diet is oil made from seal blubber. The blubber is cut into chunks, stuffed into a seal poke, and allowed to ferment. This amber-colored oil is eaten at all meals. It is never heated or used in cooking; it is a sort of vinegary smelling sauce into which every bite of food is first dipped. The oil is mixed with berries for dessert and a small quantity is taken as a drink before meals. It is a major source of Vitamin A and essential fat in the Eskimo diet. Seal oil is also a medium for preserving other foods.

Plants

Plant foods are consumed mainly in spring and summer, when the Eskimos gather them in the woods and along the riverbanks. There is a large variety of these plants but not much quantity. The favorites are wild onion, wild sweet potato, Indian potato, groundnuts, woolly lousewort, water sedge, wild celery, mare's tail, mountain sorrel, wild rhubarb, and sourdock. Willow leaves are also picked in early spring. These plants are usually eaten raw as a sort of salad or added to soups. When the plants are available, they are frequently the only thing the Eskimos eat. If the season is good and the wild plants plentiful, many are stored in seal pokes with the seal oil. They make a delicious treat in winter.

Berries are extremely popular with the Eskimos, who have no other fruit. Wild blackberries, red currants, blueberries, low bush cranberries are gathered by the whole family and eaten fresh, dried, or preserved in seal oil. The dried or fermented berries are mixed with snow in winter to make agutuk, Eskimo ice cream. Cranberries, the most popular berry gathered, contain a factor that helps digest a heavy protein meal. They are also a good source of iodine if they have grown near the ocean.

Wildfowl

Because so many areas of Alaska are breeding grounds for migratory wildfowl, birds of various kinds are an important part of the Eskimo diet in early spring. At that time, their supply of salmon caught the year before is nearly depleted and the arrival of the nesting birds often means the salvation of an Eskimo village. Some of the most important food birds are ducks, geese, snowy owls, ptarmigan, cormorants, puffin, and auklets. The usual method of preparing the wild birds is by simmering them for a soup. If the catch is large, many of the birds may be stored for winter use. One method is to skin and clean them and put them into a seal poke. The breasts may be boned and dried or sometimes the flesh is salted. Birds that stay in the area all year, like the snowy owl and the ptarmigan, may be preserved by freezing. They are then eaten raw, half-frozen, feathers and all. The feathers furnish oil, Vitamin D, and bulk in the diet.

Eggs

During June and July, the bird eggs are harvested by the thousands. They are often eaten raw, especially if they are well along in incubation. Some of the eggs are preserved by cooking them whole and storing them in seal oil, while raw eggs are occasionally allowed to decompose before eating.

Eggs are one of man's best foods. They contain all of the nutrients necessary to nurture the growing bird embryo including Vitamins A and D and iron. The protein of the egg is the most perfect source of protein for man.

Other Meats

From time to time the Eskimos along the Kuskokwim may hunt caribou or polar bear. These are important foods for the northern and inland groups but only occasionally are they eaten by the coastal villagers. Polar bear, which has a strong, unpleasant flavor, is never eaten raw or half-frozen; it is always boiled, usually with the addition of some fat. The caribou is eaten entirely; the stomach and its contents, the intestines after careful cleaning, the liver, and the fat and muscle around the eyes. The bones are cracked to extract the marrow, which is eaten raw or added to a stew. Frequently, the flesh of the polar bear and caribou will also be used to feed the sled dogs.

Other Foods

In the fall the Eskimo women gather "mousenuts." These are not really nuts, but any sort of food the field rodents have stored in their underground nests for the winter. One or two large sacks may be collected by a family for use during the winter. The usual mousenuts are tender seedlings of native grasses as well as bits of root and seeds from various tundra plants. This stolen cache is added to soups.

Eskimos gather kelp from the shore and eat it raw, cook it in the soup, or store it in the seal poke. One ounce of kelp supplies 25 milligrams of Vitamin C and 273 milligrams of calcium, equal to that in a glass of milk. Kelp is one of the best sources of iodine and other trace minerals.

Blood

When a sea mammal is caught, the blood is carefully saved, to be frozen into convenient-sized chunks and stored. When needed, a chunk of frozen blood will be added to boiling water and this, along with perhaps some mousenuts or roe, makes a thick and nourishing soup. While it seems that this soup would be an excellent source of iron, actually most of the iron in hemoglobin cannot be metabolized by the human body.

DINING WITH AN ESKIMO FAMILY

Entering an Eskimo home in the middle of their long, dark winter is something of a shock. Entry is through a narrow tunnel that effectively keeps out the wind and prevents heat loss, but as soon as the visitor stands up, he is assailed by the heat. The interior is practically tropical. Outer clothes are quickly shed and hung on wall pegs. The heat comes from whale oil lamps and stoves and the snow makes a fine insulation.

During the days and weeks of miserable weather, when no one ventures out to fish or hunt, the men used to spend their time carving beautiful dishes and utensils from wood, bone, or horn. This practice is all but abandoned, and these lovely artifacts can now be found only in museums. Many families still boast an intricately carved wooden meat tray but china and plastic are used now. Some Eskimos still cling to the old practice of having individual dishes and cups for various family members, a custom going back to ancient times, when a beautifully carved bowl would be given an infant to be his dish throughout life.

Mealtimes consist of a very light breakfast, a meal at about eleven a.m., dinner at five or so, and a late evening snack. Frequently the same food will be served at all meals.

The first procedure in preparing dinner in Kuskokwim is to go outside and climb the platform where the frozen fish and seal pokes are kept. This requires two people, one to fetch the food, the other to beat off the sled dogs, who willingly grab whatever they can. After the careful selection of a number of frozen fish and perhaps a chunk of blood, the food is carried inside to thaw. When the fish have defrosted a bit, the heads and tails are removed to be cooked separately for the children, who eat earlier than their parents. The fish is then put in a pan with just a bit of water. When it has barely come to a boil, it is removed from the heat and allowed to cool. The Eskimos prefer to eat even their cooked food cold.

Berries preserved in seal oil and a little "sweet" fermented seal liver will finish off the meal.

The Eskimo of the past sat on a fur-covered bed to eat. The food was placed on a low wooden platform in front of him. The women served the fish to each diner with their hands. After selecting just the right piece of fish, the server would squeeze it over the pan so that no liquid would drip onto the fur bed covers. The bed must not get damp under any circumstances. The pieces of fish were held in the hand and skillfully cut off at the lips with a bone knife. No plates were used. When the fish had been eaten, the soup was passed from diner to diner in a large dipper from which each sipped noisily.

If soup was not served at a meal, a little melted snow usually was offered. The berries and greens that had been stored in the seal oil were removed from the oil with the fingers.

Cooking holds a very secondary place in the Eskimo life and usually iron pots or discarded cans of the traders are used for cooking vessels. In the old days, clay pots were used and often the hot stone method of cooking was employed.

Naturally, in summer everything is quite different. Fresh foods are enjoyed and most of the time the family eats out-of-doors. Life must be especially pleasant in summer as the gentle twilight that never turns to night lengthens the evenings. The family gathers around the fire, the old tales are told and retold. The adventures of the day are recalled and the old people recount tribal legends.

AN ESKIMO DINNER PER INDIVIDUAL

BLACKFISH, 1¼ pounds
FISH BROTH,
   groundnuts and onions, 2 ounces
   kelp, 1 ounce
CRANBERRIES, 1 cup
SEAL OIL, 2 tablespoons
"SWEET LIVER", 1 ounce

AN ESKIMO DINNER FROM YOUR KITCHEN

FISH SOUP
SOURDOUGH RYE BREAD (spread with bleu cheese and butter)
CRANBERRY RELISH (on greens)

The Eskimo menu is changed because few Americans would eat over 1 pound of nearly raw fish, bitter cranberries, and fermented liver. Sourdough bread is included because sourdough has been practically a staple food for many Eskimos since the gold miners brought it to Alaska in 1896. The Eskimos, who carefully maintain their starters, often make pancakes with it.

The chief sources of nutrients in the Eskimo meal are:

PROTEIN	fish
FAT	seal oil
CARBOHYDRATE	cranberries
CALORIES	fish
VITAMIN A	seal oil, whole fish, and "sweet liver"
VITAMIN B₁	fish
VITAMIN B₂	"sweet liver"
NIACIN	fish
VITAMIN C	kelp and cranberries
CALCIUM	fish bones
IRON	whole fish
FIBER	cranberries

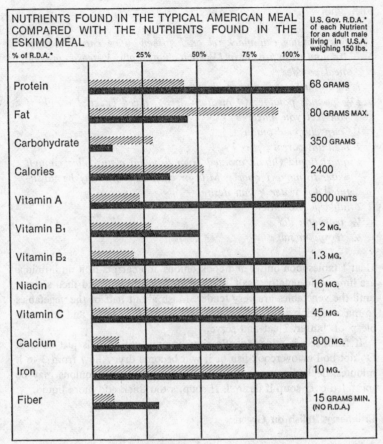

NUTRIENTS FOUND IN THE TYPICAL AMERICAN MEAL COMPARED WITH THE NUTRIENTS FOUND IN THE ESKIMO MEAL	U.S. Gov. R.D.A.* of each Nutrient for an adult male living in U.S.A. weighing 150 lbs.
% of R.D.A.* ··· 25% ··· 50% ··· 75% ··· 100%	
Protein	68 GRAMS
Fat	80 GRAMS MAX.
Carbohydrate	350 GRAMS
Calories	2400
Vitamin A	5000 UNITS
Vitamin B₁	1.2 MG.
Vitamin B₂	1.3 MG.
Niacin	16 MG.
Vitamin C	45 MG.
Calcium	800 MG.
Iron	10 MG.
Fiber	15 GRAMS MIN. (NO R.D.A.)

*R.D.A. is the recommended daily nutrient allowance intended to meet the needs of a *healthy* individual.
Diagonal lines represent the American meal.

Fish Soup

*1 fifteen-ounce can mackerel or 1 fifteen-ounce can salmon or
1 pound fresh fish cut in 1½-inch chunks, plus ½ teaspoon bone
meal powder*

1 eight-ounce can minced clams

*1½ pounds potatoes (4 medium-sized), diced (peel skin only if
you feel you must)*

½ cup chopped onion

2 medium carrots, sliced

*1 quart liquid (liquid drained from fish and clams, plus enough
water to make 1 quart). Milk or chicken broth may be substituted for water if you desire.*

2 tablespoons butter

½ teaspoon dill

½ teaspoon salt

Heat 1 tablespoon butter and cook onions and carrots in it until onions
are limp. Add potatoes, salt, and liquid. Bring to boil and then simmer
until the vegetables are very tender. Mash about half of the vegetables
to make a thick soup. Add clams and fish. Salt to taste, and add 1 tablespoon butter. Heat and serve.

If fresh fish is added, gently simmer only until fish is just cooked.
Do not boil or overcook fish or it will become dry. Allow from 3 to 8
minutes, depending upon the fish. Chopped raw green onions may be
sprinkled over soup if desired. If soup is too thick add more liquid.

Cranberry Relish on Greens

*2 cups raw unsweetened cranberries, fresh or frozen. Use blue-
berries or other berries if cranberries are unobtainable.*

*2 small oranges, peeled with vegetable peeler (leaving white
membrane on), and quartered (orange skin may be used if it
hasn't been dyed)*

2 small, unpeeled apples, cored and quartered

1 tablespoon honey, or to taste (relish should not be sweet)

Wash fruit and put through fine cutter of food grinder or chop in a
blender. Add honey to taste. Allow relish to stand in the refrigerator a
few hours so that the flavors will blend and sauce will thicken. If using
berries other than cranberries, grind only ¾ cup. Fold remainder,
whole, into ground fruit.

Mixed Greens

Tear a small amount of an assortment of greens into small pieces. Romaine lettuce, watercress, young dandelion, and chopped parsley would be good. Toss with a little oil and vinegar mixed with honey. Serve cranberry relish on top of greens.

Sourdough Rye Bread

> 1 cup starter (you can make your own with the recipe following, or you can buy it)
> 2 cups lukewarm water
> ½ to 1 cup whole wheat flour
> 2 cups rye flour
> 2 tablespoons blackstrap molasses
> 3 tablespoons butter, melted
> 2 teaspoons salt

Mix all the ingredients together, using only enough flour (about ½ cup) to make a sponge. Let batter rise in a warm place, about 70 degrees, overnight or for about 12 hours. Then add sufficient rye and wheat flour (about 3 cups) to make a stiff dough. Turn dough onto a floured board and knead it until it is smooth. Form into a loaf and place on an oiled baking sheet. Brush with oil and sprinkle with cornmeal if you wish. Or place dough in an oiled bread pan and brush with oil. Cover bread and allow it to rise until doubled in bulk, about 3 to 4 hours. Bake in a preheated 400° oven 10 minutes, then reduce oven temperature to 350° and bake until crust is nicely browned and the loaf sounds hollow when tapped. It should take 1 hour or more.

Sourdough Starter

> 1 tablespoon brown sugar
> 1¼ cups warm water
> 1 cake bakers' yeast
> 2 cups unsifted whole wheat flour

Dissolve sugar in warm water. Add yeast and stir until dissolved. Add enough flour to make a stiff batter. Stir well, place batter in a 1-quart stone crock or glass bowl. Cover and allow to stand at room temperature, about 70°, 2 to 4 days. Stir down occasionally, at least once a day. When some starter is used, replace with equal amounts of flour and water. This starter may be stored in the refrigerator indefinitely. When you want to use some starter, allow it to stand 24 hours at room temperature first.

Bleu Cheese and Butter Spread

> 3 ounces bleu or Roquefort cheese
> 2 tablespoons butter

Mash bleu cheese with a fork. Blend in butter to make a smooth paste. Place in a small crock or bowl and chill. Garlic powder may be added if desired. Each diner can spread it on his warm sourdough rye bread. Or you can spread it on the sliced bread, reassemble the loaf, place it in a paper sack fastened with a paper clip, set it on a pan, and heat in the oven until the butter has melted.

Sourdough Hot Cakes

> ½ cup sourdough starter (you can buy it or make your own; see page 155)
> 2 cups whole grain flour
> 1 tablespoon molasses
> 2 cups potato water (water in which potatoes have been cooked)
> 2 eggs, well beaten
> 2 teaspoons double-acting baking powder
> 2 tablespoons melted butter
> ¾ teaspoon salt
> Blueberries in season

The night before you want to serve hot cakes, mix starter, liquid, flour, and molasses. Let stand covered in a warm place overnight. Next morning replenish your jar of starter with ½ cup of the new batter. Mix eggs, salt, and baking powder and add to the batter along with the melted butter. Blend well with as few strokes as possible. Do not beat hard. Drop batter by tablespoonfuls onto a lightly oiled griddle or frying pan. Sprinkle blueberries over batter. Brown on both sides. Serve with butter and maple syrup or honey. Hot cakes may be eaten cold as a bread.

Kidney Stew

1½ pounds kidneys
2 cups broth: meat, chicken, or vegetable
4 medium potatoes, scrubbed and cut into 1-inch pieces
1 medium onion, cut into chunks
½ cup raw cranberries or ¼ cup red wine
2 tablespoons parsley, minced
½ bay leaf
⅛ teaspoon dill, ground
⅛ teaspoon tarragon, ground
2 tablespoons butter
8 medium-sized raw mushrooms, quartered
Salt to taste

Add bay leaf, dill, tarragon, onion, and cranberries to broth. Bring to boil and simmer 20 minutes. Add potatoes and cook until they are tender. Thicken gravy, slightly, if you desire by mashing some of the potatoes or mix a paste of cold water and whole grain flour and stir into gravy. Simmer 5 minutes. Remove all white membrane from the kidneys. Cut kidneys into ¾-inch cubes and add to the stew. Simmer gently only until they lose their pink color, or about 4 minutes. Season to taste with salt. Add butter, parsley, and mushrooms. If kidneys are cooked at too high a temperature or overcooked, the odor of ammonia is sometimes released. To prevent this all the white membrane must be removed before they are touched by water. The kidneys should be cooked as short a time as possible, at low heat. If an acid is added to the cooking liquid, the odor will be neutralized. This odor is not caused by urine but by enzymes in the kidney that produce ammonia from nitrogen.

Liver Paste

1 carrot, thinly sliced
1 onion, thinly sliced
1 pound liver
Salt to taste
2 to 4 tablespoons butter

Sauté carrot and onion slices in a little butter until onion is transparent. Add liver and a very small amount of water or chicken broth. Cover and steam liver over low heat about 4 minutes, or just until it loses its pink color. Put liver and vegetables through a meat grinder 2 or 3 times or chop in a blender. Add salt to taste plus any juices left from steaming the liver and from the grinding. Blend in enough soft butter to make a spreadable paste. If it is too soft, add powdered milk, whole grain bread crumbs, or toasted wheat germ to firm it. Garlic, sage, or other spices may be added to taste. Chill. Liver paste is good spread on whole grain bread or fresh raw vegetables.

Baked Roe

Choose 1 pound of any fish roe. Roll roe, with membrane unbroken, in melted butter or vegetable oil seasoned with lemon juice, then in toasted whole grain bread crumbs. Bake on a flat oiled baking dish in a preheated 300° oven, 30 minutes, or until a meat thermometer registers 150°. Serve with melted butter seasoned with ground fresh cranberries or lemon juice and chopped chives.

Sun-Dried Fish

Thread fresh fish fillets on long thin sticks with sharpened ends. Place in the sun on a rack to dry. Care must be taken to protect the fresh fish from insects and to cover them at night to keep them dry.

Steamed Dried Fish

Cut dried fish into serving size pieces. (You may substitute fresh fish if you desire.) Place in a pan on top of some sliced onions and kelp or parsley sprigs. Add just enough water, broth, or white wine to produce steam—about ¼ cup. Fish should not touch broth. Cover pan and simmer gently 15 minutes or just until fish is tender. Remove fish and vegetables from pan. Add plenty of seal oil or butter and crushed cranberries or lemon juice to the remaining broth. Heat broth and pour over the fish.

If using fresh fish, it will cook in much less time. It is very important not to overcook fish as it quickly becomes dry. Fish is done just as soon as it looks solid white.

Cranberry Ice and Ice Cream

> *4 cups raw cranberries*
> *2 cups water*
> *1 cup honey, or to taste*

Cook 2 cups of cranberries in water until soft. Force mixture through a sieve or liquefy in a blender. Mix honey with the resulting juice. Heat slightly, if necessary, to blend in honey. Grind the remaining 2 cups of cranberries in a food grinder or chop in a blender using some of the juice in the blender. Combine the chopped cranberries with the juice. If mixture is not sweet enough, add more honey (it should not be too sweet). The flavor is improved by adding the juice of 1 lemon. Place mixture in a large, shallow pan and place in the freezer. When 1 inch of ice has formed around the edges of the mixture, remove it from the freezer. Place it in a bowl and beat it with a mixer to break up the ice crystals. When the mixture is smooth and about the consistency of cake batter return it to its freezer pan, cover, and refreeze. Repeat the beating process when the ice is about ¾ frozen. If it is very icy, beat it again when you serve it so that it is like a mush. If cranberry ice is not too sweet, it is good served as a relish with the main course. While the Eskimo often whipped caribou fat into his "ice cream," most of us prefer whipped cream. To make ice cream, carefully fold 1 cup of heavy cream, whipped, into the cranberry ice after you have beaten it the first time to break up the ice crystals. Omit the second beating. If you wish to use other fresh fruit to make fruit ice or ice cream omit the water and the cooking. Reduce the honey to taste. Mash any soft berries or fruit, add honey, cover, and allow to stand ½ hour to draw juices from the fruit. Vanilla or almond extract enhance the flavor of the fruits.

To make one serving of real ice cream, add the whipped cream to the mashed fruit syrup. Place ¾ cup of the chilled mixture into a clean tin can. Set can in a large bowl filled with layers of chopped ice and rock salt. Use 3 parts ice to 1 part rock salt. Mix ice cream with a wooden spoon until it hardens.

THE LIGHT BITE, ESKIMO STYLE

A QUICK MEAL: Canned salmon or liver paste (page 157), whole grain bread and cranberry relish (page 154).

A SNACK: Frozen berries mashed in a blender with just enough yogurt to liquefy. Flavor with honey and vanilla extract to taste. Any raw fruit may be frozen whole, chopped, and placed in the blender with yogurt to make instant "frosties."

The Chinese,
Relentless Survivors

China—magnificent, mysterious, and remote—is the home of 800 million gourmets. The whole country is populated with gastronomic experts whose uncompromising attitudes about food have conquered invaders, caused revolutions, and established standards of excellence in food preparation that are the envy of chefs all over the world. Nowhere else is food—its selection, preparation, seasoning, and eating—such a major preoccupation. Lin Yutang writes: "If there is anything we are serious about it is neither religion nor learning, but food. We openly acclaim eating as one of the few joys of this human life." Chinese greet each other with "Have you eaten?" expressing the hope that a meal can be shared. A grand epic poem was written about a feast in the third century B.C. The poet, Ch'u Yuan, went into some detail about the various courses, how they were prepared and presented, but overlooked the occasion for the feast. Undoubtedly the first real cookbook listing the quantities of ingredients as well as instructions for preparation was written by a Madame Wu from Kiangsu during the Sung dynasty. In the tenth century A.D., the first physician to concern himself with nutrition on a quantitative basis detailed a specific diet for an ailing emperor. While 300 years before, in the seventh century, a book called *Thousand Golden Prescriptions* described how rice polishings could be used to cure beriberi, a Vitamin B_1 deficiency disease. About twelve centuries later, the cure for beriberi was discovered in the West.

Food as a weapon was utilized by the Chinese in a very unusual manner. During a time of unrest, an extravagant empress was so self-indulgent that great numbers of peasants were required to import exotic foods from distant provinces for her table. By way of protest a dish called *Kweifei* chicken was named after her, an insulting likeness of the woman herself. The recipe called for a plump, white chicken to be marinated in wine, then stewed in wine, and finally served in a rich wine sauce. The political implications, not to mention the ridicule, proved too much for the emperor, and the downfall of the Tang dynasty followed.

Invaders brought their food preferences and made futile efforts to retain their own eating style, with predictable results. To the Chinese, Mongol food was considered beneath contempt—barbarous, disgusting, and inedible, consisting mainly of great hunks of meat thrown right into the fire. Even while the Mongols ruled China, the Chinese ruled the kitchen and refused to prepare Mongol food. Eventually these invaders became absorbed into the mainstream of Chinese life, victims of the "Kitchen Victory." They probably conceded that Chinese cooking was better than Mongol anyway.

Because of their early development of writing and printing, the Chinese had an advantage over most of the world. This ability to write down ideas and so make them available to anyone no doubt accounted for the incredible list of Chinese discoveries and inventions that dominate every aspect of civilized life. From astronomy and a fairly accurate clock, to crop rotation, to printing and paper-making, nearly everything in our daily lives was first developed by the Chinese. The only possible exceptions are the wheel and fire, and a study of ancient China could cause some speculation about those.

A look at these ancient Chinese shows them to have been brilliant and sophisticated, living in harmony with nature, even though nature often betrayed them by bringing floods or droughts with relentless regularity. It was during times of famine that the Chinese discovered that carp tongue, shark fin, sweet pea vine, and swallows' nests were edible. These foods are now considered great delicacies.

Principles established by their greatest spokesman, Confucius, a firm and practical realist, dominated their lives. Preaching order, decency, and self-control, he was a great moralist who preferred to be regarded as a teacher. With a simple philosophy and a conviction that there was a right way and a wrong way to live, he traveled throughout China during his lifetime, from 550 to 478 B.C., bringing wisdom and serenity to his followers.

Chinese agriculture began so many centuries ago it is impossible to pin down a date. Somewhere between ten to fifteen thousand years ago fields were first planted, crops harvested, and towns established. Rice culture, dominant in the south of China, accounted for the early development of an elaborate social order. The enormous amount of water needed to grow rice led to the creation of complicated series of canals, dams, and levees. It was impossible for one family or even one clan to construct these huge systems, so a central government evolved that could solve the problems and provide the manpower. It is possible to travel great distances by boat along the canals and through the lakes created by this massive irrigation system. In his journals, Father Ricci, a sixteenth century Jesuit, tells how, in 1590, he traveled from Nanking, the southern capital, to Peking, the northern capital, by boat—a somewhat hazardous trip but far easier than on foot. The vigorous health of the Chinese was also noted by Father Ricci who wrote: "The Chinese are longer-lived than the Europeans and preserve their physical powers up to seventy or eighty years of age."

For centuries the Yellow River, the curse of China, was partially contained by the superhuman effort of thousands of coolies building ever-higher levees to hold back the floods. As the river silted up and rose higher, so did the walls of the levees until in some areas they reached as high as 70 feet. Eventually, of course, the river would break through and another disastrous flood, followed by years of famine, would debilitate the population of northern China. In spite of these fearful floods and famines that occurred with depressing regularity (over 1,800 in 2,000 years) the people's health remained amazingly good. Most illnesses were related to malnutrition resulting from famine but given even the smallest quantity of their usual food, on a regular basis, the Chinese could and did accomplish astonishing feats. The Great Wall was built by men who ate little besides rice and cabbage. This simple diet, however, is nutritious due to the marvelous qualities of cabbage. Of all of nature's bounty, the lowly cabbage is probably the most universally consumed vegetable in the world. Every culture eats cabbage, raw, cooked, or preserved. It contains a good deal of Vitamin C, in fact, as much as in a comparable quantity of citrus fruits. Unlike that in most foods, the Vitamin C in cabbage is not destroyed by cooking. Throughout history, cabbage has been known as the poor man's vegetable, for very few foods give such a great return for so little effort. In contrast to rice, which needs constant attention during its growing, cabbage is planted, ignored, and then harvested.

The amazing stamina of the Chinese, their strength and their endurance, came not only from their food but from the way they prepared it. The staple food of southern China was polished rice. With most of the nutrients removed, it would have been a poor diet indeed were it not for the various combinations that were served with the rice, an enormous variety of vegetables, freshwater fish, pork or duck in small but essential quantities, and perhaps most important, soybean products. Even in winter, fresh vegetables were available from various sprouted seeds. Mineral-laden and enzyme-rich, sprouts provided high quality food at a time when it was most needed, winter and early spring. In addition, these healthful and nutritious foods were prepared in an almost ideal manner. They were stir-fried over a hot fire of grass or charcoal in a tiny amount of fat until heated through but still crisp and flavorful. Foods cooked in this manner retain most of the properties of raw foods.

The Chinese preoccupation with food developed some unbending rules. Each dish must have four textures: crunchy, soft, crisp, and hard. Each meal must have four flavors: sweet, sour, salt, and acid. A banquet or company meal—and it was a poor day indeed that didn't include some sort of festive meal with friends—was arranged following rigid tradition. Each guest had a bowl of rice in front of him (women never ate at the table with the men), his chopsticks, and a porcelain soup spoon. Arranged on the table, but not always in reach of each guest, were four (simple, low-key), eight (pleasant, but not lavish), sixteen (getting on to a banquet), twenty (a festive feast), or more dishes featuring the qualities required in Chinese cuisine. There were usually three or four soups, pickled or salted vegetables; duck, pork, and fish dishes. Each guest ate some rice and "pushed it down" with a tidbit of food from one of the many dishes on the table. Reaching for what you wanted was expected and the meal was frequently interrupted by elaborate toasts from the host, the guest of honor, friends— anyone at all. Toasts were drunk from thimble-sized cups filled with rice wine, a rather mild, pleasant-tasting drink. The meal lasted for hours.

One unusual feature of Chinese cuisine is the manner in which the food is prepared before cooking. Each type of vegetable has a special way it must be cut, while meat is cut with or against the grain depending upon the dish being cooked. Nothing must be larger than one bite. Lin Yutang has an interesting theory behind this elaborate chopping and cutting of food. In every Chinese household are numerous women—aunts, nieces, unmarried daughters, and daughters-in-law—and tasks must be found for them or quarrels would be incessant. Hence, all that chopping. As if to confirm this, he describes a dish of nearly a dozen finely chopped ingredients that requires constant stirring for about two hours. The Chinese are guilty of few undesirable practices where food is concerned, but vegetables that are chopped hours ahead of time and left out in the air and light suffer serious nutritional destruction. Over half the vitamins are lost. The best Chinese cooks prepare their vegetables just before cooking them.

There are three major cuisines of China: Cantonese, regarded by many as the very finest; Peking, hearty and filling; and Szechwan, spicy and flavorful.

The major division of China into north and south is quite abrupt. North of the Yangtse, the Peking area, the people eat wheat, millet, and maize; their food is steamed, their soups are hearty, and they eat more meat than the rest of their countrymen. Rice is not a major part of their diet. Peking meals feature great bowls of steaming noodles, the pasta that Marco Polo took back to Italy. Robust flavors are favored and even the most sophisticated dishes retain the bold simplicity of peasant food. The people are distinctive too. They are tall, muscular, and large-boned with wide handsome faces. Cold and snowy, the climate of the Peking region has no doubt influenced its food. Meat-filled dumplings, savory and rich, contrast sharply with the delicately flavored dishes of the warm and tropical south. Farming on a monumental scale occupies most of the people of the north, concentrated on wheat, millet, soy, and maize. More pork is eaten, but duck is the legendary favorite. The beauty and exquisite flavor of Peking duck are world renowned.

In the south, rice is the staple food. Although it is much more difficult to raise (an old saying is that the rice spends more time in the farmer's hand than in the ground), has a smaller yield per acre, and poorer nutrition quality than the grains of the north, there is little question that it will ever be replaced. Fish is an important item in the southern diet, both along the coast and inland. Chinese seem to prefer freshwater fish to saltwater varieties and have developed elaborate hatcheries to raise and improve the breeds. Each farm has a pond well stocked with carp. The dozens of coastal islands that are sprinkled along the China Sea shelter countless tiny fishing villages that supply the major cities with octopus, shellfish, cuttlefish, and mollusks, not to mention the all-important kelp.

The southerners are small, slender, willowy people, attractive and doll-like. Most of the Chinese in this country are from the Canton area, recruited in the 1800s to work on the railroads or the mines of the West Coast.

Cantonese food is the *haute cuisine* of China. With its subtle blending of flavors, its delicate sauces and stunning varieties of vegetables, there is little question that Cantonese food is a culmination of the culinary art. The climate is favorable, mild, almost tropic, and every imaginable fruit and vegetable is grown. In the coastal provinces of Chinkiang and Kiangsu lived the gastronomic snobs of China. In this languid, semitropic area, food was a serious topic and a major preoccupation. Tiny villages became famous for certain products they sold. Without Chinkiang vinegar or Yangchow noodles, a meal was a disaster. Bean curd was prepared in dozens of ways, an example of Chinese ingenuity. On gaily decorated floating restaurants, a simple dish of carp and noodles delicately flavored and superbly cooked would be served as a sort of between-meal snack. The whole effect of the lantern-lit, flower-bedecked barges was charming and frivolous and so essentially Chinese.

Szechwan, with its moist and gentle climate, forms a great triangle in the heart of China. Startling scenery, perhaps the most dramatically beautiful in all the world, is the major feature of this little kingdom, which developed in virtual isolation.

Szechwan food is a brilliant freak that breaks all the rules and gets away with it. Hot, hot, hot red peppers, garlic, and ginger are combined with sweet foods and various fruits. The result is a cuisine as pugnacious and peppery yet good-humored and straightforward as the people themselves. The Szechwanese are noted for their small stature and feisty dispositions; even their horses and dogs seem to have acquired these tendencies. Szechwan ponies are irascible and hard to train. The cuisine features a wide variety of relishes and sauces to combine with the hot foods; pork is cooked until hard and crisp; Szechwan chicken, a spicy and eye-watering dish, is a great favorite. Fish, beef, and duck are not popular.

The garlic, ginger, hot peppercorns, and tiny peppers that flavor so many Szechwan dishes give them a spice and tang unique in the world. Garlic, used extensively in the cooking, has a number of therapeutic, if antisocial, qualities. Chinese who eat lots of garlic rarely suffer from high blood pressure and biochemical tests have shown that garlic actually has the ability to lower blood pressure. Interestingly, after sugar feeding, a 12 percent drop in blood sugar was noted among rabbits who were given twenty-five grams of garlic extract. Liberal intake of garlic has long been noted as responsible for controlling intestinal worms. Medicinally, garlic is a diuretic, stimulant, antibiotic, expectorant, and sweat promoter. Russian scientists have isolated a natural antiseptic substance in the aroma of garlic. We now know that the strong smell and the health-giving properties go hand in hand. Chewing a couple of sprigs of parsley after eating heavily garlicked food can remove most of the offending odor; but when a very large quantity is consumed, the odor comes from all the pores in the body.

Garlic and other herbs had an important role in the folk medicine of China and every village featured an herbalist who was wise in the ways of plants. Ginseng, a strange and rather rare root that grows in a human shape, has for over 5,000 years been considered one of the most potent plants in the Chinese pharmacopoeia. Recent analysis has shown that it has particular medicinal value as a stimulant and heart rejuvenator. It is also an effective placebo. Many of the strange and exotic roots, plants, and barks that make up a Chinese medicine store do indeed have tremendous medicinal value, and these ancient remedies are now taking their place alongside modern antibiotics in contemporary China.

In spite of their land's immense size, its regional and climatic differences and geographic barriers, and its multitude of local dialects, all Chinese share many common attitudes and customs. Perhaps the strongest and most enduring is family unity. Children have always represented the wealth of the family, boys especially. They were adored and doted upon, indulged and petted, with never a cross word directed at them. Daughters, not as highly favored as sons, didn't fare as well. They had pretty much to fend for themselves. This parental indifference produced an interesting woman, strong and self-willed, practical but inscrutable and generally unscrupulous, willing to go to any lengths to attain her goals. Such women have proved to be a major asset and moving force in the creation of new China. They took their new equality as a matter of course; for centuries they had been doing most of the work anyway. As children, when they were old enough, they were expected to help with the chores.

Since more than 80 percent of all Chinese lived in rural areas and worked in agriculture, farm life dominated the society. The house surrounded a courtyard and made it an integral part of the family life. All doors and windows opened to the courtyard and much of the day's activities took place in this garden. One of their favorite foods was carp and there was usually a pond where they swam. (China raised more freshwater fish than the rest of the world put together.) Except for the very wealthy, little in the way of decoration or artistry was found in the home; the rooms were plain and simply furnished. As the sons married and brought home their new wives, additional rooms mushroomed around the original dwelling until it began to resemble a compound or tiny village, which indeed it almost was. All ages, from infants to the very old, lived together, sometimes to the sounds of shrill voices and loud arguments, but always with the security of a closely knit family. The women ruled the kitchen and rural food was simple, straightforward and filling, but always beautifully prepared. Even the most sophisticated palate sometimes longed for a bowl of *congee,* a rice gruel eaten daily by peasants and coolies. Frequently an elaborate banquet would feature a simple peasant dish as if to remind the guests of their origins, but also because it tasted good.

Regardless of area—cold, snowy north, tropic south, or mountainous west—soybeans are a major crop and a staple food everywhere in China. They are pressed for oil; they are fermented for bean curd; the major flavoring comes from soy sauce; and one of the chief sources of protein in the Chinese diet is the ubiquitous soybean.

Probably one of the oldest crops in the world, the soybean is considered by the Chinese as one of the sacred grains. For centuries, Asians have cultivated the soybean because it is meat, milk, cheese, and bread in one small, round kernel. It is the best source of protein in the vegetable kingdom (40 to 45 percent); it contains more iron and calcium than any other grain or legume and is an excellent source of unsaturated fat as well. Beyond question it is the most versatile of the grains and takes so many forms it is hard to believe all the foods that come from this one plant. Chinese bean curd and Japanese *tofu* are the same thing, a cheese made of soy milk. The only type of cheese ever eaten by the Chinese, it is a smooth-textured, soft but firm cake that the Chinese call "meat without bones." It is high in protein and calcium, low in fat and with infinite variations for serving. Cut up in small cubes and added to soup is about the simplest.

A less widely known but equally important benefit is the two-and-a-half percent lecithin content in soybeans, one of the few foods that contain this elusive nutrient. The importance of lecithin in the diet is still being studied but Pottenger and Krohn found, after tests on 122 patients, that the blood cholesterol showed a marked decrease in 70 percent of those who took lecithin. Indications are that heart disease and hardening of the arteries could be ameliorated by soybean lecithin.

During the nineteenth century, Western influence became a factor in Chinese life. As this influence increased, over the violent objections of the rulers, drastic changes occurred. One of the most disastrous was the outcome of the great Opium War. At issue were the vast opium fields of India, which were vital to that country's economy. Britain, which controlled India, needed customers for this crop and turned to China. The trade concessions won by the British made them immune from prosecution for breaking local Chinese laws. As a result, opium addiction became epidemic and created a serious health problem. Equally as serious was the appalling venereal disease rate, spread throughout the cities by thousands of infected prostitutes. In addition, the usual famines took their toll and reduced resistance to disease. Over 80 percent of the calories in the Chinese diet came from grains, with only bits of meat, beans, and vegetables. When their food supply was short, their diet lacked the protection the vitamins in such foods as eggs, fresh fruits, and leafy vegetables provided. They were extremely susceptible to disease if their usual diet fell below a certain quantity.

By the 1920s, China was called "the sick man of the Orient." From a life expectancy of over eighty years, the average Chinese now could look forward to living to thirty-four years old, if lucky.

Infant mortality was alarmingly high, 160 infants per 1,000, and deficiency diseases due to undernutrition accounted for over 50 percent of these deaths. Health care was inadequate and the people suffered terribly under corrupt officials and burdensome taxes.

Opposing factions fought each other viciously and, as a result, were ill-prepared to defend their country from the invading Japanese in the 1930s. The Civil War ended after World War II with the Communists clearly victorious. Faced with the monumental task of revitalizing their ruined country, they have succeeded in a way that defies belief.

In 1950, two major problems vied for attention and priority: Food production had to be increased and in some areas reestablished, and public health had to be restored. The first step was to lower the standard of living in respect to food, clothing, and life style. Suddenly it was unpatriotic, if not treasonable, to eat refined rice and other fine foods. Coarse-ground millet and grain bread became the symbols of the revolution. The well-being of the farmers demanded immediate attention but the great majority of Chinese doctors lived and practiced in the cities. The communist solution was to send the doctors to the farms, where they established clinics, inaugurated sanitation programs, and trained paramedics under a village health committee.

It was discovered that nearly 11 million people had schistosomiasis, a debilitating and ultimately fatal disease that rages all over Africa and Asia. It is carried by a type of snail that lives in the rice paddies and canals. The snails bore into the flesh to lay eggs and, as the larvae develop, they cause the destruction of tissue in the human host which leads to a wide variety of ailments, including sterility, before eventual death. Night soil, used all over China for fertilizer, recycles the parasites. A massive program of treatment for the victims as well as eradication of the snails has resulted in control of schistosomiasis throughout most of China. It remains a serious problem, however, in Africa.

Equally significant was the communist regime's brutal but effective solution to the world's worst drug problem. With the state controlling every aspect of life, it was a simple matter to halt the sale, use, and distribution of opium. Addicts unable to resume a normal drug-free life simply disappeared. Less drastic but equally impressive were the methods used to control venereal disease. Prostitution was eliminated. Everyone worked for the state and prostitution was not considered a productive job. The stigma of the prostitute was removed by convincing the women they had been victims of imperialism. Treatment, long unattainable, eliminated active venereal disease in the urban areas and brought it under control throughout the rest of the country. This massive program made China the first country in the world to contain these ancient and fatal diseases.

In twenty years, through adequate diet and vigorous public health measures, the Communists made China one of the healthiest nations in the East. Life expectancy rose nearly 50 percent, from 34 to 52 years, and is still rising. The infant mortality rate fell 75 percent, from 160 per 1,000 to 39 per 1,000. Reports from nutritionists who have visited China today state that the people look healthy and are obviously well fed. There is no sign of dietary deficiency in modern China.

The agricultural programs, however, were less successful. Disastrous crop failures, caused as much by political interference as bad weather, nearly brought down the government. Subsequently, the communes were reorganized with local cadres in charge, and realistic work goals were established by commune committees.

The two major goals of Red China, improved public health and increased food production, are still an important consideration of the country's leaders. Public health is the only type of medicine in China; there is no research of any significance, no national or international medical meetings, no papers published. Doctors undergo three years of training and no particular preparation is necessary, just the desire to become a doctor. Next in the hierarchy of the health program are the paramedics who run the local clinics. They diagnose, prescribe medicines, inoculate, and do simple surgery. Finally, in each village are the so-called barefoot doctors. They take a six-month course that includes learning emergency first-aid and the teaching of nutrition, sanitation, child care, and methods of birth control. These barefoot doctors are also expected to work four hours a day in the fields. In addition they may tend an herb garden and grow many of the folk medicines frequently used. Fully half the work that makes up the daily routine of doctors in the United States and many other countries could be done by someone trained as the barefoot doctors are, leaving the highly trained physician free for more serious problems.

The barefoot doctor on the commune is the first person to examine someone who is ill. If he cannot treat the problem, the patient is taken to the nearest clinic, where the paramedics decide the best course. If the situation requires more than simple surgery, acupuncture, or treatment with drugs, the patient is sent on to a major hospital in the nearest urban area. All of this treatment is not free, but it is very inexpensive. China's enviable public health system includes possibly the best infant care program in the world. All pediatric care is free and this includes the broadest spectrum of immunization, nutrition education for the mother, and frequent clinic visits to keep track of the baby's health and development. Children, as always, are China's greatest treasure.

Family life underwent violent change in the years following the revolution. In an effort to free women for work, children were placed in child care centers shortly after birth. The infant mortality rate among these institutionalized children rose so alarmingly that changes were quickly made. The working mother now has about two months' leave for childbirth and can take longer if she wants. The children are then kept at home and tended by a grandparent. Institutions for the elderly had also proved to be a mistake. The older folks were needed at home by the family. When the child is about four, he is sent to day school. In spite of changes of government, family life in China is much the same as before, with several generations making up the household and the family unit still strong and viable. Of course, the family is now part of the commune and has a responsibility to the goals of this larger group. Family members must attend frequent meetings where these goals are constantly being reinforced by cadre leaders.

With the control of disease and drug addiction, the health of the Chinese has improved dramatically but little change has taken place in their diet or methods of food preparation. In this the communist leaders have shown practical common sense. Their food has always been excellent and no change would bring any improvement. Small garden patches are still a feature of most rural homes. These privately owned and tended bits of land have proved to be a tremendous asset as each family can grow much of what it eats, thus releasing for the cities food grown on the communes.

Farmers get all the exercise they need, but Chinese office and factory workers as well as shopkeepers are as sedentary as anywhere else in the world. To combat this and keep everyone at the peak of physical fitness, a massive program of community exercise has everyone, young and old, out in the parks each morning doing *Tai Chee,* a simple but stimulating set of exercises. Wearing soft-soled shoes, next best thing to bare feet, they all gather in the parks and perform the stretching, jumping steps of Tai Chee. Keeping muscle tone in legs and feet is the beginning of good health, according to the late Dr. Paul Dudley White. Visitors to China are encouraged to join in the daily Tai Chee and, between that and the wholesome fresh foods eaten daily, the tourists have discovered they feel better and better as their trip progresses. As T. K. Cheung wrote: "In sharp contrast with packaged tours of the West or Japan, China is a totally different experience. Walking in clean, smog-free air, combined with fresh vegetables, additive-free food and brown rice, apparently contributed to the gradual improvement of our physical condition as the tour continued."

The dramatic changes taking place in China seem to be without parallel, but that is not the case. Throughout the long history of China, dynasties have come and gone; governments have risen and fallen; rulers have instituted land reform, set prices, nationalized trade and commerce, provided for the old and sick, de-emphasized the classics, and ruled the country with an iron fist. Always in the past, the people have eventually grown tired of living under such rigid control and have forced reforms or overthrown the government. They yield for a brief time to change and then resume their lives again in the enduring pattern of China, the eternal family. This pattern cannot be destroyed or permanently altered because the Chinese are relentless survivors and through the centuries survival has depended upon the basic elements of Chinese life: the family unit, the small family-owned farm, and the family-owned business. China is very old and the West is very young, and there is much we can learn from them.

FOODS OF CHINA

The Chinese rarely eat anything raw; however, their method of cooking not only kills harmful bacteria but also preserves most of the nutrients of the raw food. The bite-sized pieces of vegetables, meat, or fish are quickly stir-fried in just enough very hot oil to coat each piece, and just long enough so they can be easily chewed. Because they are stir-fried, all the vegetables in a Chinese dish must be at the peak of perfection. Limp celery and tired peppers can be added to soups or stews with little or no damaging effect, but if lightly sautéed these vegetables look sickly and spoil the dish. Many varieties of foods are cooked together to achieve the qualities desired in the dish, a contrast of textures and flavors. Very light sauces are often added to enhance the flavors of the food.

CHIEF SOURCES OF NUTRIENTS
IN THE SOUTHERN CHINESE DIET

PROTEIN	rice, with some meat, poultry, fish, or beans
FAT	soy oil and peanut oil
CARBOHYDRATE	rice
CALORIES	rice
VITAMIN A	greens
VITAMIN C	greens
VITAMIN B_1	pork, poultry, fish, and rice
VITAMIN B_2	pork, poultry, fish, and greens
NIACIN	pork, poultry, fish, and rice
CALCIUM	greens, soybeans
IRON	greens, soybeans
FIBER	vegetables and rice

Food preservation in China is done mostly by salting, and brine-preserved vegetables are a part of every meal. Wind drying of meats and vegetables is also common and many courtyards feature a clothesline strung with eggplant peelings, radishes, mushrooms, chicken, and fillets of fish, all drying in the breeze. They will be reconstituted when needed and added to an array of different dishes.

Beans and Bean Products

Navy, lima, black, and many other beans are dried by the Chinese. They are a good source of the incomplete proteins, iron, B vitamins, and amino acids, which are low in polished rice. When eaten with rice the rice–bean combination increases the protein quality by 43 percent over these same foods if eaten separately and also raises the protein quality to that of meat. Two favorite snacks are made from beans. Raw beans are roasted, salted, and eaten as nuts, while cooked beans are mashed, sweetened, and made into tiny cakes.

Soybeans, as mentioned before, are considered by the Chinese to be one of the five sacred grains. They are the finest source of protein in the vegetable kingdom. Their protein quality is 61 percent, making them nearly as good a source of protein as meat, in which the quality varies from 63 percent to 70 percent. Because they have no starch, their carbohydrate content is low. They contain more iron and calcium than other beans and they are rich in lecithin, potassium, and essential fatty acids found in their unsaturated oil. Soybeans contain Vitamin B_{12}, a vitamin often lacking in vegetarian diets. Bean curd is the most popular form in which soybeans are prepared. It is made by cooking and mashing the soybeans, and adding gypsum, which causes the mixture to ferment. When calcium sulfate (gypsum) is added to the soybeans, their calcium content doubles, making bean curd an excellent source of calcium. The fermentation of the soybeans renders their protein and calcium easier to assimilate and adds enzymes to the diet. Bean curd has a delicate flavor, and is added to soups and other dishes or dried for future use. Soy milk is made from soybeans either by pressing the beans or pounding them into flour and adding water. Though it is used as an infant food, it doesn't contain the amount of calcium found in cow's milk. Peanuts are often added to soy milk to improve the flavor.

A nutritional comparison of 100 grams of human, cow, and soy milk and bean curd follows:

	Protein (grams)	Calcium (mg.)	Iron (mg.)	Calories
Human milk	1.1	33	.1	77
Cow's milk	3.5	118	trace	65
Soy milk	3.4	21	.8	33
Bean curd	7.8	128	1.9	72

Soy milk and human milk contain lecithin and Vitamin E, but none is found in cow's milk.

Soy sauce, a dark brown, pungent liquid, is the most important flavoring agent of the Orient. Small bowls of soy sauce are always on the table so foods may be dipped into it. It is never poured over rice. Soy sauce is made by adding salt to cooked soybeans and allowing the mixture to ferment. It is important in the Oriental diet because a harmful enzyme found in raw fish and which destroys Vitamin B_1 is destroyed by fermented foods. Four teaspoons of soy sauce contain one gram of protein. A type of soy sauce made from red beans has a sweeter, sharper flavor than others. Westerners sometimes have trouble digesting soybeans. Over the years, the Orientals have developed an intestinal flora capable of quickly and easily digesting soy products. Pressed soybean oil is the most frequently used oil in China.

Green mungo beans are another kind of legume also used in a number of ways; they are the beans most commonly sprouted and they are also pressed for milk. They can be ground into powder and the starch precipitated from the powder. This starchy flour is mixed with water to form a thin paste, poured into a vessel that has many small holes like a sieve, and then held over boiling water. As the starchy paste dribbles into the water, it cooks into a translucent vermicelli-like product called "long rice." This is served with a savory sauce or mixed with pieces of pork and rolled into a flat, pancake-like steamed bread.

Grains

In addition to rice, wheat, corn, buckwheat, and sorghum are other grains eaten by the Chinese. They are used to make steamed bread, noodles, or dumplings. Noodles are a popular food all over China, particularly in the north. They are sometimes flavored with dried shrimp or green tea. They range in size from threadlike to wide, flat sheets. They are boiled, deep-fried, stuffed with filling, simmered in soup, and are also a favorite snack.

Rice

Brown rice has the highest biological protein value of all the grains, higher than that of meat and equal to that of cheese, but in smaller quantities. For instance, the protein in one and one half cups of cooked rice equals that in one ounce of cheese. Rice is not a complete food and cannot support life; Vitamins A and C are missing and the calcium and iron content is low. When rice is polished by removing the brown coating, the protein quality is reduced 40 percent and most of its B vitamins are removed. The B vitamins are essential for the body to digest carbohydrates. Most of the digestive problems reported to be suffered by the early Chinese were undoubtedly caused by their large consumption of polished rice. Rice polishing started when Confucius introduced it and instructed all of his followers to polish their rice before eating it. This custom soon became a status symbol in both China and Japan; only very recently is the trend being reversed. Rice is served at every meal and, in combination with a bit of fish or meat and vegetables, it provides a well-balanced meal. Rice is made into a gruel called congee that is usually eaten at breakfast or for a late evening snack. This congee is a thin rice soup with any sort of food added, shredded greens, bits of pork, liver, onions, pickles, or raw fish slices. Rice is also made into flour or fermented into vinegar. It even makes a delightful wine.

Vegetables—Leafy Greens

The most frequently served greens are spinach, broccoli, cauliflower and its leaves, kale, turnip greens, cabbage (all varieties), Chinese celery, and watercress. They are chopped into small pieces and cooked just long enough to make them safe to eat but not so long that they lose their crisp texture, nutritional quality, and pleasing color. Greens supply the vitamins and minerals lacking in the high-grain diet—A, C, iron, and calcium.

Cabbage

There are numerous varieties of cabbage grown by the Chinese. Several different kinds are preserved by salting. They were making sauerkraut as far back as 200 B.C. It not only has a high Vitamin C content and a stimulating effect upon the digestive system, but its iron and calcium are also easier for the body to assimilate. Celery cabbage has a delicate taste, not as strong as other varieties. It is an attractive plant, with wide leaves forming an elongated head edged with a frilly ruffle. Chard cabbage, *bok toy,* looks like a cross between celery and swiss chard. It is a popular favorite in many Oriental dishes. Mustard cabbage, *gai choy,* is milder than mustard greens but has the same distinctive flavor. It consists of a clump of fat, apple-green stalks ending in a dark green leaf. This is the most nutritious variety and contains 165 grams of calcium and 3,100 units of Vitamin A in an average serving, compared with common cabbage with 43 grams of calcium and 150 units of Vitamin A.

Other Vegetables

Eggplant is one of the few vegetables eaten raw. When it is peeled, the skin is dried for future use. The meat of the eggplant is cubed and served as a side dish. It is often pickled or gently steamed. The high water content of eggplant makes it a good food to balance a heavy meal. It is a fine source of undigestible fiber, which makes it very filling and also good for the intestinal system. Chinese eggplant is long and thin.

White radish, *lok baak,* is shorter and more fibrous than the Japanese variety. It is very crisp and tender, mild and sweet, more like a turnip in flavor. It is used as a garnish and as a tasty addition to a salad. The leaves have a rather strong flavor and are eaten in small quantities.

Snow peas, or edible-podded peas, add color and texture to many Chinese dishes. They are crisp and delicately flavored. Because the pods have no parchment-like lining as regular peas do, they can be eaten pod and all. They are a good source of calcium, Vitamin B_1, iron, and Vitamins A and C.

Bamboo shoots are another vegetable that adds a crisp texture to dishes. They are often used in soups and in vegetable dishes. Fresh shoots must be peeled.

Water chestnuts are something like a narcissus bulb; they have a sweet, crisp flavor when fresh.

Broccoli is an extremely good food that is often overlooked in the United States. The flowers, stems, and leaves are an excellent source of Vitamins A and C, calcium, potassium, and iron. One cup contains 2 milligrams of iron (as compared to .2 milligrams in a cup of spinach), 190 milligrams of calcium, 5,100 units of Vitamin A and 105 units of Vitamin C.

Fruits

The Chinese use only small quantities of fresh fruit. A single piece of fruit may occasionally be served at the end of a meal, but more often it is eaten as a snack. Some of the fruits commonly eaten are oranges, tangerines, pineapples, dates, figs, apples, apricots, cherries, grapes, peaches, pears, persimmons, strawberries, plums, and loquats.

Melons

Melons similar to squash or gourds are a favorite vegetable and the Chinese grow many varieties. Bitter melon, *foo gwah,* about the size of a cucumber and a brilliant green, has a slightly bitter flavor and is often added to meat dishes or soups. Most people have to acquire a taste for it. Fuzzy melon, *mok gwah,* is a sweet-flavored oval shape with green fuzzy skin. It is often added to soups or quickly stir-fried. Most people like the taste after the first bite. Winter melon, *doong gwah,* looks like a large watermelon but the flesh is white and firm. Though it has a bland taste, it is used in the preparation of one of the most delicious dishes in Chinese cuisine, winter melon soup. It is usually the first course of an elaborate banquet and deserves all the praise it receives. The top of the melon is removed and some of the flesh is scooped out. A mild but flavorful stock made with pork, duck gizzards, mushrooms, lotus seeds, water chesnuts, bamboo shoots and other delicacies is then steamed inside the melon. As the soup is served, some of the melon is scraped from the sides and added to the bowl.

The high water content of these melons makes them a good balance to a heavy starch meal. They are very easy to digest and are fairly high in roughage, making them an excellent food for the elderly.

Melon rinds are pickled and combined with other vegetables or served as a garnish and the seeds of melons are dried, roasted, and eaten as snacks.

Fish

Fish, especially freshwater fish, is eaten frequently in China. When it is eaten raw, soy sauce and mustard are served as accompaniments. Onion or fresh ginger is added to cooked fish to reduce any heavy fish flavor. Over 100 varieties of fish are eaten and prepared in countless ways. Of the freshwater fish, carp and goldfish are the great favorites and most families have a fish pond where they raise carp. Older Chinese are devoted to salted fish and eat it at every meal. It is usually soaked, seasoned with fresh ginger root, and steamed on top of rice. Ocean fish are usually dried and later added to soups or eaten as crunchy snacks. Fish cakes are made by pounding fresh raw fish into a paste and combining it with ham, shrimp, and water chestnuts. The mixture is then shaped into balls and added to soups or stuffed into vegetables like peppers or mushrooms.

Meat

Pork is the principal meat consumed by the Chinese and it is used in small quantities in many dishes. It is added mainly for flavor or, when crisply fried, for texture. Most meals will include a pork dish. Pork contains more B vitamins than beef or lamb, and these B vitamins are important to the Chinese because their polished rice diet is low in them. Only a small amount of pork is needed to add enough protein to the meal. All parts of the hog are used in some manner, but the organs and entrails are more highly prized than the flesh. The skin is fried crisp, the fat is rendered, and the feet are pickled. When bony parts of an animal, such as pigs' feet, are pickled, a single serving may supply as much calcium as three quarts of milk. In northern China, pickled pigs' feet are traditionally served to pregnant women.

Seeds and Nuts

The Chinese are very fond of all sorts of seeds and nuts: melon seeds, sesame seeds, cashews, and many other varieties. They are a major snack food and find their way into some of the most elegant dishes in Chinese cooking. Slivered almonds are used to enhance vegetables. Like all nuts, they are an excellent source of B vitamins and unsaturated fat, and provide good amounts of iron, potassium, and incomplete proteins. Almonds contain three times more calcium than most other nuts and seeds. They can be pressed for their milk, which the Chinese often feed to babies. They are the only nut that contains Vitamin D. The protein quality in cashews is highest of all the nuts and their softer texture makes them easier to digest. Cashews are used for texture and flavor in many chicken dishes.

Lotus

The lotus is a type of water lily and one of the most versatile plants in China. The root, stems, and seeds are eaten. Gathering lotus is a messy job. Men must wade into a muddy swamp where the lotus grows and feel for the roots with their toes; then, still using their toes, they grasp the root and pull it up. Worth all the trouble, the lotus is an unusual vegetable, looking like a string of fat, brown link sausages when pulled from the mud. But after it is washed, peeled, and sliced crosswise, it is pure white and reveals a snowflake pattern. These slices are eaten raw or added to many dishes. The stems of the lotus are also eaten raw, or stuffed with vegetables and meat and then steamed. The leaves are used to wrap foods for steaming. The pod, a large flat circular bowl dotted with seeds, isn't eaten but the seeds are. When young, they are eaten like candy. As they mature, the seeds are steamed or dried and served as a sweet.

Fats

The Chinese use a variety of fats to cook their foods. Soy oil is the most common, but peanut oil is used in deep frying, and sesame seed oil and pork lard are used for flavoring.

Seaweed

Although many types of seaweed are eaten in China, the most popular variety is *kai choy kou*. It is sold in long strips in the markets and is quite gelatinous. It is used much like animal gelatines; that is, it is added to warm water or fruit juice and sweetened with honey or powdered dried fruit. When it cools, it becomes firm and is a popular snack or dessert. The seaweed contains a wide variety of trace minerals.

Spices and Herbs

All sorts of spices are used lavishly but carefully in Chinese cooking. From garlic and onion to ginger and peppers, every dish is enhanced with some sort of spicy flavoring. Ginger root is used raw or cooked. It is very hot but a small amount can work wonders with a simple dish. Ginger resembles a light brown iris root. It is also pickled or preserved and served as a garnish. Coriander—cilantro—resembles parsley and is also used frequently as a garnish. The Chinese are fond of blending spices to achieve unusual flavors. *Heung New Fun* is a blend of cloves, fennel, licorice root, cinnamon, and star anise and is called five-spice. This, and another called seven-spice, is used as a marinade for meats.

A white powder derived from dried, fermented wheat gluten has been made for centuries in many Chinese households to add flavor to their foods. "Taste powder" is now manufactured from hydrolized gluten. Called monosodium glutamate (MSG), it is liberally used in most Chinese cooking in the United States. It enhances the natural taste of various foods. However, many persons are allergic to MSG and suffer "Chinese Restaurant Syndrome." The symptoms include chest pains, flushing of the face, and headaches, all of which disappear when the food leaves the stomach.

Luxury Foods

Chinese use the eggs of duck, goose, pigeon, and chicken although they are not an important part of their diet. Eggs are often fried into thin, flat omelets and cut into strips to be used as a garnish. Occasionally, eggs will be added to fried rice. The most prized eggs are the so-called thousand-year-old eggs, which are actually about five months old. Duck eggs are encased in a paste of lime, salt, wood ashes, and black tea. At the end of five months, they have fermented into an amber-colored jelly-like white with a dark yellow, solid yolk. They are eaten raw and served with pickled onions and pickled ginger. Visitors do not usually enjoy thousand-year-old eggs.

The nest of a specific sea swallow is used in the famous bird's nest soup. The nests are made of a combination of tiny fish and saliva from the bird's salivary gland, which makes a sticky adhering substance. After they are gathered, at some risk because the nests are found high on rocky coastal cliffs, they are soaked and patiently picked over strand by strand. Any foreign material is discarded and the nests are then simmered in chicken broth. As they simmer, the nests flake apart and become practically transparent. Occasionally, the nests are made into a sweet dish, but the soup is the favorite. It is practically all protein and said to be potently nourishing.

Shark's fin soup is very complicated to prepare and is a great favorite at banquets. In old times it was considered an aphrodisiac. Shark is one of the few saltwater fish preferred to freshwater varieties by the Chinese.

The Chinese are fond of all poultry—duck, chicken, and squab—but they are considered luxuries and are usually eaten only at fairly elaborate feasts. Duck is the favorite by far and most farms have a flock of ducks.

DINING WITH A CHINESE FAMILY

In China, mealtime is taken seriously. Even an afternoon snack of tea and dot hearts is prepared and presented with elegance and a flourish. A coolie's simple meal is consumed with style. He may carry his bowl of rice and its bit of meat or fish to a spot that offers a lovely view or gather with friends and pretend they are enjoying a banquet.

But between the elaborate feasts of the prestigious and the simple fare of the peasant, the vast majority of Chinese enjoy their delightful food in a traditional and unchanging manner that follows ancient rules. Often all three meals are the same, consisting of boiled rice accompanied by several dishes.

In the kitchen, foods are chopped into bite-sized pieces with cleavers of various sizes and weights. Working so quickly their hands are practically a blur, cooks chop huge varieties of fresh vegetables for a particular dish. The principal cooking utensil is a *wok,* a circular metal pot with sloping sides and a round bottom. It sits on a ring to stabilize it. The wok comes in all sizes—from tiny ones six inches in diameter used to prepare some type of garnish or sauce to the huge two-footers for steaming rice and other foods. Steaming trays of loosely woven bamboo have flat bottoms and two- or three-inch sides. They stack on top of each other so several foods can be steamed in the same wok. The wok is an almost perfect pan; only a tiny amount of oil is enough to sauté foods. Because of its sloping sides, the foods all slide to the center, hottest part of the pan. To stir-fry the foods so everything cooks uniformly, a sort of kitchen ballet takes place. Rapidly moving hands and arms quickly agitate the food in the wok, and the stirring and tossing involves prancing fancy footwork by the cook. If, as is usually the case, several dishes are being prepared at the same time, the tempo increases to the point where an observer is overwhelmed by the disorganized mayhem and apparent insanity going on in the kitchen. All this frenzy is accompanied by shouted orders, calls for special ingredients, and voices raised in praise of a particular dish. Somehow, in spite of all the confusion, an elegant and delicious meal will be carried out to the diners.

The dining table is usually round, covered with a beautifully embroidered cloth, and arranged with a place setting for each diner. The setting consists of a bowl of rice, a boat-shaped ceramic spoon for soup. Rice, served at every meal, is considered the fruit of the sweat of your fellow man, and while leaving some food in the serving dishes is not frowned upon, to leave one grain of rice in your bowl is a serious offense.

The seating arrangements follow an unchanging precedent. The guest of honor sits facing the door, the most desirable spot, and the host sits near a corner of the room, the least desirable location. All the serving dishes of food are placed on the table in a circle. Placing them in rows of straight lines invites the spirits to dinner. Each diner takes some rice and "pushes it down" with a morsel from one of the dishes. It is considered quite proper to reach as far as you can for whatever food appeals to you. It is not necessary to excuse yourself, but if you want to be demure, you limit yourself to the dishes in front of you.

Bites of food are dipped into one of the several bowls of soy sauce on the table; soy sauce is never added to food at the table. The Chinese find the custom of putting several foods that have been cooked separately on the same serving dish absolutely barbaric. Dishes are made of wood or porcelain, and food is eaten with bamboo chopsticks. Chopsticks are used to convey food from the serving dish and the more fastidious use the clean ends. Hot soup, congee, or noodles are best when sucked in with as loud a noise as possible, while a belch at the end of a meal is a compliment to the host's fine food.

Soup is not served first. After the rice bowl has been emptied, it is filled with soup. Tea accompanies every meal and the Chinese enjoy a variety of herbed and scented teas. Weak tea is favored, and the best tea results when the leaves are steeped the second or third time.

Hot, scented towels are offered before and after the meal.

A CHINESE DINNER PER INDIVIDUAL

GUY GON TONG
chicken broth, ¾ cup
chicken liver, ½ ounce
chicken gizzard, 1 ounce
spinach and green onions,
   2 ounces

CHOW HAAK LOOK
shrimp, 1½ ounces
pineapple, ¼ slice
green pepper, ⅛
onion, ⅙ medium
carrot, ⅛ medium
oil, ¾ teaspoon
sesame seeds, ¾ teaspoon

CHICKEN ALMOND
chicken breast, 1 ounce
celery, ¼ cup
peas, ¼ cup
onions, ⅛ cup
mushrooms, 1 ounce
almonds, ⅛ cup
chicken broth, ¼ cup

BRAISED BROCCOLI
broccoli, 3½ ounces
onions, 2 ounces
oil, 2 teaspoons

BROWN RICE, 1¼ cups cooked

A CHINESE DINNER FROM YOUR KITCHEN

CHICKEN GIBLET SOUP
SWEET AND SOUR SHRIMP
CHICKEN ALMOND
BRAISED BROCCOLI
BOILED BROWN RICE

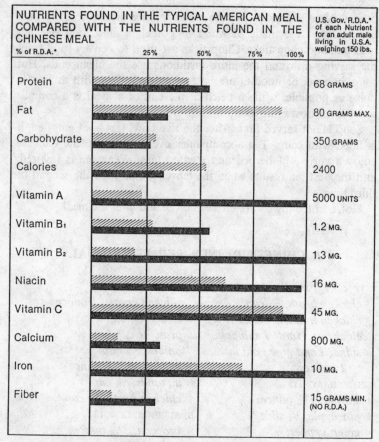

NUTRIENTS FOUND IN THE TYPICAL AMERICAN MEAL COMPARED WITH THE NUTRIENTS FOUND IN THE CHINESE MEAL					U.S. Gov. R.D.A.* of each Nutrient for an adult male living in U.S.A. weighing 150 lbs.
% of R.D.A.*	25%	50%	75%	100%	
Protein					68 GRAMS
Fat					80 GRAMS MAX.
Carbohydrate					350 GRAMS
Calories					2400
Vitamin A					5000 UNITS
Vitamin B₁					1.2 MG.
Vitamin B₂					1.3 MG.
Niacin					16 MG.
Vitamin C					45 MG.
Calcium					800 MG.
Iron					10 MG.
Fiber					15 GRAMS MIN. (NO R.D.A.)

*R.D.A. is the recommended daily nutrient allowance intended to meet the needs of a *healthy* individual.

Diagonal lines represent the American meal.

The chief sources of nutrients in the Chinese meal are:

PROTEIN	shrimp, chicken liver, chicken, and rice
FAT	peanut oil
CARBOHYDRATE	rice
CALORIES	rice
VITAMIN A	chicken liver and broccoli
VITAMIN B_1	rice
VITAMIN B_2	chicken liver
NIACIN	chicken liver, chicken, and rice
VITAMIN C	broccoli
CALCIUM	broccoli
IRON	chicken liver
FIBER	broccoli

HOW TO USE CHOPSTICKS

Learning to eat Oriental fashion takes Westerners a little time. By eliminating metal spoons and forks, you can enhance the flavor of these delightful cuisines and experience a bit more of the venerable cultures they reflect. The following directions should help you become adept with the wooden chopsticks and increase your enjoyment of Chinese and Japanese foods.

The lower chopstick is held firmly by the base of the thumb pressing the chopstick against the base of the index finger, while the underside of the end of the ring finger presses outward against the chopstick. The upper chopstick is flexible. It is held between the end or upper underside of the thumb, across the underside of the index finger down to the first knuckle and the side of the middle finger between the knuckles and the tip on the side nearest the thumb. The tip of the chopstick is opened and closed by pressure from either the index or middle finger, while the thumb tip acts as a pivot. Even bites of seafood and chicken can be separated when the opening and closing motions are done firmly enough.

Chicken Giblet Soup, "Guy Gon Tong"

> 2 chicken livers, each cut into 4 pieces
> 4 chicken hearts, cut in half
> 2 chicken gizzards, each cut into 4 pieces
> 3¼ cups chicken broth
> ½ package chopped frozen spinach or 6 ounces fresh spinach,
>   shredded
> 2 teaspoons chopped green onion bulbs; save tops for garnish
> 1 teaspoon soy sauce or to taste

Simmer gizzards, hearts, and chopped onion bulbs in 1¼ cups chicken broth until gizzards are tender, about 30 minutes. Add remaining chicken broth, spinach, liver, and soy sauce. Simmer only until liver loses its pink color. Serve with raw chopped onion greens floating on top in individual bowls. You may vary giblets with what you have available.

Sweet and Sour Shrimp, "Chow Haak Look"

> 4 ounces medium or large shrimp, cooked. If using large shrimp,
>   cut each shrimp in half lengthwise. You may substitute firm
>   hunks of any cooked fish or cooked pork.
> ½ medium green pepper, seeded and cut into 1-inch squares
> ¼ medium carrot, sliced diagonally into ⅛-inch slices
> ⅛ medium onion, cut into 1-inch chunks
> 1 slice of pineapple, cut into 16 pieces
> 1 tablespoon oil

Heat oil and stir-fry onion and carrot 1 minute. Add pepper and stir-fry vigorously 2 minutes or until vegetables are crisp and tender. Add shrimp, pineapple, and sauce (see below). Heat and serve garnished with toasted sesame seeds in a flat china serving dish.

Sauce for Sweet and Sour Shrimp

1 tablespoon ketchup   *1 teaspoon cornstarch*
1 tablespoon soy sauce   *¼ cup plus 2 tablespoons pineapple juice*
½ tablespoon vinegar   *½ small clove garlic, minced*
½ tablespoon honey

Mix ketchup, soy sauce, vinegar, garlic, and honey. Cook over low heat 3 minutes, stirring frequently. Mix cornstarch and 2 tablespoons pineapple juice. Add to sauce remaining pineapple juice and then cornstarch mixture. Stirring constantly, simmer 2 minutes or until sauce thickens slightly.

Chicken Almond

1 tablespoon vegetable oil
*½ pound chicken breasts (2 small or 1 large); remove bones and
   cut into narrow strips about ⅛ inch thick and 1 inch long*
2 tablespoons soy sauce
1 cup celery, cut diagonally into thin slices
1 cup peas
½ cup onion, chopped
¼ pound mushrooms
1 cup chicken broth
1 tablespoon cornstarch
2 tablespoons water
*½ cup toasted almonds (toast almonds in a 350° oven until lightly
   browned)*

Heat oil and stir-fry chicken pieces about 3 minutes or until chicken turns opaque. Add chicken broth, soy sauce, celery, peas, onions, and mushrooms. Cover and simmer 2 minutes. Mix cornstarch with water and add to mixture. Simmer uncovered, stirring until mixture thickens. Add salt or more soy sauce to taste. Fold in almonds. Serve in a bowl with low sides.

Braised Broccoli

1 pound broccoli, cut into 1-inch-long pieces
½ pound onions, cut into narrow strips
1½ tablespoons oil
2 tablespoons soy sauce
¼ cup boiling chicken broth

Heat oil in a skillet. Stir-fry onions and broccoli 4 minutes. Mix soy sauce and chicken broth. Pour over vegetables. Cover and cook over low heat 5 minutes, or just until broccoli is crisp and tender. Serve in a common serving bowl.

Boiled Brown Rice

The same as for the Japanese meal (page 221). Serve in individual bowls.

Peking Duck

1 domestic duck, about 6 pounds
2 scallions or onions, chopped
½ cup boiling chicken broth

Fasten neck of the duck with a skewer. Place scallions and broth in the duck cavity. Close opening with skewers. Rub duck with oil or unsalted melted butter. Place it, breast side up, on a rack in a shallow roasting pan. Roast in a 300° oven 30 minutes to the pound or until a meat thermometer inserted into the thigh muscle registers 185°. Forty-five minutes before duck is done, baste it with the following sauce:

2 tablespoons soy sauce
3 tablespoons honey
2 tablespoons pan drippings
1 teaspoon ground cinnamon

Mix all ingredients and heat sauce. Baste duck every 15 minutes for the remaining roasting time. In Peking the duck is sliced into very thin slices, each slice with some skin. The meat is dipped in a sauce and wrapped in a doily (like a wheat tortilla) or a lotus bun (recipe follows) with a thin slice of scallion and eaten like a sandwich. It is usually served with a big soup, made from the previous customer's duck bones, and celery cabbage. As few Chinese homes have ovens, Peking duck is a special restaurant meal.

Lotus Buns

 2 cups whole wheat flour
 ½ package of bakers' yeast
 ¾ cup lukewarm water
 Melted butter or vegetable oil

Dissolve yeast in water. Mix in the flour and knead to mix well. Divide dough into 8 pieces. Roll pieces into 3-inch circles with a rolling pin. Brush each piece with melted butter. Fold circles in half to form semi-circles. Score the tops of the buns with fork tines from the center of the straight side to form 3 equal arcs. The bun should look like half of a lotus leaf. Let rise for 45 minutes, then steam on a steaming tier for 15 minutes. Serve hot.

To improvise a steamer, support a rack such as a cake-cooling rack at least 2 inches above simmering water in a large kettle with a lid. You can rest the rack on a tin can that has had its ends removed. Place the buns directly on the rack. There must be at least 1½ inches from the top of the buns to the lid. To absorb moisture, put a cloth or dish towel over the top of the kettle before putting on the lid. The water should simmer just enough to produce steam but should not boil vigorously. Do not remove the lid while food is cooking.

Since the condiment sauces are very salty, no salt is used in making lotus buns. You may add ½ teaspoon of salt.

Condiment Sauces

Usually plum sauce and *hoisin* sauce (both available at specialty stores) are served or the following sauce can be used.

 4 tablespoons chopped onions   ½ cup soy sauce
 4 tablespoons chopped celery   2 teaspoons honey
 ½ teaspoon cinnamon   2 tablespoons sherry, beer,
 ½ teaspoon anise   or saké

Simmer 30 minutes. Strain sauce before serving.

Stir-Fry Liver

> *1 pound liver*
> *2 tablespoons soy sauce*
> *1 tablespoon sherry, beer, or saké*
> *½ teaspoon honey*
> *Dry bread crumbs*
> *⅓ cup chicken broth*
> *2 teaspoons cornstarch*
> *1 tablespoon water*
> *2 tablespoons butter, chicken fat, or oil*
> *1 scallion, thinly sliced, or 8 green onions, chopped*
> *⅓ pound snow peas (Chinese pea pods); break off tips and remove strings*
> *¼ cup toasted sesame seeds*

Cut liver into narrow strips. Toss in a sauce of soy sauce, wine or beer, and honey. Roll liver in bread crumbs. Allow coating to dry 5 minutes. Heat fat in a skillet; sauté the liver 2 minutes, stirring frequently. Add the scallions and snow peas; cook over low heat 3 more minutes or until the liver is light pink inside (pork liver must be cooked until no pink remains). Mix cornstarch and water. Add the remaining sauce used to coat the liver and chicken broth to the cooked liver. Stir in just enough of the cornstarch mixture to thicken the sauce slightly. Be sure to scrape any browned bits of bread or liver from the bottom of the pan.

Place liver and vegetables on a serving dish and sprinkle with sesame seeds.

Szechwan Bean Curd

> *2 pounds fresh bean curd (4 cakes), cut in ¾-inch slices*
> *2 tablespoons soy sauce*
> *4 cloves garlic, crushed*
> *2 slices ginger root*
> *1 scallion or onion, cut in ¾-inch pieces*
> *½ teaspoon honey*
> *½ teaspoon hot pepper sauce or cayenne pepper, to taste*
> *2 tablespoons peanut or vegetable oil*

Sauté garlic, ginger, and scallion in hot oil 2 minutes. Push to side of pan. Add bean curd and cook until lightly golden. Using a spatula, carefully turn bean curd to brown other side. Add soy sauce and honey, season with hot pepper sauce to taste, and serve immediately.

One pound of cooked meat, poultry, or seafood cut in pieces ¼ inch by 1 inch by 2 inches may be substituted for all or part of the bean curd. Garlic, ginger root, and hot pepper sauce may be omitted and 1 cup of peas may be substituted.

Congee

1 cup short grain brown rice
3 quarts water or thin stock

Bring water to a boil and add rice. Lower heat and simmer, uncovered, approximately 2 hours or until the rice is thoroughly broken up and mixture has the consistency of thin oatmeal. Stir occasionally to prevent congee from sticking to the pan and add more boiling water if necessary. When done, the congee should be thick and creamy. Add soy sauce to taste. Congee is served very hot either for breakfast or for a snack late at night. It is sipped from the bowl. Just before serving, bits of cooked meat, poultry, seafood, or vegetables can be added. For a nourishing breakfast, a beaten raw egg is stirred into each hot serving. Another favorite congee is made by putting thin slices of raw fish into the hot cereal. The heat from the congee cooks the fish. Chinese parsley and sliced ginger are favorite garnishes.

Pickled Pigs' Feet

4 pigs' feet
1½ cups vinegar
1 tablespoon whole cloves
4 bay leaves
¼ teaspoon ground cinnamon
1 clove garlic, chopped
¼ cup soy sauce
1 small onion, sliced

Scrub the feet and cover with ½ cup vinegar and boiling water. Simmer slowly until the meat begins to fall from the bones (about 3 hours). Place the pigs' feet in an earthenware or glass container. Remove fat from the broth and combine 3 cups with cloves, bay leaves, cinnamon, garlic, soy sauce, and onion. Add enough vinegar to the mixture to make it quite tart. Cover feet completely with the broth mixture. Cover lightly and refrigerate 3 to 5 days before serving. Be sure to serve the liquid with the feet as it is an excellent calcium source. Backbones, spareribs or small oxtails may be substituted for pigs' feet.

Cooked Noodles

You can buy whole grain noodles or make your own (recipe follows).

Drop 3½ cups of noodles (8 ounces) into 6 cups of boiling chicken, meat, or vegetable broth. Cover pan and simmer noodles until tender, 15 to 20 minutes. Toss cooked noodles and any remaining broth with ¼ cup soy sauce and 2 tablespoons sesame seed oil or butter. Add chopped green onions, toasted sesame seeds, pieces of cooked meat, fish, poultry, vegetables, legumes, or chopped hard-boiled eggs—any and everything but always onions. May be eaten piping hot or cold, with or without a small amount of broth.

To Make Noodles

    2 eggs plus 1 yolk, beaten
    1 teaspoon soy sauce
    ¼ cup milk or potato water
    2 cups any whole grain flour
    ½ cup sesame seeds, ground (powdered
        dry shrimp, dried vegetables or green
        tea are also used)

Combine eggs, soy sauce, milk, and sesame seed meal. Add enough flour to make a stiff dough. Place dough on a floured board, divide into half and roll each half very thin. Let stand 20 minutes. Roll up dough like a jelly roll and cut into strips of desired width. Open strips out and cut into desired lengths. Let dry 2 hours or more. Store in an airtight container in the refrigerator.

Almond Cookies

    2½ cups rice flour   1 cup butter
        (whole wheat flour   1 egg
        may be substituted)   2 tablespoons ice water
    1 teaspoon baking powder   40 whole almonds
    1 cup brown sugar
    2½ cups finely ground almonds

Mix dry ingredients well. Cut in butter and then work it in by hand. Add the egg and 1 tablespoon water. Knead the dough, adding more water only if needed. Form into small balls and place well apart on a greased cookie sheet. Press down slightly and put an almond in the center of each cookie. Bake in a 375° oven 5 minutes; lower heat to 325° and bake until cookies are golden brown, about 8 to 12 minutes.

ARHANT'S FAST OR VEGETARIAN'S TEN VARIETIES*

The Arhants are Buddhist Saints. Hence this dish is "food for the saints." Arhant's Fast consists of a number of specified vegetable ingredients, some of which are dried materials. There are, however, some local variations depending upon availability. In this dish, many of the ingredients have to be prepared separately before they are put together. Here are the separate and ensemble steps in the cooking.

A. Hair vegetable. This is a black hair-like seaweed. Get about 40 cents' worth in Chinatown. Soak in hot water for ½ hour, rinse several times to get rid of all the sand. Pull it apart into small groups (this step is optional).

B. Dried tiger lilies. Get ⅙ pound in Chinatown. Soak in hot water ½ hour and rinse clean.

C. Peastarch noodles. These are a kind of transparent noodles, made of the starch of a kind of tiny green peas, the same kind from which pea sprouts are raised. They are very common in China and can be got in Chinatown. Put ¼ pound in a pot full of boiling water and cook over low fire for ½ hour. Then turn off fire and let it stand and cool off.

D. *Ginkgo* or *paak-kwo* in Cantonese. Get ⅙ pound in Chinatown. When bought, they have white, hard shells outside. Crack shells with nutcracker. Soak nuts in a big bowl of hot water and peel off inner skin.

E. Mushrooms. Get ¼ pound. Properly you should use dried mushrooms, which are more savory than fresh ones. . . . Cut vertically into thin slices. It is possible to dry fresh mushrooms and later soak them, but that takes days.

F. Gluten of flour, or skin of bean curd. Get ⅙ pound, both from Chinatown. If you get gluten of flour, cut it into pieces of 1 cubic

* Buwei Yang Chao, *How to Cook and Eat in Chinese* (New York: Vintage Books, 1972). By permission of the publisher.

inch. If you get bean curd skin, put it in a pot of boiling water and keep boiling for ½ hour. Then cut into 1½-inch wide strips.

G. Chinese cabbage; 3 pounds. Either Chinese green cabbage or celery cabbage (which you cut into pieces about 2 inches long).

H. 1 package of frozen peas. Thaw them out.

I. ½ can winter bamboo shoots. Cut into slices of about 1 square inch.

J. Fried puffy bean curd; 6 pieces (or 12 pieces if small). Get in Chinatown. The best is to get them ready-fried, but if you cannot, get 1 pint fresh bean curd and cut each into 4 pieces and fry it in deep vegetable oil until it is brown.

Cooking material:

4 teaspoons vegetable oil   2 teaspoons taste powder
2 teaspoons salt   2 cups water
½ cup soy sauce

Direction for ensembles:

Heat the vegetable oil in a pot (not necessarily heavy, but big), put the cabbage in first (item g) and stir for 1 minute. Then add in everything from (a) to (j); then also add in the soy sauce, salt, taste powder, and water. Boil together for 20 minutes.

This can be a main dish on meatless days. It looks rather complicated, but as you practically get everything in Chinatown, you need make only one trip to shop for these things. When you give the salesman the list, he will immediately know what you are making and may give you some suggestions and tell you why his combination is certainly better than mine.

If you cannot get some of the items from this list, you can add in something of your own, such as chestnuts, string beans, carrots, etc. Sometimes we do not use so many things. As few as four or five kinds are sometimes used and the dish is still called Vegetarian's Ten Varieties. But better have things nearly right to taste nearly right.

A beauty of this dish is that it can be kept as long as one week without losing flavor.

THE LIGHT BITE, CHINESE STYLE

A QUICK MEAL: Noodles with about a cup of broth, chopped green onions, sesame seeds, and pieces of cooked fish, poultry, meat, bean curd, or eggs. Complete the meal with a wedge of cabbage, an apple, or other fruit. Noodles will keep warm very well in a thermos bottle or can be eaten at room temperature.

A SNACK: Roasted soybeans. To prepare soybeans, soak a cup of dry soybeans in 1½ cups of water in an ice cube tray for 2 hours, then freeze overnight. The next day drop them into ½ cup hot, salted water and simmer for 30 minutes or until they are as tender as peanuts. Drain the soybeans and dry them on paper towels. Spread on a shallow pan and roast in a 350° oven 30 minutes, or until they are brown. Stir several times so that they will brown evenly. Toss in melted butter or vegetable oil, if desired, and salt to taste. The Chinese fry the soaked soybeans a few at a time in 350° deep fat. The beans are then drained on absorbent paper and sprinkled with salt while still warm.

Soy nuts are eaten like nuts, or they can be ground and used in place of nuts in many recipes. When added to cereal, they boost its protein quality as well as adding a good flavor.

Japan, A Land
of Harmony

The unique dichotomy of Japan is difficult for visitors to understand. Ancient traditions and urgent progress live side by side. A shop selling computers is next to one featuring hand-painted fans. This strange double life, however, doesn't confuse the Japanese, who take it remarkably in stride.

An attractive young Japanese woman in a smart pants suit leaves her office in Tokyo, scrambles aboard a crowded subway and heads for her home in the suburbs. Once there, she changes into a lovely, soft silk kimono and begins to fix dinner. As sophisticated, modern, and well-educated as anyone in the world, once she slides the *shoji* screens of her home shut, her world slips back hundreds of years to an age of *shoguns* and *samurai*. The meal she serves her family is the same as that eaten by generations of Japanese and it will be presented with the same care. Even the room where it is eaten looks like an ancient Japanese print—low tables and *tatami* mats, soft cushions to kneel on—and dominating the room, its only ornaments, a delicate painting and a vase containing a single flower. In fact, the only distinction between this room and its counterpart of 300 years ago is the color television in the corner. The Japanese are avid TV viewers, yet the traditional Kabuki Theater performances are always sellouts. Young Japanese ride motorcycles, march in protest, and go to rock concerts, but they marry the person their parents select. In Japan the divorce rate of arranged marriages is half that of the love marriages. Common backgrounds and a clear understanding of each partner's role in marriage contribute to the stability of family life. From supermarkets to factories, nearly everything in Japan is automated, but in the countryside women still plant rice by hand, standing knee-deep in mud. Japanese honor and live by their past while surging headlong into the future.

Smaller than California, with a population of over 100 million, the Japanese archipelago stretches roughly across the same latitude as our Maine-to-Florida coast, and the weather is similar also, with the ski areas in northern Hokkaido, and beach resorts and hot springs in southern Honshu. The problems of feeding this huge population are enormous. Only about 17 percent of the land can be farmed because of the mountainous terrain, yet the need for food continues to increase. Hillsides are terraced and farmed, every suburban home features a tiny vegetable garden, and ever-increasing quantities of food are being imported.

With at best only a tenuous hold on their trembling land, the Japanese have made living in harmony with nature a religion. They revere the beauty of their mountains. The changing seasons are subjects of poetry and song. In a country beset by some of the worst industrial pollution in the world, depersonalization in overcrowded cities, and the frantic competition to succeed, the Japanese could not survive without beauty and harmony. They need it, they seek it out, they honor it. Their food reflects this feeling for they would never dream of eating something out of season. Although they wait impatiently for the first bamboo shoots of spring, for only then will they be served, it would never occur to them to freeze or can them to make them available all year round. The shoots represent an important aspect of the new season, something to anticipate with pleasure.

Their delight in the changing of the seasons is understandable. In spring Japan becomes a fairyland, and each of the other seasons brings its particular beauty to the land. The breathtaking loveliness of their island home is a source of constant pleasure to the Japanese all through the year, and groups of hikers can be seen everywhere enjoying a day in the mountains or picking their way along a rocky beach. Their love of music is prodigious and their taste uninhibited. From rock and country Western, to jazz, to symphonic, to the atonal sounds of the *samisen*, music surrounds the Japanese.

This unique mix of old and new, the bewildering combination of modern technology and ancient custom, is delicately balanced, a balance maintained by enduring family traditions that have never changed and probably never will. Nowhere is this more apparent than in the Japanese eating habits.

In preparing a meal, the people of Japan place great emphasis on its appearance. Artfully cut vegetables are arranged to create a picture. Color and texture are carefully studied to produce just the right effect—a cloud over a mountain, tiny fish swimming in a rocky pool—all "drawn" with crisp, fresh vegetables and finely sliced pieces of fish. To a Japanese family, appreciation of a meal starts with how it looks. The woman of the house graciously accepts compliments on her attractive creation and only then is the first bite taken. The food is served in small dishes of china or lacquer (metal is never used), and the dishes are selected to complement the food they will hold. Wooden chopsticks are used because wood is organically closest to food. The meal, served on individual lacquer trays, will consist of a clear soup, a bowl of rice, fish prepared any one of a number of ways, fresh and pickled vegetables. Although this is the basic pattern, variations produce meals of exquisite flavor and beauty.

Because of their limited land resources, it was to the sea that the Japanese turned for food and it has been bountiful. The waters around Japan are the richest on earth. As a result fish is served at every meal, as a soup, in delicately fried tempura, cooked whole and beautifully garnished, served raw as *shashimi*, dried, salted, sautéed, hot or cold. The variety of ways to serve the fish is second only to the variety served. Octopus, eel, tiny minnows, huge swordfish, shellfish and mollusks of all sorts, reef fish, deep sea fish (the Japanese fishermen are among the most determined and courageous in all the world), tuna, shark, anything that lives in the sea finds its way to the table and that includes seaweed.

Rice, eaten at every meal, is lacking in many nutrients, especially if it is polished. But in combination with seafood, it becomes a major source of protein, making an extremely nutritious meal. Unpolished rice is gaining popularity among nutrition-conscious Japanese and the rice-fish meal is even more wholesome as a result. Dr. Sanford Siegal in his new book, *Dr. Siegal's Natural Fiber Permanent Weight Loss Diet* (Dial Press, 1975), tells how prisoners of war in Japan, men who lived under incredible stress, were fed a diet of rice and rice polishings, the high-fiber bran that the Japanese ordinarily feed to farm animals. In camps where prisoners were fed this bran, none of them developed ulcers. In the camps where the rice bran was discontinued, duodenal ulcers became rampant. The nutritional value of the rice bran combined with its high-fiber content make it an important food.

Iodine, found in all seafood, is mysterious, elusive, and essential for health. Lately it has been the object of increasing attention from doctors and scientists. It has long been known that sufficient iodine prevents goiter, but recent studies have shown that iodine is one of those elements absolutely essential to humans. In the *National Health Federation Bulletin,* Dr. Emory Thurston states that a deficiency in iodine may be the cause of low resistance to infection, a tendency to obesity, loss of tone in the circulatory system, and poor or faulty development of the reproductive organs. He further states that inorganic iodine, the sort found in iodized salt, is no substitute for the real thing, the iodine found in all seafood. The body retains this natural element longer than the synthetic, and only organic iodine can function as a catalyst for stabilizing calcium metabolism. With their enormous intake of seafood, the Japanese probably ingest over 100 milligrams of iodine daily, far in excess of the recommended daily amount, but their marvelous health is the best testimonial to the importance of this essential element. Their mortality rate from degenerative heart disease is the lowest of seventeen industrial countries surveyed; approximately 51.8 per 100,000 compared with the United States rate of 312.9. Breast cancer is rare in Japan and recent studies have shown that breast tissue deprived of sufficient iodine is more susceptible to cancer. Obesity is virtually unknown—try to picture a fat Japanese. Except for the huge *sumo* wrestlers, who may weigh up to 300 pounds, Japanese are uniformly slim and wiry, for which credit can go to their fish, rice, and vegetable diet.

The Japanese appreciation of the harmony of life is most evident in their gentle way with vegetables. The markets offer a stunning array to choose from: mushrooms, huge white radishes, cucumbers, an incredible variety of greens, carrots, beans, eggplants, all carefully grown and picked just at the peak of ripeness. The word "cooking" does little justice to the Japanese manner of preparing food. A Japanese meal reflects the very essence of these cultivated people, their love for disciplined beauty and their appreciation of all forms of artistry; the way they cook their vegetables is almost an art form in itself. Cut into bite-sized pieces, they are stir-fried in sesame seed or peanut oil until barely heated through.

For the clear soup of Japan, they are added raw. In making tempura, each piece is dipped into a rice flour batter as light and gauzy as silk and quickly deep-fried. The batter turns golden brown but the vegetable is scarcely cooked. Each food retains its color, flavor, and texture and, most important, its food value. These crisp, delectable vegetables are a perfect complement to the bland bean curd called *tofu,* served with most meals.

Soybeans, the source of tofu, have long been a major food of the Japanese. They can be picked immature and cooked in the pod or shelled and cooked. Mashed and fermented, they make the tofu; and they are also pressed for their juice and fermented to make soy sauce. Soybeans, rice, and fish are the main protein foods of the Japanese. Traditionally, very little beef was eaten because the Japanese, along with many other cultures, found cattle ate more food than they produced. With their limited land resources, food grown for human consumption took priority. In Kobe, beef of a very special sort is raised, however. The animals are kept in pens adjacent to the home and fed fermented mash; they are massaged daily and rarely does any family raise more than one or two at a time. Kobe beef is considered the best in the world but it is incredibly expensive, as much as thirty dollars per pound. For very special occasions, a Japanese woman may buy several paper-thin slices of Kobe beef and prepare an elegant *sukiyaki* right at the table.

Eating habits have changed to some extent since the war, especially in the major cities. Inevitably, American meat-eating ways influenced the Japanese and they are now the major importer of American beef. In urban areas, where foreign influences are most quickly felt, affluent Japanese now serve beef quite often. This, along with a generally higher standard of living, has led to an interesting phenomenon. Today's young Japanese are six to ten inches taller than their grandparents. There is some debate as to whether increased stature is desirable in the Japanese but the fact remains that the young people tower over their elders. While this change is most noticeable in Oriental families, children the world over are growing taller. In addition, they are reaching sexual maturity with a rapidity previously unknown throughout the history of man. Dr. Hugh Trowell of England, who has devoted many years to the study of nutrition and health, feels that this alarming trend of early sexual maturity is due to the large amounts of protein that babies receive from cow's milk and the processed foods that are part of the infant diet.

The work ethic and vitality of the Japanese are formidable. EVERYONE works. Only the very old, who have already spent many years laboring in field or factory, can devote their time to pleasure and relaxation. Even then they are expected to act as guardians of the young, and advisor and referee for the rest of the family. In rural areas the wife and daughters work in the fields while the husband and sons fish. Urban women have jobs outside the home. Because of the long school day, children often get home after their parents, so they rarely have time for an outside job. With few exceptions, the very young and the very old, work is their life and the energy and stamina of the Japanese are legendary. Centuries ago Chinese visitors remarked on the health and vitality of the Japanese. They were especially impressed by the fact that Japanese lived so long; persons over 100 years old were fairly common. Even today they have few of the degenerative diseases of other industrialized countries. Both atherosclerosis and diabetes are rare. There is little arthritis and few disorders of the nervous system. An increase of colon cancer seems to be evident in areas where meat-eating is on the increase, but it still ranks low as a cause of death. The largest mortality figures are from high blood pressure related to their enormous intake of salt. In the north, where salted fish is a big part of the diet, high blood pressure is a problem and accounts for the most deaths. The most serious defect in the generally excellent health of the Japanese seems to be poor eyesight. Nutritionists believe this is a result of their low-fat diet. To metabolize Vitamin A, a certain amount of fat is needed. The average Japanese diet generally contains plenty of Vitamin A, but not enough of the fat necessary to utilize it. At any rate, the general health of the Japanese ranks second to none among the industrialized countries. Credit for this goes to their sensible eating habits certainly, but a closer look reveals something else of great importance.

The quality of the food they eat is extraordinarily high. Japan is the most efficient food producer in the world. They not only feed more people now than they did a decade ago, they feed them better. This is possible because of the type of fertilizer used. For centuries Japanese farmers have fed their fields with human excrement, the humble and much-maligned "night soil." Now Japanese scientists have found a way to convert this all-too-available product into a sterile and odor-free fertilizer that produces more, better quality, and faster growing crops than those produced by chemical fertilizers. Healthy, vigorous plants are more resistant to disease and insects so pesticides are rarely used, and in many cases they are banned. The high nutritional quality of vegetables grown in organically fed soil cannot be discounted as a major factor in the enviable health of the Japanese. For many centuries the Japanese have continuously cultivated their land with no apparent soil exhaustion, in contrast to the United States, where thousands of acres have been depleted in the last 200 years. At one time chemical fertilizers were tried in Japan in an effort to increase per acre tonnage, but the cost in terms of depleted soil ruled out extensive use of these products. The Japanese government has now banned their use.

Of course, not all is tofu and shashimi. Fried chicken has arrived along with colas and hamburgers. The major cities feature Western fast food shops alongside the Japanese version, tempura stands. Actually, tempura is faster to prepare than a hamburger. Patrons at a tempura stand sit or stand at a counter while the cook keeps presenting them with deep-fried morsels of fish and vegetables. But the novelty of fried chicken is overpowering to the inquisitive Japanese. Cola drinks, packaged cereals, along with candies and cookies with little or no nutritional value are claiming increasing amounts of the family food yen and the young people outdo themselves to follow Western ways. As a result, tooth decay in Tokyo is about the same as in the United States, intolerably high, while in the rural areas it ranges from 50 percent to zero.

For centuries Japanese farmers have gathered the seaweed swept onto their beaches to use as a compost for enriching the soil. As a fertilizer it is unparalleled. It contains no seeds or spores to compete with the growing plant, deteriorates rapidly, and is free. Then, sometime in the sixteenth century, the Chinese, who seem to have invented everything, introduced the Japanese to seaweed as a food. From that time on, seaweed in one form or another has become a staple in every Japanese home. It is eaten dried, fresh, or pickled with nearly every meal. The six varieties of seaweed eaten by the Japanese make up about 10 percent of their diet and are served in dozens of ways. A leaf of dried seaweed is softened and laid out flat. Very thin slices of sea bass are placed on the leaf, which is then tightly rolled and sliced into one-inch pieces. Seaweed is an ingredient in *sukiyaki; yosenabi,* a delicious seafood and vegetable dish; *shabu shabu,* a beef and vegetable dish; *sumashi,* a bean curd and shrimp soup. It is eaten just about as often as we eat lettuce. The Japanese version of a sandwich is cooked rice balls stuffed with fish and vegetables and wrapped in a seaweed leaf. They make a delectable seaweed soup and dried shredded seaweed is added to many dishes. It is surprising that seaweed has not achieved the same popularity throughout the rest of the world. However, it seems to be rather hard for Westerners to digest. Presumably, the Japanese have developed an intestinal flora capable of digesting the seaweed carbohydrates.

Because it has no root system (seaweed attaches itself to rocks), the leaves of the plant contain all the nutrients and minerals of seawater, which means it has them in about the same ratio as do the internal fluids of mammals. Seawater has even been used successfully as a substitute for whole blood in emergency transfusions at sea. In addition, seaweed contains over forty trace elements, Vitamins A, B, and C, and some varieties even contain a fair amount of protein. Contrary to popular belief, it does not have a huge sodium content. Commercially processed seaweed is used extensively in the United States as a suspension for pharmaceuticals, and a stabilizer for dairy products, cosmetics, toothpaste, and bakery products. It also has many industrial applications, but it never appears in its natural form on our table. As it is extremely rich in iodine as well as other nutrients, people who eat large quantities of seaweed have been found to have fewer teeth and gum problems and less susceptibility to colds; and they are also generally more free from arthritis and breast cancer.

For centuries kelp, algae, Irish moss, and all varieties of sea plants have been used for medicinal purposes. Agar, a derivative of seaweed, is an excellent colloidal and is found in many remedies for stomach disorders, constipation, respiratory problems, and as a protection for wounds. Seaweed is the major source of iodine and has a far higher concentration than seafood. In areas where fresh seafood is unavailable, many nutritionists believe kelp in tablet or powder form should be taken daily. About .15 milligrams is recommended. However, in areas that are subject to radiation fallout, Dr. K. M. Saxena, reporting in *Science,* felt that daily doses of up to 2 milligrams offered protection from strontium poisoning.

The late Professor Cavanaugh of Cornell University did a survey of the effects of kelp on the healing of fractures. He analyzed the calcium, phosphorus, iron, and iodine in the blood of patients with fractures at different intervals during convalescence. He found that when daily doses of kelp were added to the patients' diets, the level of calcium in their blood was raised and healing time of fractures was reduced by 20 percent.

Iodine found in the thyroid gland serves as an aid to burning up excess fuel in the body. If the fuel (food) isn't used in energy, it is stored in the form of fat. An efficiently functioning thyroid, one that has sufficient iodine, burns up the excess and helps avoid obesity. Drinking chlorinated water (and what water isn't chlorinated today?) leaches iodine from the system, so supplemental kelp tablets help maintain the iodine level so necessary for good health.

Few industrialized nations have been able to retain their ancient culture to the extent that Japan has. Strong and viable, the family unit has clung to old traditions in this rapidly changing country. Even in the most modern Japanese home, furnished in European style, one room will still feature tatami mats, low tables, and sliding walls. Lovely and serene, a traditional Japanese home impresses Caucasians with its simplicity. Soft cushions on the floor, the complete absence of clutter in both design and interior, ease the mind and calm the spirit. Homes of the wealthy are beautifully hand-crafted creations, but even a humble farmer's home has a graceful form. In the kitchen, just about the only difference between an urban and rural home is the number of electrical appliances. The charcoal *hibachi* is now electric, as is the deep-fryer. Few kitchens feature an oven because the Japanese rarely bake their food.

To the Japanese, bathing is almost as important as eating. Scrupulously clean, they bathe daily and in ancient times while water was plentiful, the fuel to heat it was not, so—practically enough—communal baths became a national custom. The procedure for a Japanese bath is quite sensible; in fact, it seems preferable to ours. Prior to entering the bath, a large pool of heated and scented water, everyone washes thoroughly with soap and rinses completely. It would be unthinkable either to wash in the bath or enter it dirty. No one feels any embarrassment about nude communal bathing, but it is considered extremely rude to stare at other bathers. The Japanese are not breast conscious; in fact, they feel the feet are the most appealing part of the feminine form. The entire family bathes together and they enjoy the opportunity to greet friends and neighbors, to visit and gossip while soaking together in the warm water. Instead of viewing it simply as a necessity, the Japanese have made bathing a relaxing social event.

The Japanese have been able to maintain their equilibrium in their headlong pursuit of material wealth. Law enforcement agencies throughout the world have marveled at the low crime rate in Japan. Does the strong family unit account for this, or the Japanese work ethic that makes idleness almost a sin? Or is their well-balanced diet that keeps them so healthy the reason for this enviable record? Whatever the answer, Japan has the highest literacy rate in the world, the lowest crime rate, and the best health of any industrialized nation. The other side of the coin is the appalling increase of pollution and contamination that seems to go hand-in-hand with rapid technological development.

Located on Kyushu Island, the fishing village on Minimatu Bay hugged the shore of one of the most beautiful harbors in Japan. This tiny, almost land-locked bay, surrounded by towering hills, protected the fleet that fished the local waters daily. On the far side of the bay, nearly hidden from view, was the Chisso Chemical plant that produced vinyl chloride used in the manufacture of plastics. Mercury-laden waste from the plant poured into Minimatu Bay in huge quantities and about ten years ago a strange phenomenon began to occur. The local cats started going crazy and then died. Soon these same ghastly symptoms began to affect the villagers. First there were severe emotional changes. These usually calm, serene people began to show signs of extreme anxiety. This was followed by loss of memory, impaired vision, ulceration of the gums, crippling of the limbs and, finally, death. Japanese scientists launched a thorough investigation of Minimatu Bay and its unhappy inhabitants and quickly discovered that the fish eaten by the villagers were so loaded with mercury that they were actually poisonous. By this time nearly 200 people had died, and many more were crippled for life. Further checking showed that 194 plants in Japan were dumping mercury into bays and streams. At the urging of a newly formed citizens' group called the Public Hazards Countermeasure Council, mercury dumping was banned all over Japan and the victims of Minimatu Bay were paid a huge compensation.

Life, however, is over for the village. The level of mercury saturation is so great that plans are being discussed to fill in the entire bay, bury it and its poisonous fish under tons of rock and dirt. The Japanese, who have so successfully avoided the terrible degenerative diseases of other industrialized nations by adhering to their traditional and healthy diet, find themselves victims of that very progress they so desire. Solutions are being sought, laws are being passed, and it is hoped they will be effective.

FOODS OF THE JAPANESE

Almost as important as the foods the Japanese eat is their manner of preparing them. When a food must be cooked, it is cooked just long enough to make it safe while still retaining the qualities of raw food. Cooking utensils consist of the *wok* for stir-frying; the griddle for sautéing; the hibachi, often used right at table to charcoal broil; and the deep-fryer. Steamers are also used, mainly for cooking breads, custards and, occasionally, rice. Ovens are not popular and are rarely used. Unlike the Chinese, the Japanese usually cook the foods individually and serve them separately.

Grains

Rice is the mainstay of the Japanese diet, and is generally served boiled at all three meals. Formerly, nothing but polished rice was considered edible in the homes of the wealthy, but brown rice is becoming increasingly popular as the Japanese learn more about good nutrition.

CHIEF SOURCES OF NUTRIENTS
IN THE JAPANESE DIET

PROTEIN	seafood
FAT	peanut and sesame oil
CARBOHYDRATE	rice
CALORIES	rice
VITAMIN A	greens
VITAMIN C	greens
VITAMIN B_1	rice
VITAMIN B_2	seafood
NIACIN	seafood
CALCIUM	greens
IRON	greens
FIBER	rice and vegetables

Sushi, a popular Japanese snack, is made of cold vinegared rice and various ingredients such as cucumber, dried gourd shavings, fried egg, octopus, or shrimp rolled up in a sheet of seaweed and cut into small pieces. Though the Japanese are primarily a rice-eating people, they occasionally serve other grains. Whole barley is steamed and served in place of rice. Barley is a good source of the B vitamins when its bran coating is not removed. For centuries the Japanese have favored a thin noodle made of buckwheat and a wider one made from wheat. They are always served steaming hot in a broth of bonito and soy sauce. Bowls of steaming noodles are a popular snack for office workers.

The green soybean is picked and steamed, pod and all, before the beans are shelled, or the beans may be shelled first and steamed. Served with rice, the combination contains a good ratio of most nutrients. Soybeans are rich in protein and are a good source of the B vitamins lacking in polished rice. *Miso,* a fermented bean paste, is often combined with fish, vegetables, or tofu, and is made by grinding cooked yellow soybeans with fermented rice and salt. The mixture is then stored in wooden vats and served at least once a day. Tofu is made in the same way the Chinese make bean curd. This method of making tofu increases its calcium content so that it becomes a major source of calcium in the Japanese diet. It is served in countless ways: cut up in soup, combined with vegetables, deep-fat fried, or stuffed with fish or vegetables for a popular picnic item. Another byproduct of soybeans is *shoyu,* the Japanese-style soy sauce. It is made by adding toasted wheat to soybeans and fermenting them together. It is slightly sweeter than Chinese soy sauce and is used as a seasoning for Japanese foods. Beans and fish are often simmered in it.

Sweetened paste is made from mashed black beans, limas, or red beans combined with dried persimmons, honey, or sugar. They are eaten as little cakes.

Vegetables

Popular favorites among the vegetables include bamboo shoots, cucumber, *daikon,* eggplant, several varieties of cabbage, carrots, celery, spinach, edible podded peas, long beans, lotus root, mushrooms, sweet potatoes, white-flowered gourds, and yams. Eggplant, carrots, cucumbers, and daikon are the only vegetables the Japanese consider safe to eat raw.

Daikon is a huge white radish. It is shredded and used as a bed for other foods.

Mushrooms find their way into many Japanese dishes. Several varieties are grown and used dried or fresh. The favorite is the straw mushroom called *nameko,* a tiny, slippery variety. When cooked it makes a jelly-like liquid that is used to thicken soups. Mushrooms are a source of protein and Vitamins D and B. Raw, they also contain important enzymes and are easily digested. Their protein is of as high a quality as meat, with four large mushrooms supplying three grams of protein.

The high water content of eggplant makes it a good food to balance a starchy meal. It is high in fiber and low in calories. Eggplant can be "cooked" by marinating it in soy sauce or lemon juice. Raw, marinated eggplant cubes are a delicious snack. Eggplant is a good source of Vitamin B_1, the vitamin essential for the digestion of starch. B_1 is removed from rice when it is polished.

Pickled vegetables or fruits are served with nearly every meal; they are made by packing the fresh produce in salt brine, sake mash, or mustard. These pickles include cucumbers, celery cabbage, daikon, eggplant, melons, greens, plums, and turnips. The minerals in pickled foods are easier for the body to assimilate and they aid in the digestion of other foods.

Seaweed

Seaweed is often used for seasoning; it is also very nutritious even in small amounts. It is the richest source of trace minerals known. Occasionally the Japanese eat seaweed fresh as we eat lettuce, but it is usually dried. The Japanese tie fresh seaweed into interesting shapes and simmer them in their soups. Dried seaweed is ground and sprinkled on food like salt or pepper. Several varieties of seaweed are used by the Japanese. Among them are:

Kombu, a tough, gray, dried tangle. It is an essential ingredient in *dashi,* a broth basic to many dishes.

Nori, this dark brown, broad-leafed seaweed is dried, then soaked in water when needed. It is used as a wrapping for rice rolls and, when toasted, make a delicious garnish for many dishes.

Wakame, used as a complement to cucumbers and miso, is tender like raw spinach and the best-tasting seaweed. It is generally served with vinegar or in soup.

Kanten is the pectin of Japan. It congeals at room temperature and the resulting gelatin is used in making desserts and bean jellies.

Meat

Beef is the most popular meat in Japan although it is served only occasionally. A favorite dish, of peasant origin, is *sukiyaki.* Paper-thin strips of beef are cooked on a very hot griddle, right at the table. Then various chopped vegetables are quickly added and stir-fried, one at a time. Soy sauce is added so the vegetables simmer just a bit. The smell of sukiyaki cooking is almost irresistible. It is said the dish originated with farmers who used to cook their food out in the field, using the metal part of the plow as a griddle. *Suki* means plow and *yaki* means broiled.

Poultry

Chicken is the favorite variety of poultry in Japan. It may be cooked and added to custards or cut in small pieces and barbecued. It is not, however, a widely used meat.

Eggs

Fresh eggs may be poached in soup stock occasionally, but most frequently eggs are beaten and fried into a flat omelet. This will then be cut into interesting shapes and used as a garnish. A popular dish, made of soup stock and eggs, is steamed to make a custard and served as a main dish.

Spices

Spices are used sparingly, as most foods are seasoned with shoyu (soy sauce). Some foods are grated and dried and used as a spice. These include parsley, citrus peel, daikon, and some varieties of seaweed.

Oil

Sesame and peanut oil are those most frequently used in cooking. Both oils are excellent sources of the essential fatty acids found in unsaturated fat. Sesame is the most stable of the oils and adds a good flavor to all foods. Cut vegetables are coated with oil as they are stir-fried. This prevents oxygen from destroying some of their vitamins. Except for stir-frying little oil is used by the Japanese.

Nuts and Seeds

Walnuts, chestnuts, and hazel nuts are popular in Japan but by far the most widely used is the sesame seed. In a diet that is mainly grains, sesame seeds are an important mineral, fat, and protein source. Sesame seeds are the only seeds that complement grains. When they are eaten with rice their total usable protein increases by 21 percent. Toasted whole, they are sprinkled on various dishes as a garnish, and they are added to many foods to improve the flavor. Sesame seeds are a storehouse of iron, B vitamins, and essential fatty acids; and they are the only seed to contain a large amount of calcium. It is important, however, to eat the seeds that are brown in color. The white seeds have had the skins removed and most of the nutrients are gone. For anyone who is apt to have a calcium deficiency due to lack of milk, sesame seeds may be the answer. They can be liquefied and used in place of milk.

Following is a nutritional comparison of whole milk and sesame seeds:

	Protein (grams)	Calories	B_1 (mg.)	B_2 (mg.)	Niacin (mg.)	Calcium (mg.)	Iron (mg.)	Unsaturated Fatty Acid (grams)	Total Fat Grams
¼ cup sesame seeds	4.5	140	.2	.05	1.35	290	2.6	5.5	12
1 cup whole milk	8	165	.08	.43	.2	285	.1	1	10

Fruits

Fruits are generally eaten raw by the Japanese. Sometimes they are served at the end of the meal but usually they are eaten as a snack. Fruit is an important part of the diet, as most kinds are a good source of Vitamins A and C as well as iron. They provide roughage and their sugar content makes them a quick energy booster. Oranges are of course known for their high Vitamin C content and when the Japanese eat the peeled fruit, including the white membrane, they obtain a considerable quantity of bioflavonoids, "Vitamin C's co-worker." Fruits commonly eaten by the Japanese include oranges, oriental pears, mandarin oranges, white peaches, persimmons, strawberries, mulberries, watermelon, and plums. Frequently, plums or white peaches are pickled and eaten as a relish or side dish, but most often the fruit is eaten fresh. While the Japanese prefer white peaches to yellow varieties the former do not contain the nutrients found in yellow peaches. Persimmons are known as the apples of the Orient. They are by far the richest source of Vitamin A for the Japanese, who dry and powder them and use them like sugar to sweeten foods. A ripe persimmon, soft to the point of mushy, is sweet as honey—almost too sweet for some tastes. If it is eaten before it is fully ripe, it has an unpleasant flavor and causes the mouth to pucker. Overripe persimmons can be frozen whole and eaten like sherbet. They are truly delicious.

Fish

The mainstay of the Japanese diet and one of the best-known protein sources, fish is eaten at every meal and as a between-meal snack. Thinly sliced raw fish, served on a bed of grated daikon and seasoned with soy sauce, is called *shashimi*. Fish is often simmered in soy sauce or barbecued on the hibachi. Finely chopped shark or swordfish is mixed with water, sugar, and salt, molded into various shapes and steamed. The outsides are then painted with food coloring and these fish cakes are called *kamabako*. Minute shrimp are dried and added to soups for flavoring, while bonito is dried and flaked and used in many ways. A broth called *dashi,* made by boiling dried bonito fish and seaweed, is an essential ingredient in many Japanese dishes. Tiny fish, some less than an inch long, are either dried or deep-fat fried and added to many foods. Called "crispy things," they add an interesting texture to soups, or vegetable dishes and also make a crispy snack. They are eaten whole and are very nutritious. Eel is widely regarded as a delicacy. It is often dipped into soy sauce, grilled over charcoal, and served on top of hot rice. Eel is a rich source of Vitamin A and fat. Anything that lives in the sea is eaten by the Japanese; jellyfish, sea cucumbers, and octopus are highly relished. They are eaten dried, fresh, or salted. A popular breakfast dish is made by placing salted fish on top of a bowl of rice as it steams.

DINING WITH A JAPANESE FAMILY

The elegant simplicity of a Japanese home reflects their love of disciplined beauty and this same simplicity is apparent in their food. In comparison with the Chinese, who feel that a meal must have at least four different dishes and each dish must consist of several ingredients, a Japanese meal is almost austere. Rice, soup, pickled vegetables, and some sort of fish or meat are served three times a day, day after day. Subtle flavorings and imaginative combinations prevent Japanese food from being dull. It is, in fact, anything but dull.

The dining area of a typical Japanese home has sliding shoji screens that can be opened to afford the diner a view of the exquisite garden. Here again, disciplined beauty is the keynote. Artfully arranged stones, a tiny pond with a miniature waterfall, and the absolute minimum of greenery give a Japanese garden a look of serenity. The dining room floor is covered with padded tatami mats and soft cushions surround the low, lacquered table where the diners will sit. The walls of the room are rice paper panels which are movable, making the modular rooms very adaptable. One wall may feature a delicate painting and each room has a niche where a beautiful vase or carved piece of statuary is displayed. Somewhere in the room there will be a lovely and understated flower arrangement in the *ikibane* style. The interior wall of each room slides open to reveal a storage area where bedding, cushions, and other utilitarian items may be kept out of sight.

The dining table is a large, square, lacquered and decorated showpiece. The diners recline on cushions around three sides of the table and the meal is served to them artistically arranged on individual trays. Dishes are made of china or lacquered wood, and come in many sizes and shapes. Each dish complements the single food served on it. Soup is drunk from bowls while other food is eaten with wooden chopsticks. There is a dish of soy sauce on each tray and food is dipped into it bite by bite. On the fourth side of the table is the portable hibachi. It is usually a small table with a charcoal pit in the center. Either a grill or griddle, depending on what will be cooked, is placed over the coals and the dish is prepared in front of the diners.

Green tea, served in tiny cups with no handles or saucers, is drunk throughout the meal; warmed sake, a fermented rice wine, will mark a special occasion. Regardless of the meal, the Japanese like to finish the meal with a bite of pickled food.

In the past, only the men dined, while the women served them, and then ate later, usually in the kitchen. The main utensil in a Japanese kitchen is the wok, used in a manner similar to the Chinese. The Japanese also have bamboo steaming trays and use a wok with high sides for deep-frying. It has a rack that attaches to the side where the cooked foods stay warm while draining. Japanese kitchens do not have ovens.

A JAPANESE DINNER PER INDIVIDUAL

SUIMONO
chicken broth, ¾ cup
bean curd, 1 ounce
mushroom and
green onion slices

SUNOMONO
cucumber slices, ½ medium
sole, 1 ounce
oil, 1 teaspoon
radish and onion slices

HALIBUT
3½ ounces
oil, 1 teaspoon

EGGPLANT
½ Oriental variety
oil, ½ teaspoon

HITASHIMONO
mustard greens, 3½ ounces
sesame seeds, 1 tablespoon
nori, 2 sheets

BROWN RICE, cooked, 1¼ cups

GREEN TEA

A JAPANESE DINNER FROM YOUR KITCHEN

SUIMONO (clear soup)
CUCUMBER-FISH SUNOMONO
TERIYAKI FISH STEAK
GRILLED EGGPLANT
HITASHIMONO (cooked greens)
BOILED BROWN RICE

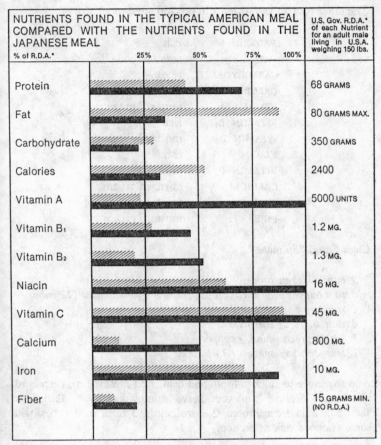

NUTRIENTS FOUND IN THE TYPICAL AMERICAN MEAL COMPARED WITH THE NUTRIENTS FOUND IN THE JAPANESE MEAL	U.S. Gov. R.D.A.* of each Nutrient for an adult male living in U.S.A. weighing 150 lbs.
% of R.D.A.* 25% 50% 75% 100%	
Protein	68 GRAMS
Fat	80 GRAMS MAX.
Carbohydrate	350 GRAMS
Calories	2400
Vitamin A	5000 UNITS
Vitamin B₁	1.2 MG.
Vitamin B₂	1.3 MG.
Niacin	16 MG.
Vitamin C	45 MG.
Calcium	800 MG.
Iron	10 MG.
Fiber	15 GRAMS MIN. (NO R.D.A.)

*R.D.A. is the recommended daily nutrient allowance intended to meet the needs of a *healthy* individual.

Diagonal lines represent the American meal.

The chief sources of nutrients in the Japanese meal are:

PROTEIN	fish
FAT	sesame seed oil
CARBOHYDRATE	rice
CALORIES	rice
VITAMIN A	mustard greens
VITAMIN B_1	rice
VITAMIN B_2	mustard greens
NIACIN	fish
VITAMIN C	mustard greens
CALCIUM	mustard greens
IRON	mustard greens
FIBER	mustard greens

Clear Soup, "Suimono"

3 cups chicken broth
3 to 4 ounces bean curd or tofu, *cut into ½-inch cubes (12 cubes)*
4 small raw mushrooms
8 thin slices of carrots
1 whole green onion, chopped
1 teaspoon soy sauce or to taste

Add soy sauce to chicken broth and heat. Add mushrooms, bean curd, and carrots. Simmer 2 minutes. Serve in individual bowls. Each bowl should contain 1 mushroom, 2 carrot slices, 3 bean curd cubes, with some chopped onions on top.

Cucumber–Fish, "Sunomono"

¼ pound fresh white-fleshed fish or scallops (not halibut or cod)
¼ cup soy sauce
¼ cup vinegar
1 tablespoon sesame oil (optional)
1 teaspoon honey
¼ cup minced onion
1½ cucumbers
6 red radishes

Slice fish very thin. Combine soy sauce, vinegar, honey, and onion. Add fish and mix well. Let stand 2 hours in the refrigerator. Mix again after it has stood for an hour. Cut cucumbers lengthwise and slice into thin slices. Slice radishes thinly. Toss with oil. Pour fish mixture over vegetables and marinate a half hour longer, covered and in the refrigerator. The fish will actually have cooked. Serve on small individual plates or bowls. Garnish with parsley sprig.

Teriyaki Fish Steak

> ¾ to 1 pound fish steak, ¾- to 1-inch thick (halibut or similar fish)
> 3 tablespoons vegetable oil
> 3 tablespoons soy sauce
> 12 to 16 small raw button mushrooms (optional)

Mix oil and soy sauce. Marinate fish and mushrooms 1 hour on each side. Barbecue fish on a charcoal grill, or broil. Baste with marinade occasionally. Turn fish when half the thickness has become solid white. Allow 15 minutes total time for a steak 1-inch thick. Heat the mushrooms in the marinade, but do not cook. Serve fish and grilled eggplant (recipe below) together. Pour sauce over both and sprinkle a little chopped parsley over all. Garnish with a green onion and several lemon wedges sprinkled with paprika.

Grilled Eggplant

> 2 Oriental eggplants (4 if they are very small), unpeeled or 4 slices ¾ inch thick from a regular-sized eggplant
> 2 tablespoons soy sauce
> 2 tablespoons oil

Cut Oriental eggplants in half lengthwise. Mix soy sauce and oil. Marinate eggplant slices 2 hours. Broil or barbecue over charcoal on both sides until tender, about 10 minutes. Brush with marinade occasionally. Mix remaining marinade with fish marinade, to be served on the fish and eggplant.

Hitashimono

> *1½ packages frozen chopped collard greens, or 1 pound fresh*
> *greens, chopped*
> *4 tablespoons soy sauce or to taste*
> *2 tablespoons chicken broth*
> *4 tablespoons sesame seeds; grind 3 tablespoons of the seeds,*
> *leave 1 tablespoon whole*
> *8 nori sheets or egg wrapper (recipe follows)*

Simmer greens in chicken broth just until tender. If you need more liquid to cook greens, add more chicken broth. If too much remains after the greens are cooked, remove greens and reduce liquid by boiling. Return greens to pan. Add ground sesame seeds and soy sauce to taste. Steam nori sheets to soften. Wrap greens in nori sheets, jelly roll fashion. Place ⅛ of the greens in the center of a sheet from top to bottom and fold the sides around. Set the rolls, seam side down, on individual plates. Allow 2 per person. Sprinkle with toasted sesame seeds.

Egg Wrapper

> *2 eggs, beaten*
> *1 teaspoon soy sauce*
> *2 tablespoons chicken broth*

Mix ingredients. Heat a lightly oiled 7-inch frying pan and add ¼ of the egg mixture. Tip pan so that egg covers the bottom completely. Cook over low heat until done underneath and firm on top. Remove pan from heat. Cut egg wrapper in half, thus making two wrappers, and carefully remove each half from the pan. Place ⅛ of greens mixture in the center of the wrapper extending from top to bottom of the short sides. Fold the ends over the greens and place seam side down on individual plates. You should have a cylinder 3½ inches tall and about 1½ inches in diameter. Sprinkle the cylinder with toasted sesame seeds. If you do not wish to wrap greens, the Japanese also just serve them in a saucer and sprinkle them with the toasted sesame seeds.

Boiled Brown Rice

1⅓ cups brown rice   *Soy sauce, to taste*
4 cups boiling water   *Butter or sesame oil, to taste*

Add rice to boiling water. Cover and lower heat to simmer or just low enough so that water does not boil over. Cook rice 1 hour or until tender. If water becomes absorbed before the rice is cooked, more boiling water may be added while the rice is cooking. If the rice is too moist after cooking, reduce the liquid by boiling without the lid. Next time use less water. Season with soy sauce and a little butter or sesame oil. Serve in individual bowls.

Sukiyaki

1 pound boneless tender beef such as sirloin or tenderloin. Trim off fat and slice meat crossgrain into paper-thin slices about 1 inch by 2 inches (slightly frozen meat is easier to slice). Chicken breast or seafood may be substituted.
2 medium onions, cut into ¼-inch slices
1 cup fresh mushrooms, sliced ¼-inch thick
1 cup celery, cut diagonally ¼-inch thick
1 cup bamboo shoots, sliced ¼-inch thick
12 green onions including green tops, cut into 1½-inch lengths
1 pound spinach, stems removed and chopped (leave leaves whole)
½ pound soybean cake (tofu), cut into ¾-inch cubes
6 ounces cooked udon (flat noodles); or cooked whole grain spaghetti, cut in half
4 tablespoons vegetable oil
4 to 6 raw eggs, beaten until very smooth

Sauce

½ cup soy sauce
½ cup beef broth
¼ cup sake, beer, or dry sherry

Combine ingredients for the sauce and heat in a saucepan.

In preparing sukiyaki each kind of food is kept separate as it cooks and as it is served. You may cook it at the table in an electric frying pan. It is best to make one half of it at one time and then repeat when the first half is about eaten. Heat oil in a 12-inch skillet. Stir-fry meat in the oil until it is light pink. Push to one side of the pan and pour ½ cup of the sauce over it. Add onions, celery, bamboo shoots, and mushrooms; simmer 3 minutes. Keep the vegetables in separate areas in the pan. Pour remaining sauce into pan. Add green onions and spinach; push them into the liquid and turn them frequently. When the spinach is wilted, push it into a mound. Add bean cake and spaghetti or noodles, pushing aside the other foods still in their little piles to make room. Turn to absorb heat and broth. To serve, either dish food onto plates or let each guest help himself from the cooking pan. Those who like may dip each bite into the beaten raw egg, which is served in individual bowls.

Tempura

Assemble some or all of the following foods on a large tray.

> Fish or shellfish; cut boneless fish or lobster into bite-sized pieces. Leave small fish whole (remove heads if you desire). Cut large scallops in half; remove shells from shrimp but leave tails on for dipping.
>
> Eggplant, cut into slices ¼-inch thick and 1-inch square
> Carrots, cut into thin diagonal slices
> Leek or onions; cut leek into thin slices; quarter onion and separate sections
> Green onions, cut into 1-inch lengths
> Sweet potato, scrubbed and unpeeled; sliced into disks ⅛-inch thick
> Green pepper, cut in quarters, then crosswise into ¼-inch slices
> Green beans, cooked and cut in half
> Fresh mushrooms, cut in half if large
> Spinach; use small leaves and leave ¾ inch of stem for dipping
> Snow peas (edible pea pods); remove tips and string; leave whole
> Bean curd (tofu), cut into ¾-inch squares

Tempura Batter

> 2 eggs, beaten
> ¾ cup rice flour (whole wheat flour may be used)
> 1 teaspoon soy sauce
> 1 cup broth or water

Mix eggs, broth, and soy sauce until frothy. Fold in the rice flour, mixing as little as possible.

Tempura Sauce

> *1 cup* dashi, *or clam juice*
> ⅓ *cup sake, sherry, or beer*
> ⅓ *cup soy sauce*
> ½ *teaspoon honey*

Mix all ingredients together and heat to a boil. Remove from heat and serve warm in individual bowls. To cook tempura, pour vegetable oil (at least part should be sesame oil) into a deep-fat fryer or an electric frying pan to a depth of 2 to 3 inches. Heat oil to 350°. It is important that this temperature be maintained. Dip food into batter. Let the excess drip off a little, then place the food in the hot oil. Fry on both sides until golden brown. Serve at once. Remove pieces of batter that have dropped from the food into the oil so that they do not burn. Tempura can be served as appetizers for a party or with rice as a complete meal. Each diner dips his piece of food in the tempura sauce, lemon juice, freshly ground or prepared horseradish, mustard, or grated daikon. You may substitute equal parts of grated red radish and grated turnip for the daikon.

Sushi

> *2 cups cooked brown rice*
> *1½ tablespoons vinegar*
> *1½ tablespoons honey*
> *¾ teaspoon salt*
> *Tidbits of cooked vegetables, meat, poultry, fish, or nuts*

Combine vinegar, honey, and salt. Heat only enough to liquefy honey. Mix into warm cooked rice. Make little rice balls with your hand, placing a bit of food in the center of each. Pack tightly into small containers such as nut cups or an empty plastic egg carton. Cover and chill at least one hour. Eat the sushi with soy sauce. In Japan they roll the rice and tidbits up jelly roll fashion in a seaweed wrapper and then slice the rolls into 1-inch pieces. You can also wrap them in egg wrappers (page 220).

Pickled Mixed Vegetables, "Tsukemono"

½ pound cabbage
1 bell pepper
½ carrot
½ onion
½ cup vinegar
2 tablespoons soy sauce
1 tablespoon honey
¼ teaspoon celery seed
¼ teaspoon powdered mustard

Finely chop or shred the vegetables. Combine remaining ingredients and add the vegetables. Mix well. Place in a crock or glass jar, cover, and refrigerate one week. Use in small amounts as a relish.

Pickled Mushrooms

16 small fresh mushrooms
2 tablespoons soy sauce
4 tablespoons vinegar
1 tablespoon honey
⅓ cup minced onions

Combine soy sauce, vinegar, honey, and onions in a saucepan. Bring to a boil, then cool. Pour cooled dressing over washed mushrooms. Marinate mushrooms 24 hours in the refrigerator. Serve 2 mushrooms on a bamboo skewer. Save marinade and use it for salad dressing.

Main–Dish Custard, "Chawan–Mushi"

½ cup or 4 ounces cooked chicken, sliced wafer thin
8 medium shrimp, cooked, peeled, and deveined
4 medium mushrooms, cut in half
4 water chestnuts, finely diced
¼ cup frozen peas
½ cup spinach, chopped
5 eggs, well beaten
3 cups dashi, clam juice, or chicken broth
2 tablespoons soy sauce, or to taste
1 or 2 lemons

Divide chicken, shrimp, and vegetables equally among 4 *chawan-mushi* bowls, custard cups, coffee cups, or individual casseroles (1½-cup size). Thoroughly mix eggs, liquid, and soy sauce. Pour mixture into cups. Cover the cups with lids or aluminum foil. Set in a kettle of warm water. The water should reach to about half the height of the bowls. Cover the kettle or steamer but leave the lid slightly ajar. Steam custard in water just under boiling for 20 to 30 minutes until it is just set and a toothpick inserted in the center of a custard comes out clean. Serve hot in the cups with a piece of lemon rind on top for garnish. Fresh lemon juice may be poured over each custard if desired.

Fried Rice

4 cups cooked rice
1 package (10 ounces) frozen peas, defrosted
1 cup mushrooms, coarsely chopped
½ cup green onions, including green tops, chopped
2 tablespoons soy sauce, or to taste
2 eggs, slightly beaten
3 tablespoons sesame oil or butter

Heat oil in a frying pan and sauté green onions until limp, about 2 minutes. Add rice, peas, mushrooms, and soy sauce. Stir until mixture is heated and rice is slightly brown. Add eggs and continue stirring until they are just set. If mixture seems too dry, add a little heated chicken broth. Diced cooked meat, poultry, fish or raw bean sprouts may be added.

Carrots and Kidney Beans in Tofu Sauce

2 large carrots, cut in half and then into long, thin strips
½ cup cooked kidney beans
2 tablespoons honey
1 tablespoon soy sauce or to taste
½ block tofu (¼ pound); ½ cup yogurt may be substituted
¼ cup sesame seeds, toasted

Simmer carrots in a small amount of water or chicken broth seasoned with soy sauce until crisp tender. Add kidney beans and heat. Liquefy tofu in a blender; add honey and soy sauce to taste. Serve vegetables in individual dishes, with sauce and sprinkled with sesame seeds. Carrots are often cooled before serving.

Bean Paste, "Kinton"

> *1-pound can of kidney beans, lima beans, or other legumes (you*
>   *may also use sweet potatoes) and their liquid*
> ¼ *teaspoon salt*
> ¼ *cup honey*
> ⅛ *teaspoon almond extract (in Japan chestnuts or dried per-*
>   *simmons are often used for flavor)*
> *Food coloring*

Press cooked beans through a coarse strainer or reduce to a paste in a blender. Combine bean paste, bean liquid, and salt. Cook uncovered over low heat, stirring often until mixture forms a ball and begins to pull away from the sides of the pan. Mix in honey, flavoring, and enough food color to make a bright color (green for lima beans, red for kidney beans, and so forth). Roll paste into small balls about the size of a marble, and let dry, uncovered, at room temperature 1 or 2 hours. Serve 2 balls on a bamboo skewer placed on a small plate. Store extra paste, covered, in the refrigerator. Kinton is often formed into a loaf and sliced into thin pieces or used as a filling for steamed buns. It is served as a tea delicacy, not as a dessert.

THE LIGHT BITE, JAPANESE STYLE

A QUICK MEAL: Sushi, tofu cubes in soy sauce, and a sliced orange or yellow peach.

To prepare tofu, cut it into ½-inch cubes and marinate in soy sauce. Chopped onion and garlic may be added. In Japan the cubes would be skewered on wooden toothpicks with a small shrimp, onion, radish slice, or other dainty morsel.

A SNACK: A hot or cold steamed sweet potato.

Mexico, A Land
of Contrasts

Contemporary Mexico is a land of fascinating contrasts. Mexico City, glittering like a jewel on the velvet of its valley floor, sparkles in the evening shadows. Surrounded by towering mountains, this exciting city is one of the most cosmopolitan urban areas in the Western Hemisphere. The cultural, educational, and economic nucleus of Mexico, it is a delightful combination of ancient Aztec superstition and urbane Spanish formality.

But out in the surrounding countryside, clinging to the steep mountainsides or baking on a treeless plateau, are thousands of small villages that have remained virtually unchanged since the Conquest. Wars and revolutions, political upheavals and secular disputes have swept across Mexico for centuries with little effect upon village life. In these hamlets, the ancient ways prevail. The language is Nahuatl, the ancient Aztec tongue, not Spanish. Architecture strongly reflects the Spanish influence, but the kitchen is pure Aztec. Since the Spanish invaders were all men, it is reasonable to assume that the architecture, religion, and transportation would have been greatly affected by the conquerors, but the women ran the kitchens and the Spanish exerted no influence in that department. The *metate,* the grinding stone; the *tlequil,* the hearth; the *comal,* the griddle that sits upon the hearth; and the *ollas,* the pots in which the food is cooked, have not been modified in form or function since pre-Columbian times.

The many foods grown by the Indians with their highly advanced horticulture greatly intrigued the Spanish. Some of the foods indigenous to Mexico and now part of our daily fare include tomatoes, avocados, sweet and white potatoes, squash, pineapple, papayas, vanilla, corn, beans, and chiles, all grown for hundreds of years before the Spanish came. One food in particular attracted the Spanish—a bean or seed that was ground and mixed with water to make a drink. These cocoa beans were highly regarded by the Aztecs. They were used as currency, and the drink made from them had royal or religious status; only men of high rank were allowed to drink it. The invaders added sugar to the otherwise bitter drink and cocoa became popular all over Europe.

Europe during the Dark Ages was in turmoil, with barbarians sacking its cities, while in the Americas, Mayan, Olmec, and Aztec cultures were flourishing. Here, one of the most accurate calendars ever developed was in daily use. Incredible cities and temples dominated the countryside, built by craftsmen whose work easily rivals the best of Egyptian achievements. Agriculture was successful, communications were fast and dependable, good roads traversed the country. But details of social and religious structure are obscure, the devastation wrought by the invading Spanish was so complete. To establish their total domination over the people and their religion, the Conquistadors destroyed the Aztec, Olmec, and Mayan temples and erected Spanish structures, usually churches, on the ruins. Recently, the systematic looting of pre-Columbian sites by unscrupulous collectors has made reconstruction of these ancient cultures almost impossible. Stelae, magnificently carved columns that told the history of a village or a temple, were removed and scattered to museums and private collections throughout the world. With the continuity of the stelae interrupted, the story they have to tell is incomprehensible.

Mexican villages and towns have a charm all their own. A typical town has a central plaza with the church dominating one end. There is usually a fountain in the center of the plaza and an ornate community bandstand that looks like the frill around a Christmas cake, where local musicians play on Sunday evenings. Around the plaza are the shops and homes of farmers and professional or semi-professional villagers. Nearly every family has a *milpa,* a small bit of land that they own and cultivate. These milpas are set out along the mountainsides in an irregular series of fields, planted in corn, chile peppers, tomatoes, beans, and squash. Many of the villagers are engaged in other activities such as midwifery, teaching, shoemaking, and so forth, but most also tend a milpa.

In the villages, Mexican homes are simple, picturesque, usually inexpensive, and extremely well adapted to their environment.

They are generally built of materials close at hand; walls of sticks or thin boards roofed with palm fronds in the tropic areas where trees are plentiful, adobe bricks and tile roofs in areas where wood is scarce. Depending upon the wealth of the owner, the home will consist of one or more detached one-room structures. Multiroomed houses are built with a windowless wall facing the street and wide openings looking onto an interior courtyard. Love of color and inherent gaiety are expressed in Mexican homes. They are painted in brilliant tones of yellow, orange, green—all the rainbow hues. Flowers and blooming plants are everywhere, inside and out, lending charm to the sparsely furnished rooms. Mexicans generally prefer to sleep on mats on the floor, though in the tropics they usually sleep in hammocks. Low benches and tables and a shelf or chest for storage make up the rest of the furnishings. Many Mexicans cling to the old idea that furniture should be low and near the ground. They feel the earth is "soft and warm" and that it is good to maintain contact with it. Low stools are safer, they feel, because if one sits in an ordinary chair for any length of time he becomes sleepy and may get an inflammation of the legs. (They are right. The pressure from an ordinary-sized chair exerted on the leg behind the knees does interfere with the circulation of blood to the lower legs. Continued pressure can cause varicose veins or thrombosis in the leg.)

The rhythm of village life is dictated by various events. Market day is of paramount importance, culturally and economically. Each village has a specific market day, usually held once a week, when people from surrounding villages come to bargain and to buy, to sell and to trade. Families from a nearby village will set up a booth at their allotted place in the plaza. This space is always reserved for everyone from that village. Further down the plaza will be the area designated for another village. These tiny territories never vary or change. Sometimes the wares are spread out on the ground, but many local governments are now providing comfortable, roofed stalls for the vendors. It is at the market that the surplus from the milpas is offered for sale. The shoes made by the *zapatero* find a buyer. The grotesque masks so much a part of every holiday are eagerly bought by young and old in anticipation of the fiesta. Meat from a recently butchered animal will be offered by a family. Market day is a time for exchanging gossip, seeing friends or family from other towns, and hearing the latest news.

Live chickens, children's laughter, shouts and greetings add to the delightful din.

Religious holidays are another major feature in village life. Scarcely a week goes by without some sort of celebration. The extent of the celebration depends upon the importance of the holiday. Some are so trivial that a token gesture is considered sufficient, a gathering of people in the plaza after sunset, for instance. Others may require days of preparation and involve tremendous efforts by everyone in the town. The Saint's Day of the village is such an event. There are music and dancing, special foods are prepared, fireworks explode the evening stillness, and large amounts of *pulque* and beer are drunk. Most of the religious, and all the secular, holidays are times of gaiety and fiesta. The only exceptions are the last three days of Lent and All Souls' Night. These are solemn and fearful occasions and are observed in a pious manner. Throughout all the celebrations there is a strong primitive and slightly pagan influence. This is an interesting acculturation of rigid Spanish church and ancient Indian rites.

Life in a small Mexican village is busy all the time. Between fiestas and market days, there are the usual events of living: birth, death, and marriage, with each event demanding its proper share of attention. The birth of a child is a joyous occasion, and even in the poorest homes a child is eagerly greeted. During pregnancy, the expectant mother is supposed to keep to herself. There are no particular food taboos, and if she wants to eat something unusual, everyone tries to satisfy her whim. Children are usually delivered by a midwife and several of these knowledgeable women live in each village. The midwife stays with the mother for about a week after delivery and rules the household during this time. When the new baby is about three days old, all the family members come visiting, bringing gifts for the child and mother. Baptism is, of course, a great event, and includes a huge feast, music, dancing, and lots of pulque. The children are breast-fed for several years and, as the Mexicans love large families—the more the better—it is not uncommon for a mother to be nursing more than one child.

Corn grown on the tiny milpas is the staple food of the Mexican diet. After harvesting, about the middle of December, the corn is dried and stored in bins. When needed, the kernels are shucked from the cob and soaked in water with fire ash. A handful of ashes from the tlequil are added to the water. No one knows the origin of the custom, probably it is felt this speeds up the softening process, but it is always done this way. After the kernels are soft, the women pound the corn in the metate until it forms a smooth, slightly granular paste. This paste is used in numerous ways. It is patted into a flat *tortilla* and toasted on the grill; spread on corn husks, filled with meat, and steamed; served hot as a mush; served as a soup; and made into a beverage. It is eaten daily in huge quantities by everyone. Interesting changes take place when corn is prepared by soaking it in fire-ash water and ground on the soft limestone metate. The iron content increases 37 percent and the calcium increases an astonishing 2,000 percent. Abrasive material introduced from the metate helps inhibit tooth decay. Studies show that because of the Mexicans' huge intake of corn, amounting to 80 percent of their daily diet, they obtain calcium levels equivalent to those in over two quarts of milk plus the correct ratio of magnesium and phosphorus necessary for its proper utilization. Dr. Michael Walsh found that Mexican Indians "starving" by our standards had a calcium intake equivalent to eight quarts of milk a day. Ample Vitamin D is obtained from the sun, as they spend nearly all their waking hours out-of-doors. The enormous intake of these minerals and Vitamin D account for the strong bones, beautiful teeth, and dental arches of Mexicans living on their traditional diets. In addition, the crude cornmeal, like other whole grains, furnishes a good fiber that helps proper digestion and reduces the cholesterol levels in the blood. Substituting tortillas for bread in the daily diet could prove to be an advantage for people with high cholesterol problems.

It is a delight to watch a Mexican woman make tortillas on her metate. This is a broad, flat stone with a lip at one end and uneven legs. The low part slopes away from the woman. She grinds the corn with a stone pestle, rather like a rolling pin. When the meal has reached the correct consistency, a mystery to all but the tortilla-maker, a lump about the size of an egg is separated from the rest. The patting begins—slap, slap, slap—and the dough is flattened between the palms until it is paper-thin. Trying to copy one of these agile experts can lead to frustration and disaster. The patty disintegrates if it gets too dry; it also falls apart if it is too moist. A perfect, round tortilla, just the right thickness, is the product of skill and practice and the women begin learning the art as children. The flattened tortilla is tossed onto the hot griddle until it is lightly toasted on both sides. It is then ready to eat as is or become an ingredient in countless dishes. There is no limit to the ways the versatile tortilla can be used in the preparation of a meal. After it is grilled, it can be fried until very crisp and then layered with beans, *chorizo* (the Mexican sausage), avocado, lettuce, and grated cheese. A piece of cheese wrapped in a tortilla can be cooked in a sauce or eaten plain. The tortilla serves as an edible container for meat or cheese, a scoop for beans, and can be carried off to the milpa for a snack. Virtually everything served includes tortillas fixed in some manner, and tortilla-making goes on almost constantly in a Mexican kitchen.

The balance of the diet is primarily chiles, beans, greens, fruits, cheese, and rice. Some variety of beans is eaten at every meal: pinto, kidney, dried limas, or black beans. A bubbling pot is always on the stove in a Mexican kitchen. These beans, eaten with corn or some other grain, provide the same quality protein as meat. Not much meat is eaten except on fiesta days, but these occur so frequently that meat, mostly chicken or pork, must be considered part of the diet. Most families raise a hog. When it is slaughtered they will keep the tail, feet, head, and fat for their own use. Rendered hog fat is used to deep-fry tortillas or as a flavoring in their beans, and is the main source of fat in their diet. The skin may be crisply fried and eaten as a snack. Very little of the meat is kept by the family; most of it is sold on market day for money to buy necessities. The poorer the family, the more dependent it is upon beans, corn, and chiles.

The Otami Indians live in one of the bleakest areas of Mexico, a high and arid desert. Except for frequent rainfall, there is no water supply and the Otami must depend on wild plants and what few vegetables they can manage to grow. Their only drink is pulque. Into this desolate area came a Rockefeller Foundation team to survey the health of the Otami. Their findings were astonishing.

Among these Indians they found there was no high blood pressure, no heart disease, no cancer, no crime or insanity, and few dental problems. In fact, 80 percent of the children had perfect teeth. With no water for bathing, they seemed to have no body odor. Analysis of their diet showed that while they ate practically no meat, their corn, bean, chile, and wild green diet provided all the elements needed for good health. The findings in this study of the Otami Indians were by no means unique. Nutrition experts have examined the health and dental condition of children in other remote Mexican villages and their results were surprisingly similar.

Prior to his work in Mexico, Dr. Robert S. Harris, of Massachusetts Institute of Technology's Nutrition Biochemistry Laboratory, had completed a study of the health of 800 school children in a middle-class suburb of Michigan. He found many of them to be suffering from serious nutritional deficiencies and 92 percent had dental caries. Then, a few years later, he examined the health of several hundred extremely poor Mexican children as part of a school lunch program being established by the Mexican Federal Government. To his amazement, he found that the poorest of the Mexican children had little or no nutritional deficiencies and their dental health was far superior to that of the middle-class children in the Michigan survey.

Without drinking milk, the Mexican children had a higher calcium intake than their United States counterparts, thanks to the calcium-laden tortillas. Their protein levels were well above accepted minimums, with the addition of pinto beans. Iron, phosphates, in fact all the necessary minerals were uniformly high on their diet of corn, beans, and chiles. Dr. Harris established the lunch program for the Mexican government, but he stuck with the foods already consumed by these healthy, vigorous children. They didn't need better food; they simply needed more of it. The meals were prepared by local women in the old traditional manner.

Most Mexicans have quite a variety of foods they eat and enjoy. Several agronomists, in a survey of plant food resources, collected and analyzed 224 plants eaten frequently by Mexicans. They discovered that many of them are richer in certain essential nutrients than any of the 98 food plants ordinarily eaten in the United States and listed in the U.S. Dept. of Agriculture's official compilation of United States plant foods. The most valuable plant in the Mexican survey was *malva,* a bushy plant of the mallow family and close relative of the hibiscus. It grows wild in great abundance all over Mexico and, when cooked, resembles spinach or chard. An ordinary portion of malva leaves, about 100 grams, contains 40 percent of the calcium, 90 percent of the iron, 140 percent of the Vitamin A (as carotene), and 60 percent of the ascorbic acid recommended as daily allowances for an adult male. Malva is beyond question the most nutritious single green plant food found to date anywhere in the world. In addition, it grows like a weed in nearly barren soil and needs little moisture. When it is served with tortillas and beans, all the nutritional requirements of the body are met.

Fortunately, the Mexicans have few food taboos. Many of their highly prized dishes seem unpalatable to sophisticated tastes. Iguana, a large lizard of the area, is a great favorite. It tastes like chicken and is served for special occasions. Their "caviar" is mosquito larva paste. Flower blossoms, cactus worms, and algae from lake shores are all consumed and enjoyed. Freshwater algae are being studied by scientists all over the world as a protein source for humans and animals in the worsening world food crisis. Some varieties are 70 percent protein compared with 12 percent in wheat flour and 25 percent in beef. Algae, easily cultivated in artificial lagoons, could eventually produce 20,000 pounds of protein per acre, compared with protein yields of 135 pounds for wheat and 27 pounds for beef. In addition to protein, algae are a rich source of many minerals and vitamins.

Chile peppers, mild, medium, hot, or explosive, are eaten with everything at every Mexican meal. The chiles are dried, ground, and added to cooked foods as a seasoning. Mild chiles are eaten raw as a vegetable or stuffed with cheese and cooked. Some chiles are added to salads and some are pickled in brine. Delicious sauces are made by chopping raw chiles, tomatoes, and onions and a variety of these sauces is always on the table ready to be poured over the food. One bowl may have a tangy sauce with just a touch of piquancy; another, made with hotter chiles, can bring tears to the eyes of novice chile eaters. The next bowl is for the pros—one tiny nibble can paralyze taste buds for hours and leave the victim gasping and crying. Contrary to general opinion, Mexican food isn't hot; the sauces are. A little restraint and testing can make the meal enjoyable.

Chiles have been cultivated in Mexico for centuries. Cortés reported that Montezuma ate cooked chiles for breakfast. They have been used extensively in folk medicine, and there is verification of their therapeutic qualities from the Max Planck Institute for Nutritional Physiology. Work there has shown that chiles promote the circulation of blood through peripheral vessels and lower the density of the coagulation compound. The increased blood flow may account for the beneficial effects of chiles on head colds and sinus headaches. They also have an extremely high vitamin and mineral content. The U.S. Department of Agriculture states that: "100 grams of raw red chile pepper (about three peppers) contains 21,000 units of Vitamin A."

As it is not uncommon for Mexicans to eat four to six chiles a day, this means they could consume about 45,000 units daily. Vitamin A isn't the only nutrient in chiles, however; the Vitamin C runs about 123 milligrams per pepper and the white membrane in the pepper is one of the richest sources of the bioflavonoids. Taking into account that the chiles are usually served with tortillas and beans, cheese, or meat, the combination is dynamite.

The average meal of a middle-class rural Mexican family will feature several tortillas eaten plain, like bread; a few tortillas cooked with cheese and a mild chile sauce, garnished with fresh greens and sliced radishes; a portion of pinto beans cooked with a bit of lard or salt pork; garbanzo beans; lightly cooked malva or some other green; and sliced avocados. For dessert, they will have fruit such as guavas, mangos, or bananas, peeled and generously sprinkled with fresh lime juice. The lime juice stimulates hydrochloric acid in the stomach and aids digestion.

This meal, eaten in the middle of the day, is followed by the traditional siesta, a marvelous and healthy custom. The usual pattern of a heavy evening meal followed by eight hours of sleep is very hard on the body's digestive system. Everything slows down at night, as our diurnal rhythms lower our heart beat and circulation. All the biological systems of the body are reduced. Undigested food stays longer in the gastrointestinal tract causing distress. On the other hand, strenuous exercise is almost as bad. After finishing a large meal, a quiet, restful and relaxed period of about two hours is considered ideal. This may not be possible in our eight-to-five society, but young children and retired people can and should follow this routine.

Now it is fiesta time and frenzied preparations are under way. It is not uncommon for the women of the house to work forty-eight hours straight preparing the elaborate meals that are so much a part of these holidays. Meat, rare in the daily diet, is featured on the fiesta menu. In an incredibly long and tedious process, tamales are made. First the filling must be cooked. This is usually chicken, pork, or beef stewed in a sauce of tomatoes, chiles, onions, and herbs. It takes all day. Then the cornmeal is spread on steamed corn husks, the outer leaves of the ear. The filling is spooned over the cornmeal and husk tightly wrapped and tied. The tamale is then steamed for several hours. The average family may eat a hundred tamales during a fiesta so the preparations take days. Another dish that makes its appearance only on special occasions is *mole poblano*. This pre-Columbian dish is exotic and complicated. It features turkey, raised by the ancient Aztecs for food and feathers, cooked in a sauce of twenty or more ingredients. The ingredient that gives mole sauce its distinctive flavor is cocoa, unsweetened, of course. To the finely ground cocoa is added a variety of chiles, spices, and herbs. Mole poblano is absolutely delicious.

For the adults, pulque is the favorite drink although all over Mexico cola drinks are fast becoming the national beverage. Pulque is the fermented juice of the *maguey* or century plant. After about six or seven years of growth, the maguey, now about four or five feet across, puts out a huge central stalk covered with flowers. Just as the stalk emerges, it is removed and the hollow center of the plant becomes a reservoir where sap collects. The plant produces an enormous amount of sap which would have been needed for the developing flower stalk and the Mexicans collect it. When they have filled an olla with the liquid, a starter of fermented pulque from an old batch is added. Fermentation takes about twelve days and the pulque must be consumed quickly or it will spoil. It has a low alcohol content, about 4 percent, but it is possible to get drunk on pulque with sustained effort. At one time, pulque production was prohibited because it was considered an alcoholic beverage, but the poorer Mexicans had nothing else to substitute; water is scarce, milk too expensive, and the pulque was free for the making. In addition, it was discovered to be an extremely nourishing drink. Being fermented, it is rich in enzymes, its Vitamin C content is significant, and it has considerable amounts of thiamine and niacin. Since the average Mexican adult drinks between two and five liters a day, large amounts of his needed vitamins come from pulque.

A treat the children enjoy drinking is the unfermented juice from the maguey called *aguamiel* (honey water). As the name implies, it is a sweet and milky fluid.

So here is Mexico, a fascinating study in contradictions. The poorer the family the more dependent they are on corn, beans, and chiles, the better their health. The more isolated the village, the better its people's chances are of avoiding processed foods and cola drinks. Ill-advised attempts at bringing progress in the form of milled flour and refined sugar to remote areas should be carefully evaluated. The conclusion of Dr. Richmond Anderson's work on *Nutrition Appraisals in Mexico* summed it up very pointedly: "While there is a need for improvement in the quality and quantity of the average Mexican diet, attempts at modification should take into account the fact that there is much of nutritive value in the food usually consumed. To try and impose the food patterns recommended for a U.S. population upon a country like Mexico . . . might lower rather than improve the nutritional status of the people."

Indeed, tampering with the traditional Mexican diet can lead to disaster. In areas where white flour rolls have replaced tortillas, where heavily sugared soft drinks are popular and beans have given way to polished rice, Dr. Walsh found faulty bone structure, crooked teeth, rampant tooth decay, and every disease he had the heart to look for. The rapid growth of Mexican prosperity has its disadvantages as the new middle class becomes status conscious and rejects its old-fashioned foods.

FOODS OF MEXICO

The food of Mexico is exciting, unusual, and varied. Savory meat dishes, piquant sauces, and imaginative desserts make it a popular favorite with many Americans who don't ordinarily care for ethnic foods. There are many regional dishes; the seafood of Vera Cruz is famous; Lake Chapala whitefish, found nowhere else in Mexico, are served in Guadalajara's finest restaurants. But the standard foods eaten daily throughout the country have their origins in ancient times and are still the most popular.

Grains

Corn is the principal food consumed by the Mexicans. Fortunately for the Mexican, whose diet would be deficient in calcium if he consumed the corn whole, the calcium content is increased over 2,000 percent when it is softened in lime water and fire ash and ground on a metate. The primary way of eating the ground cornmeal is in the form of tortillas, the flat bread of Mexico. As many as fifteen to twenty tortillas in one form or another are eaten daily. The cornmeal is also made into a porridge, fermented to make a beverage called *atole,* or steamed in corn husks to make *tamales.* While the protein quality of corn is not as good as that of many grains, when the Mexican complements the corn by eating dried beans, the protein quality in the two foods is increased by 50 percent, making their combined protein quality as good as that of meat.

Rice

The Mexicans also serve rice as an addition to the beans and corn, but not in place of them. Rice supplies niacin, a B vitamin which is scant in corn and is necessary in the prevention of pellagra. The rice, only mildly seasoned, is generally simmered with tomatoes and chiles.

CHIEF SOURCES OF NUTRIENTS
IN THE MEXICAN INDIAN DIET

PROTEIN	corn and beans eaten together
FAT	lard
CARBOHYDRATE	corn
CALORIES	corn
VITAMIN A	chiles
VITAMIN C	chiles
VITAMIN B_1	beans
VITAMIN B_2	beans and chiles
NIACIN	rice and pork
CALCIUM	cornmeal soaked in lime and ground on stone
IRON	beans and cornmeal soaked in lime and ground on stone
FIBER	beans

Beans

All varieties of beans are raised and cooked: white, yellow, pink, red, pinto, kidney, navy, brown, and black. They are served at every meal and a bean pot is always on the stove. They are simmered with a bit of lard or fat for flavor, and are mashed and served with the tortillas. Beans are an excellent protein source when eaten with grains or a bit of meat or fish. They are an outstanding source of iron, fibers, and the B vitamins. Most raw legumes contain an enzyme inhibitor that interferes with the assimilation of protein and blocks the uptake of iodine. Sprouting or cooking destroys this enzyme.

Vegetables

Mexicans usually combine various vegetables into a sauce or stew, but many are served raw as a side dish.

Cilantro, fresh coriander, is similar to Chinese parsley and is used to flavor many dishes, especially chile sauces, and makes a nice garnish. It has food value comparable to that of parsley.

Huacamotes is a variety of sweet yucca, a tall cactus plant that grows all over the western United States and Mexico. When it is cooked, the soaplike quality of the plant, arising from a substance called saponin, enables it to pass through the digestive tract without being absorbed, but like yogurt it is beneficial to intestinal flora. It helps to digest foods and prevents constipation. This saponin has been found helpful to at least half the arthritis patients at the National Arthritis Medical Clinic.

Nopales are the leaves of the prickly pear cactus. They must be peeled very carefully because of their thousands of tiny thorns; when cooked they taste a bit like green beans or okra. The flesh is firm and nopales are usually served as a side dish.

Blossoms from various squash plants are made into soup or stuffed with vegetables and cheese and deep-fried. The blossoms taste like the squash, and are an excellent source of the bioflavonoids and Vitamin C.

Verdolagas is a staple in Mexican markets. It is the common garden weed purslane. It has a mild acid taste and a mucilaginous quality that some people don't care for. It is served raw in a salad or cooked like any green. Gerard, the famous sixteenth century herbalist, said of this plant, "Raw purslane is much used in salads with oil, salt, and vinegar. It cools the blood and causes appetite."

COMPARISON OF NUTRIENTS IN CORNMEAL, KIDNEY BEANS, AND BEEF

	Calories	Protein (grams)	Iron (mg.)	Vitamin B_1 (mg.)	Vitamin B_2 (mg.)	Niacin (mg.)	Fiber (grams)	Usable Protein (grams)	Percent of Usable Protein	Fat (grams)
Cornmeal, 100 grams uncooked	355	9.0	2.4	.38	.11	2.0	1.6	4.6	51	3.9
Kidney beans, 100 grams uncooked	349	22.9	6.4	.84	.21	2.2	4.3	8.7	38	1.2
Cornmeal, 50 grams with 50 grams kidney beans	353	16.0	4.6	.61	.17	2.1	3.0	11.0	67	2.6
Rib roast of beef, 3 oz., oven-cooked	390	16.0	2.1	only a trace of B_1 and B_2		3.0	0.0	11.0	67	36.0

Fifty grams cornmeal equal about 3 tortillas, depending upon their size. Fifty grams of dried beans equal about ¾ cup of cooked beans.

When corn and legumes are eaten together their protein quality is increased 50%, making their combined usable protein 67%. A 43% increase in protein occurs when either wheat or rice is substituted for corn.

Malva is a wild leafy green plant resembling spinach that belongs to the okra and mallow family. It has the same gluey characteristic as okra and is used frequently in Mexican soups. Many centuries ago, Pliny the Elder stated, "Whoever shall take a spoonful of mallows shall that day be free from all diseases that may come to him." In a 1946 Rockefeller Foundation study of Mexican plant foods, it was found that malva is the most nutritious leafy plant in the world.

Chayote squash is only one of the many squashes, including pumpkins, consumed by the Mexicans. Chayote is light green, about the size of a summer squash, and is one of the most versatile of the vegetables. Since the flavor is mild, it is used in soups, salads, stews, and desserts. Like other squash, it is easy to digest, and is a nice complement to a heavy starchy meal. It has only one seed, which is edible in the young plant.

Tomatillos are little husk-covered, green vegetables that grow on low vines. They resemble a green cherry tomato, but taste like a slightly green plum. The skin is tough and must be removed. Tomatillos are used mainly in chile sauces.

Potatoes are usually considered a between-meal snack; they are sliced and eaten raw. Sometimes they are boiled and served on tortillas or mixed with eggs to make a dish the Mexicans call a Spanish omelet. Potatoes are high in carbohydrates and low in protein, but the protein quality is good and easily utilized. About 3½ ounces of raw potato supplies 20 milligrams of Vitamin C.

Jicama, or yambean root, is a large grayish-brown root that looks something like a turnip and tastes like a water chestnut. It is usually prepared as we fix potatoes, boiled or baked. It is popular in the western United States, where it is served raw as a snack or mixed with citrus fruits for a salad. In Mexico, street vendors sell jicama slices seasoned with lime juice and a bit of cilantro and chile powder.

Chiles, the most widely used vegetable in Mexico, come in a wide variety of shapes, sizes, and temperatures. They are used raw, cooked in chile sauces, dried and used as flavoring, stuffed with cheese and fried; just about anything can be done with a chile. Although they are served in various stages of ripening—green, yellow, or bright red—most chiles will turn red if left on the vine. The fully ripe chiles are the most nutritious. Chiles have a thin, tough membrane over the outside that must be removed. The

Mexicans rotate a whole chile over a charcoal fire until the skin is black and blistered, then peel off the skin. Chiles are extremely nutritious, and are an excellent source of Vitamins A and C, niacin and iron. They stimulate the flow of digestive juices which aids in the digestion of other foods. The juice of a hot chile pepper can cause discomfort if rubbed on the skin, and is painful if it comes in contact with the eyes. The seeds are hotter than the flesh, and a very few raw seeds sprinkled over a salad give it a flavor lift.

Other common vegetables grown by Mexicans are tomatoes, sweet potatoes, onions, carrots, spinach, chard, salad greens, beets, artichokes, celery, and cabbage.

Fruit

Avocado is a green, pear-shaped fruit with a tough skin and a large pit. It has many unusual qualities that set it apart from other fruits. It isn't sweet, doesn't look like a fruit, and has a bland, oily flesh. It is equally at home in soups, appetizers, main dishes, salads, and desserts. In fact, an entire avocado meal could be served with every course tasting different. Most often, Mexicans mash the raw avocado and mix it with a little tomato and chile and serve it as a garnish. Avocado is an excellent source of the essential fatty acids and B vitamins. It also has a small amount of excellent quality protein and easily assimilated iron. In pre-Columbian Mexico, the oil in avocado was highly prized as a skin emollient. People smeared the flesh of the fruit over their bodies. It is now recognized as one of the world's finest skin nutrients, and is also effective as a lubricant, sun screen, and natural moisturizer.

The Mexican papaya is a large melon-like fruit whose flesh ranges from pale yellow to brilliant orange. It makes an ideal dessert because of its unusual qualities. It contains an effective and potent enzyme called papain, which aids in the digestion of proteins and also contains other enzymes that assist in the assimilation of starches. Papain is the base of meat tenderizers. Papaya has more Vitamin C than oranges and is also rich in Vitamin A. It is an excellent infant food and contains no known allergens. Mexicans usually serve papaya raw, garnished with lime and chile powder. The seeds are similar to peppercorns and can be dried, ground and used as a flavoring or they may be eaten fresh. They are a good source of Vitamin E and the B vitamins. Papaya is an excellent skin freshener. After peeling the fruit, put the fleshy side of the peel all over your face and allow it to remain for about fifteen minutes. This will cause a slight drawing sensation. Rinse with cool water and the results will be a natural facial.

Several varieties of pineapple are grown in Mexico and are served as a dessert or midday snack. The plant is noted for its ability to absorb scarce trace minerals from the soil. Pineapples contain a protein-digesting enzyme. This is why gelatin won't set if mixed with raw pineapple: the enzymes digest the protein in the gelatin. Pineapples also have a healing proteolytic enzyme, bromelain, which has been found to be of value in the treatment of rheumatoid arthritis. Pineapple should be eaten raw as its enzymes are destroyed by heat.

Nopal fruit is the fruit of the prickly pear cactus. Like the leaves (see above), it must be peeled very carefully because of its many thorns, but inside is a delicious watermelon-textured fruit, which is red or yellow, sweet and juicy, and as full of seeds as watermelon. The nopal is sliced and sprinkled with lime juice and served as a dessert. An average-size fruit contains about 65 calories, and 20 milligrams of Vitamin C.

Sapote, the custard apple, is an intriguing fruit. It looks like a green apple with a round bottom and when ripe it is so fragile it cannot be shipped. It is one of the most delicately and delightfully flavored fruits in the world. It need not be peeled and tastes like a delicate vanilla ice cream. It contains Vitamins A and C, niacin, and iron.

Cherimoya is another exotic fruit of Mexico. It is heart-shaped, with a rather tough, green skin. The skin is marked with a petal-like pattern and the fruit is ready to eat when it yields to gentle pressure. The flavor resembles a combination of pineapple, strawberry, and banana, and when served very cold it is like eating a dish of particularly delicious sherbet.

Other common fruits found in all the markets are oranges, grapefruit, pomegranates, limes, many varieties of bananas, guavas, and passion fruit.

Insects

Of the many insects eaten by the Indians of Mexico, maguey worms are the favorite. The maguey worms are fried until crisp and eaten like a snack. Like all insects, they are an excellent source of protein, rich in the B vitamins, phosphorus, and iron.

Meat

Pork is the most important meat in the Mexican diet, which doesn't place much emphasis on meat. It is simmered in stews, roasted over a wood fire, made into tamales, and the fat is used to flavor beans. The skin is fried crisp and the feet are also a popular favorite. Pork supplies most of the fat in the Mexican diet. Its protein complements that of corn and beans, and it supplies niacin, the B vitamin lacking in a corn-and-bean diet.

Goat, or *cabrito,* is another favorite meat in Mexico, although the animal is mainly a source of milk. The goat's milk is sold on the hoof, the milkman leading his goats through the town and milking them to order. In Mexico, a delicious cheese is made from raw goat's milk. It is extremely nutritious, and while it is not eaten separately, it is used in many dishes, and grated over enchiladas, refried beans, and many other foods.

Poultry, Eggs, and Milk

Chicken and turkey, while popular, are eaten infrequently. They are usually part of another dish, such as chicken enchiladas, tamales, and soups. One of the famous dishes of Mexico is *mole poblano,* turkey simmered in an exotic sauce of herbs, chiles, pumpkin seeds, and cocoa. Turkey and chicken contain about 8 milligrams of niacin per 100 grams, making them, next to liver, one of the best sources of this vitamin.

Eggs, along with milk, are rarely eaten plain. They are usually part of another dish. Eggs and milk are used in *flan,* a Mexican custard. A family might make a meal of steamed tortillas with fried eggs on top, all covered with chile sauce. Milk is used to make chocolate milk and for coffee, but usually not taken straight.

Seeds

Squash seeds and sunflower seeds are toasted on the comal and eaten as snacks. They are also ground up and used as thickening in sauces. The Mexicans consume enormous quantities of seeds, nibbling on them all day long. Seeds contain protein, fiber, iron, B vitamins and unsaturated fat. Squash seeds have an unusually high iron content, while sunflower seeds are one of the few foods that contain Vitamin D. This may be because the sunflower turns its face to the sun.

Spices

No Mexican kitchen is complete without a good supply of spices. The favorite by far is cumin, or *comino*. It is used whole or finely ground. The seeds resemble caraway seeds. Cumin is added to meat dishes and is one of the major flavorings used in beans; it also blends well with many foods. Oregano is added to chile sauces and any dish cooked with tomatoes. Mexicans usually grow their own spices.

DINING WITH A MEXICAN FAMILY

Mexican mealtimes are inconsistent with those of most other cultures. Visitors to Mexico City, Guadalajara, and other urban areas may find themselves fainting from hunger as they await their elegant meal, which will not appear much before ten p.m. If the visitor has begun the cocktail hour at the customary six o'clock, serious problems can arise. The solution, of course, is to switch to Mexican custom and have a hearty lunch followed by a two- or three-hour siesta, work or play until seven or eight p.m., and eat a light supper around nine or ten. In areas that cater to tourists, the Mexicans have graciously adopted the foreigners' schedule and it is possible to get dinner at seven or eight in the evening.

The Mexicans' schedule seems much better suited to health and good digestion. First thing in the morning they have a quick snack of cocoa or coffee and leftover tortillas. A bit later they have a more substantial breakfast of eggs, beans, and tortillas. The main meal at about two is followed by a late evening supper of tortillas, beans, and any food that would be served at the other meals. The body receives energy when it needs it most, while it is active, rather than when it is ready to rest.

The midday meal of rural Mexicans usually consists of tortillas, beans, rice, and some sort of stew made with vegetables and maybe a bit of pork or chicken. So many tortillas are needed to feed a large family that frequently the mother will be making them all through the meal. The cooking utensils are pottery, the comal or griddle is a flat metal sheet, and the mortar and pestle, called *melcajete* and *tejolote,* are of stone. They are used to grind the chiles for the wide variety of sauces served at all meals. Pottery plates are used by the family and the tortilla serves as a sort of edible plate by being steamed or fried and then loaded with all sorts of food. The steamed tortillas may also be used as scoops in place of silverware. In the Indian homes, a clay brazier, or even several large stones, may serve as a stove.

In some of the Indian villages, the diners still prefer to sit on the floor to eat. The floor in one corner of the one-room house is plastered with red clay. It is swept so thoroughly that it is as clean as any table top. In an unusual example of cultural durability, even in the most modern homes in Mexico City, alongside blenders and microwave ovens, the comal or griddle is still in use. The beans are simmered in an earthenware pot and the metate (tortilla stone) is still used daily. The family will eat their midday meal at a beautiful imported dining room table, using the finest of tableware, but their meal may be the same as that served on the floor in the remotest Indian villages.

A MEXICAN DINNER PER INDIVIDUAL

TORTILLAS, 5
REFRIED BEANS, 1 cup, cooked with 1 tablespoon of lard
COLACHE

zucchini, ½	chile pepper, ½
crookneck squash, ½	tomato, ½
onion, ¼	corn, ½ ear

SAUCE
  tomato, ½
  chile pepper, 1
  green onion, 1

A MEXICAN DINNER FROM YOUR KITCHEN

COLACHE (vegetable stew)
REFRIED BEANS
HOT SAUCE (Use sauce on colache and beans.)
CORN TORTILLAS

For a special meal, add *carnitas* and *guacamole* (pork cubes and avocado sauce).

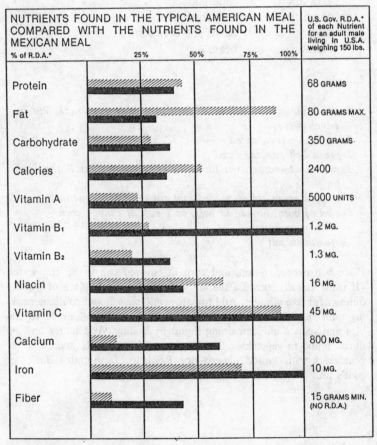

NUTRIENTS FOUND IN THE TYPICAL AMERICAN MEAL COMPARED WITH THE NUTRIENTS FOUND IN THE MEXICAN MEAL	U.S. Gov. R.D.A.* of each Nutrient for an adult male living in U.S.A. weighing 150 lbs.
% of R.D.A.* 25% 50% 75% 100%	
Protein	68 GRAMS
Fat	80 GRAMS MAX.
Carbohydrate	350 GRAMS
Calories	2400
Vitamin A	5000 UNITS
Vitamin B₁	1.2 MG.
Vitamin B₂	1.3 MG.
Niacin	16 MG.
Vitamin C	45 MG.
Calcium	800 MG.
Iron	10 MG.
Fiber	15 GRAMS MIN. (NO R.D.A.)

*R.D.A. is the recommended daily nutrient allowance intended to meet the needs of a *healthy* individual.
Diagonal lines represent the American meal.

The chief sources of nutrients in the Mexican meal are:

PROTEIN	beans and corn tortillas
FAT	lard
CARBOHYDRATE	beans and corn tortillas
CALORIES	beans and corn tortillas
VITAMIN A	chile peppers
VITAMIN B₁	beans
VITAMIN B₂	beans and chile peppers
NIACIN	beans, corn tortillas, and chile peppers
VITAMIN C	chile peppers
CALCIUM	corn tortillas
IRON	beans and corn tortillas
FIBER	beans

Colache

6 *small summer squash or 3 zucchini and 3 crookneck, cut in 1-inch pieces*
1 *medium onion, sliced*
1 *green bell pepper, sliced*
3 *medium tomatoes, cut into chunks; remove skins if they are tough*
2 *canned green chiles, seeded and cut into ½-inch strips*
3 *ears of corn, broken in half, or 1 cup of canned corn*
1 *tablespoon butter*
½ *teaspoon salt*

Place bell pepper, onion, and corn in covered pan in ¼ cup water. (If using canned corn use the liquid from the can in place of water.) Simmer for five minutes. Add tomatoes and squash and continue cooking until vegetables are just tender, about 5 minutes. Remove vegetables and reduce any remaining liquid by boiling. Add butter and reduced liquid to vegetables. Season to taste with salt. If desired, cover vegetables with grated cheese—dry Romano, fresh-grated Jack, or goat's milk cheese.

Hot Sauce, "Salsa"

> 4 medium tomatoes, finely chopped; remove skins if they are tough
> 6 canned green chiles*; remove all seeds and chop
> 6 green onions, including tops, chopped
> 1 tablespoon cilantro or parsley, chopped
> ¾ teaspoon salt
> Chile powder, chopped red chiles, or cayenne pepper may be added to taste

Mix all ingredients and allow to stand 1 hour or more so that flavors will blend.

Refried Beans

> 4 cups cooked pinto or kidney beans
> ¼ cup butter

Partly mash the beans with a potato masher, fork, or beater. Add butter and cook, stirring frequently, until beans are thickened and butter is absorbed.

Corn Tortillas

Allow 5 tortillas per person. To heat tortillas, place stacks of 10 in a covered dish and heat in a 350° oven for 10 to 15 minutes, or only until they are soft and hot. If tortillas are not available in your city, you can make corn cakes.

* To use fresh chiles, skin them by placing them under the broiler unit. Turn them until all sides are blistered and black. Remove from broiler and place chiles in a paper sack for 5 minutes. Remove from sack and catch loose skin with a knife and peel.

Corn Cakes

3 cups of cornmeal	1 teaspoon bone meal
½ teaspoon salt	About 1 cup boiling water
⅓ cup butter melted in ⅔ cup boiling water	

Mix cornmeal with salt. Add butter mixture and enough hot water to make a firm dough with your hands. Form dough into 20 cakes about ¼-inch thick. Bake on a greased cookie sheet in a 350° oven 30 to 40 minutes. Corn cakes are very good served warm with butter and honey, or with guacamole.

Pork Cubes, "Carnitas"

Cut ¾ pound lean boneless pork into 1-inch cubes. Rub the pork cubes with vegetable oil on all sides. Place on a rack in a shallow pan and bake in a 300° oven for about 2 hours, or until pork has lost all of its pink color. In Mexico they barbecue the pork over a wood fire. You can use charcoal if you wish. Turn the pork cubes often until done. Serve carnitas with guacamole and hot sauce. If you are having a special dinner, 3 ounces of carnitas could be added for each person if you reduce your refried beans to ½ cup per person and your tortillas to 2 per person.

Avocado Sauce, "Guacamole"

1 large ripe avocado
1 tablespoon lemon juice, or to taste
Salt to taste

Mash the pulp of the avocado with a fork. Blend in lemon juice and salt to taste. Let guacamole stand about 30 minutes before serving. Salsa may be added to taste if desired.

Turkey Mole, "Mole Poblano"
   (serves 6 to 8)

> *6 pounds turkey parts*
> *2 cups chicken broth*
> *1 cup hot water*
> *¼ cup turkey or chicken fat, lard or butter*
> *Chile powder*
> *Mole sauce (recipe follows)*

Sprinkle turkey lightly with chile powder and brown on all sides in hot fat (use only the amount of fat needed to brown the turkey nicely.) Arrange the browned turkey pieces close together in a single layer in a cooking pan. Pour boiling chicken broth and water over them, cover pan and simmer gently until turkey is nearly tender. Add turkey and 3 cups broth to warm mole sauce. Simmer until turkey is tender.

Mole Sauce

> *3 cups turkey or chicken broth*
> *1 large onion, chopped*
> *1 can (4 ounces) green chiles, seeded and chopped*
> *2 cloves garlic, chopped*
> *½ cup tomato sauce*
> *2 tablespoons chile powder, or more to taste*
> *⅛ teaspoon each ground cayenne and ground cloves*
> *½ teaspoon ground cinnamon*
> *½ cup toasted pumpkin seeds, ground (⅓ cup peanut butter may*
> *   be substituted for seeds)*
> *¼ cup raisins, finely chopped*
> *1 to 3 corn tortillas, toasted until dry and crushed into fine*
> *   crumbs (any whole grain toasted bread crumbs may be substi-*
> *   tuted)*
> *1½ squares (1½ ounces) unsweetened chocolate, cut in small*
> *   pieces (5 tablespoons carob powder may be substituted)*
> *Salt to taste*

Drain all but 2 tablespoons of fat from pan used to brown the turkey. Cook onion and garlic over low heat in the remaining fat until soft and lightly browned. While cooking the vegetables, scrape any browned turkey drippings from the bottom of the pan so that they flavor the vegetables and do not burn. Add tomato sauce, chiles, chile powder, raisins, spices, and ground seeds or peanut butter. Combine with 1 cup broth. Simmer 5 minutes, stirring constantly. Liquefy in a blender or force through a sieve. Add 2 more cups of broth and heat to simmer. Simmer 10 minutes and add enough tortilla crumbs to thicken mixture. It should have the consistency of very heavy cream. Add salt and more chile powder to taste. Add turkey, cover and continue simmering until turkey is tender, about 20 to 30 minutes. When turkey is tender add chocolate or carob and simmer only until chocolate is melted and blended. If sauce is too thick add more broth; if it is too thin add more tortilla crumbs.

In Mexico the meat is often removed from the bones but it is not necessary to do so.

Mole is served with rice and hot sauce. Avocado slices and corn tortillas are good additions to the meal.

Gazpacho

12-ounce can tomato juice
12-ounce can tomato cocktail drink such as "Snap-E-Tom"
2 large tomatoes, peeled and finely chopped
1 medium cucumber, peeled and finely chopped
½ green bell pepper, seeded and finely chopped
½ red onion, finely chopped
2 tablespoons vegetable oil
2 tablespoons fresh lime juice
⅛ teaspoon ground cumin
Salt and chile powder to taste

Mix vegetables with oil and lime juice. Add tomato juices, cumin, salt, and chile powder. Liquefy in a blender. Chill to blend flavors. To serve, mix well. Ladle into bowls with 1 or 2 ice cubes and serve with an assortment of the following condiments: lime wedges, avocado cubes, chopped and seeded green chiles, chopped green onions, chopped cucumbers, sunflower seeds, chopped hard-boiled eggs, croutons, and hot sauce. Gazpacho makes an ideal salad and, when served with a cooked green and a protein food, a very balanced meal.

Stuffed Squash Blossom Omelets

> *8 squash, or pumpkin, or day lily blossoms (if blossoms are very
> large use only 4)*
> *6 eggs*
> *4 tablespoons whole grain flour*
> *1½ tablespoons water*
> *¼ teaspoon salt*
> *Filling (all ingredients should be at room temperature)*
>   *½ pound Jack cheese cut into strips 1 inch shorter than blos-
>   som, ½-inch thick, and ½-inch wide, plus 1 cup refried beans, or
>   1 cup cooked shredded meat or poultry, well seasoned*
> *2 green chiles (optional), each cut into 4 strips and with seeds
>   removed*

To prepare blossoms, wash them in cold water, dry, remove stem and
stamens. Place in each blossom one chile strip, one strip of cheese, and
2 tablespoons of beans or meat filling. Lightly press blossom around
filling and twist the tips together.

California green chiles may be substituted for squash blossoms.
Remove seeds from chiles and stuff as the blossoms.

To prepare omelet, separate eggs. Beat the whites until they form soft
peaks. Beat the yolks with the flour, water, and salt. Fold into whites.
Heat a small amount of lard or butter in a frying pan over medium
heat. Make an oval mound the length of the squash blossom from
about ¾ cup of the egg mixture. Quickly lay a stuffed squash blossom
in the center of the mound and spoon about ½ cup of the egg mixture
over the blossom to encase it completely. Lower heat and cook 2 to 3
minutes; gently turn and cook until it is just set.

Serve with guacamole, sour cream, or tomato sauce (recipe below)
and a dish of hot sauce (see page 249).

Tomato Sauce

In 1 tablespoon butter sauté until soft and lightly browned 4 tablespoons finely chopped onion, 4 tablespoons finely chopped green bell
pepper and 1 minced clove of garlic. Add 1 can (15 ounces) tomato
sauce, 2 to 4 canned green chiles, seeded and chopped, ⅓ cup water,
and a pinch of crushed oregano. Simmer 20 minutes. Stir occasionally.
Serve hot.

Sweet Tamales

> ¾ *cup lard or butter*
> 2 *cups* Masa Harina (*dehydrated corn flour made by the Quaker Oats Co.; cornmeal may be substituted but it is not as good*)
> 1 *cup warm milk*
> ¼ *cup brown sugar*
> ¾ *teaspoon salt*
> 1¼ *cups corn kernels, scraped from about 4 fresh young cobs* (*If you substitute canned corn, it should be chopped in the blender.*)
> ¼ *pound dried corn shucks, soaked in warm water to soften* (*about 3 hours*)

Whip lard until fluffy. Blend in masa flour, salt, and sugar. Add corn and enough warm milk so that the dough holds together well.

For each tamale select a wide pliable corn husk. Lay on a flat surface. Place 2 tablespoons of dough on it in a rectangle about 4 by 5 inches. Allow at least a 2-inch margin at top and bottom of husk and 1 inch on the left side (rectangle should touch right side). If husks are too small, piece two together with some of the dough. To enclose the tamale, turn right side over to the center of the rectangle of dough, then fold the left side over the dough, allowing the plain part of the husk to wrap around the tamale. Fold the bottom end over the dough; then fold the top down and wrap it around the tamale if it is long enough. Tie together with a string if necessary. Lay folded side down. Steam tamales in a large kettle on a rack 2 inches above boiling water. Stack the tamales loosely on the rack so that steam can circulate freely. Cover the kettle and boil very gently. Tamales are usually steamed 45 minutes to one hour. They are cooked when dough is firm and does not stick to the shuck. To eat, remove shuck and eat hot or cold. You may enjoy a little honey or maple syrup on them. Recipe makes 30 tamales.

You can dry green shucks by placing them in a warm sunny spot about one week or until they turn yellow. Parchment paper may be substituted for corn shucks but it will not give tamales the right flavor.

To make regular tamales, omit sugar and corn kernels. Substitute water or broth for milk. Place 2 tablespoons of cooked and flavored meat, poultry, or beans in the center of each rectangle. Serve covered with mole sauce, sour cream, tomato sauce, or chile and beans.

Tortillas

If you can buy Masa Harina, you can make tortillas; cornmeal will not work.

2 cups Masa Harina
1½ cups warm water (approximately)

Mix Masa Harina with only enough warm water to form a dough. Take a lump of dough the size of a walnut and pat it between your hands, roll it between waxed paper with a rolling pin, or press it in a press to form a 6-inch to 7-inch circle ⅛ inch thick. If patting between your hands, keep a bowl of water nearby and keep hands moist. Place on a hot, slightly greased griddle and cook over medium heat, turning often until the tortilla is quite dry but still soft and lightly speckled with brown. Keep warm between towels while you make the rest.

Chicken and Rice Soup

4 cups chicken broth mixed with 2 cups water
1 cup brown rice
1 clove garlic, finely chopped
1 small onion, finely chopped
1 small disjointed chicken or parts, or ¾ pound boned, cooked chicken or turkey
1 avocado, cut into bite-size pieces and rolled in lemon juice to prevent their turning brown
4 ounces goat cheese, cut into ¼-inch by 1½-inch slices, or a 3-ounce package cream cheese, cut into ½-inch cubes
Cilantro or parsley, chopped
Onion, chopped
Canned green chiles, seeded and chopped
Lemon wedges
Hot sauce

Bring chicken broth to boil, add rice, garlic, onion, and raw chicken. Cover pan and reduce to simmer. Cook 45 minutes to 1 hour, until rice and chicken are tender. If using cooked chicken, add it to the soup when rice is tender only long enough to heat. Place chicken, rice, avocado and some of the cheese in individual bowls with the broth.

Serve cilantro, onion, chiles, lemon wedges, hot sauce, and extra cheese as condiments. The soup should of course be served with plenty of hot corn tortillas and beans.

Chiles and Cheese

> *1 seven-ounce can of whole green chiles*
> *1 small can evaporated milk, undiluted*
> *1 egg*
> *½ to ¾ pound Jack cheese*

Remove seeds from chiles and put a piece of cheese about ½ inch wide, ½ inch thick, and 1 inch shorter than chile inside. Place chiles in a greased baking dish. Mix milk and egg and pour it over the chiles. Grate the remainder of the cheese and place over top. Bake uncovered in a 325° oven until set, about 20 to 30 minutes.

Nut Cake

> *½ pound nuts, ground (In Mexico the cake is always made with*
>   *pecans.)*
> *6 tablespoons whole wheat flour*
> *1 teaspoon cream of tartar*
> *10 eggs*
> *¾ cup honey or 1 cup brown sugar*
> *1 teaspoon vanilla*
> *¾ teaspoon salt*

Sift flour, salt, and cream of tartar. Mix in nuts. Separate eggs. Beat yolks, adding the honey or sugar very slowly. The egg yolk mixture should be light in color, thick, and ultra-smooth. It is very important to beat the yolks long enough, at least 5 minutes. Stir in vanilla. With clean egg beater, beat egg whites until they hold a precise point. Sprinkle flour-nut mixture over egg yolks and mix together, pile beaten egg whites over mixture and gently fold them in. Line bottom of a 10-inch tube pan with waxed paper cut to fit. Oil the paper but not the sides of the pan. Pour in batter and level top with a spatula. Bake 50 minutes in a preheated 375° oven, or until a tester comes out clean. Invert cake on a wire rack until cool. This cake is very good toasted and spread with butter for a breakfast treat.

THE LIGHT BITE, MEXICAN STYLE

A QUICK MEAL: Corn tortillas, refried beans, half an avocado in shell, a chunk of cheese, and hot sauce.

A SNACK: Peel a cucumber, or slice a peeled jicama into ¼-inch slices. Sprinkle them with lime juice and powdered chile.

Healthy Cultures
in the United States

"For use in breadmaking the superfine flour is not the best. Its use is neither healthful nor economical. Fine flour bread is lacking nutritive elements to be found in bread made from the whole wheat. It is a frequent cause of constipation and other unhealthful conditions."

Except for the rather archaic language, this observation could have been made today by any number of nutritionists. It was, however, written in 1863 by Ellen White, one of the founders of the Seventh-day Adventist Church. Before vitamins were ever discovered, before the world of minerals became known, before nutrition deficiency diseases had been identified, this remarkable woman was establishing sound dietary rules that protect Adventists to this day.

"It is wrong to eat merely to gratify the appetite but no indifference should be manifested regarding the quality of the food or in the manner of its preparation. If the food eaten isn't relished, the body will not be so well nourished. The food should be carefully chosen and prepared with intelligence and skill.

"Those who eat flesh are but eating grains and vegetables at second hand, for the animal receives from these things the nutrition that produced growth. The life that was in the grains and vegetables passes into the eater. We receive it by eating the flesh of the animal."

Written more than one hundred years ago, these thoughts established the foundation of the dietary laws for Adventists. Food was to be eaten and enjoyed in its season. Tobacco, alcohol, coffee, tea and drugs were forbidden. Pork and shellfish and the meat of carnivorous animals were forbidden. Tens of thousands of Adventists follow these rules totally and conscientiously and something rather amazing has resulted. At the Adventist hospital in Loma Linda, California, it was discovered that Adventist men had eighty percent less lung cancer than the national average. They had seventy percent less emphysema. In addition, Adventists had fifty percent fewer deaths from heart disease, significantly lower death rates for breast cancer, leukemia and diabetes. For all types of cancer the death rate was forty percent below the national average. In addition, it was found that their children had fifty percent less dental decay.

This brief survey, covering only a small number of people, has been expanded into a definitive statewide examination of the general health and specific illnesses of approximately 100,000 Adventists living in California. The research team headed by Dr. Roland L. Phillips will pay particular attention to the significance of the vegetarian diet followed by about half the Adventists and will also note if the subject has been an Adventist since birth or a recent convert. Over a period of five years the research team will study the disease record of these healthy people and their findings will be released sometime after 1980.

Dr. James E. Enstrom, a physicist and cancer research expert at UCLA, noted some unusual figures on a cancer project he was heading. Collecting data from each state on cancer deaths, he noted that the figures hardly varied from state to state till he got to Utah. It was so far below the average he thought there had been an error in the figures, but they were correct. Utah's population is about seventy percent Mormon and it is the healthiest state in the Union. Dr. Enstrom discovered that Mormons adhering strictly to their dietary laws had approximately fifty percent less cancer than the rest of the population. Like the Adventists, the Mormon laws forbid tobacco, alcohol, drugs, coffee, and tea, and suggest that meat be eaten sparingly. Great emphasis is placed on eating whole grains and fresh foods in their season.

These figures on death rates among the Adventists and Mormons surprised many researchers. They knew that certain types of cancer were related to risk factors such as smoking and lung cancer, but felt there was no correlation to diet. Now the evidence is too clear to ignore. Living in the same environment, subject to the same pollution, sharing the stress of our industrialized society, these people don't become victims of disease at the same rate as their neighbors. The only possible conclusion is that their diet protects them.

Simple Rules
for Good Nutrition

Without exception, food preferences of primitive or unsophisticated cultures have proven to be nutritionally superior to those of the more developed societies. Nature gave humans the gift of selecting certain foods that fill nutritional requirements. The more primitive people have retained this gift to a great extent. In case after case, the general health of the groups who still have this ability is far superior to the health of highly industrialized societies. The incidence of heart disease, cancer, diabetes, vascular failure, and tooth decay—in fact, the entire spectrum of human disease—is much less, and frequently nonexistent, in these populations. Other things contribute to their well-being: The amount of exercise they get, the physical labor involved in their daily lives, and their generally stress-free social structure must also be taken into account. In some cases, isolation from communicable disease has been a major factor in their favor but, basically, diet is the principal reason for their superb health and physical stamina.

Hardly a day passes without some eminent scientist discovering in the lab new aspects of good nutrition that have been practiced by the Hunzakuts, the Tuareg, or the Eskimos for generations. It is reassuring to find scientific corroboration for these food preferences, but best of all, the food selections made instinctively by these cultures, which lead to their good health, can be followed by any supermarket shopper today.

FOOD PRESERVATION

Food preservation methods, vital to people whose crops are seasonal, vary widely throughout the world. The industrialized nations preserve grain by removing those elements that tend to spoil quickly. Unfortunately, this includes the germ, the oil, and the bran—the nutritious parts of the grain. The resulting white flour keeps well, but has virtually no food value. At best it makes a fine library paste, but in fact it feeds millions of people daily. In contrast, the Hunzakuts store their grain whole and coarsely grind only what is needed for the meal. The Digueños pounded their grains and stored the flour in clay jugs that were insect-proof. If the flour was to be stored for any length of time, the whole jug was buried, which very effectively inhibited spoiling. None of the grain growers or eaters do little more than crush the kernels to make them easier to chew. Nothing is removed. Whole grains contain a high percentage of tough fibers or cellulose. This roughage is necessary for the proper digestion of food. Dr. Denis Burkitt of the Medical Research Council of London says that most of the countries in the Western world are "constipated nations" and blames this on low-residue diets, the result of the highly refined foods that mark Western culture. When bulk and fibers are missing in the diet, food stays longer in the intestinal tract. There is mounting evidence that the lack of fiber is responsible for a whole host of ills ranging from overweight, heart disease, and hemorrhoids to varicose veins and diverticulitis. The high incidence of cancer in the colon and rectum is directly related to lack of fiber in the diet. Studies also show that cholesterol levels decrease as individuals increase their fiber intake.

The preservation of whole grain does present a problem. Rats, who always know a good thing, attack stored grain with astonishing appetite. The oils in whole grain flour turn rancid quickly. Freezing or refrigeration is the most effective method of inhibiting this reaction. The rescue of essential vitamins and minerals in whole grain flour justifies the expense and effort. In the milling and refining process, over forty nutrients are removed or partly removed from the grain. Four are then reintroduced into the finished product: three synthetic B vitamins made from coal tar, and some iron. This is called "enriching." What happens to the residue? It is used in animal feed. But only about 10 percent of the grain protein fed to animals is returned in the form of meat protein so 90 percent of this rich natural nutrient is lost.

This diagram shows the structure of the wheat grain. Other grains are similar.

Bran—the brown outer layers. They contain fiber, B vitamins, and minerals.

Aleurone layer—the area directly under the bran. It contains protein and phosphorus.

Endosperm—the bulk of the grain. It contains starch and sugar, traces of minerals, a small amount of incomplete protein, few vitamins, and little fiber.

Germ—the heart of the grain, source of new life. It contains the B vitamin complex; Vitamin E; protein with quality equal to that of meat; fat, minerals, and carbohydrates.

Refined white flour is made of the endosperm. The bran, most of the aleurone, and the germ are discarded.

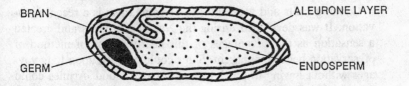

The following chart compares the nutrients of 100 grams of wheat bran, germ, and endosperm.

	Refined Wheat Flour (Endosperm)	Wheat Germ	Bran
Protein (grams)	10.5	26.6	16.0
Fat (grams)	1.0	10.9	4.6
Calories	365.0	363.0	213.0
Calcium (mg.)	16.0	72.0	119.0
Iron (mg.)	.8	9.4	14.9
Potassium (mg.)	97.0	827.0	1121.0
Vitamin B_1 (mg.)	.06	2.01	.72
Vitamin B_2 (mg.)	.05	.68	.35
Niacin (mg.)	.9	4.2	21.0
Fiber (grams)	.3	2.5	9.1
Magnesium (mg.)	25.0	490.0	336.0
Vitamin E (I.U.)	0.0	30.0	0.0

Dried foods keep very well and most cultures take advantage of this natural preservation method. Fish, meat, greens, and fruit are dried in the summer sun and stored for future use. The Eskimos live all winter on the salmon they dried during the summer. However, there is a vast difference between sun-dried and chemically dried foods. The sun-dried fruit of the Hunzakuts retains its flavor and nutritional value to an amazing degree. Of course, it takes much longer to sun-dry fruit than it does to dip it into a chemical bath that instantly removes all the moisture and flavor. To compensate for this destructive treatment, the dried fruit is dyed with more chemicals to make it attractive. The apricots are bright orange, the apples bleached white, the pears tinted a pale gold. Sun-dried fruits are often uniformly brown, not as attractive but much tastier than the artificially dried variety, and they keep just as well. In addition, uncooked chemically dried fruits are quite hard to digest, whereas sun-dried fruits, a delicious snack when eaten right out of the package, are filling and easy to digest. They supply natural sugar for energy, as well as vitamins and minerals.

Canning fruits and vegetables to preserve them is a recent innovation. It was developed during the Napoleonic Wars and created a sensation as the advantages of this nearly foolproof method of preservation became apparent. Ships could embark upon long voyages without having to put into port for fresh food. Armies could be supplied at their point of departure. They wouldn't have to depend upon the land and frequently hostile farmers who naturally resented turning over their crops to the troops.

Canned and processed foods keep quite well, but what about their food value? When food is processed there is always a destructive change in the nutrients it contains. Vital elements are sacrificed in the name of such values as shelf life, cost, appearance, and flavor. Analysis of food is far from complete. Unknown nutrients and growth factors destroyed during food processing may someday be found to be of value.

FOOD ADDITIVES

Along with what is taken out of food during processing, there is a major concern about what is added. Without exception, these manufactured foods contain either preservatives, artificial coloring, sugar, emulsifiers, or softeners—and sometimes all of these. It isn't so much whether your body can handle one or another of these chemicals; it is really a question of what their long-term effects will be. More than 700 chemicals are authorized to be used in the food we consume and of this number 428 are known to be safe. But even those designated as safe may prove dangerous as new testing methods are developed. The Russians take credit for a lot that they may or may not be entitled to, but one thing is certain. We are way ahead of them in the food additive game. Artificial flavoring and coloring of food are prohibited by law in Russia and very few additives are allowed. There is increasing evidence that artificial flavoring and coloring are extremely dangerous to health, especially that of children. Recent studies show that these two culprits are the main cause of overactive or hyperkinetic children. As youngsters, Americans are fed huge amounts of artificial flavorings and colorings, from baby foods and processed cereals to cola drinks and candy. Observers studying children of the isolated cultures have remarked on the contented, well-behaved, quiet youngsters they encountered. Their generally pure and additive-free diet cannot be discounted as a major factor in this respect.

While food additives may someday prove to be the cause of many degenerative diseases, nutritionists are also concerned about the amount of food value that is removed or destroyed in processing. The high temperatures required in commercial canning destroy protein quality, some vitamins, and all enzymes the fresh food contained, while the processes used to prepare the food remove other vitamins and minerals. Over the years these missing elements could add up to serious health problems. None of the cultures examined, nor any other culture that still follows its ethnic diet, preserve their food by canning or processing.

Frozen foods, unlike canned, retain most of their nutrients. Not all cultures are able to take advantage of this method of preservation. The Eskimos rely upon freezing to a great extent, as do most of the Arctic groups. They freeze fish, of course, but they also freeze berries, greens, and blood. Most likely the Hunzakuts freeze some meat in winter, but meat is a minor part of their diet.

FERMENTATION

By far the most popular method of food preservation among all the cultures is fermentation. Because of the abundance of available food, the Marquesans' only effort at food preservation is their practice of fermenting breadfruit, obviously a question of preference, not necessity. The only really fresh milk the Tuareg drink is early in the day. As the desert heat increases, the camel's milk rapidly changes from fresh to sour, from sour to curdled. They turn this to their advantage and make whey and curds from the soured milk, which they can't keep fresh anyway. The Eskimos ferment seal oil and fish heads. The Japanese ferment soybeans to make tofu. The Chinese are devoted to fermented vegetables and eat them daily. Soy sauce is an ingredient in most of their dishes. While fermenting is a means to an end, it is also an end in itself. Fermented foods have now been found to be an important vitamin, mineral, and enzyme source.

Fermentation, the mysterious process that changes the nature of food, is accomplished through bacterial, yeast, or enzyme action. Fermentation makes the minerals in the food more available and the protein in the food more readily absorbable. It also aids in the digestion of other foods. Fermented foods include yogurt; bleu, roquefort, camembert, and ricotta cheese; soybean curd or tofu; soy sauce; miso; sauerkraut; buttermilk; sourdough bread; pickles; kefir; wine and vinegar if they are made from naturally fermented fruit.

When unheated after fermentation, these foods are rich in enzymes. Most of them supply the lactic acid necessary for cell respiration, the mechanism whereby cells take in food and oxygen and give off waste products. They also help maintain a proper balance of acid in the colon and destroy harmful bacteria in the intestines.

The healthy human intestinal system contains billions of friendly bacteria. They keep things functioning normally. When these bacteria are present in sufficient numbers they kill harmful bacteria; they also synthesize Vitamin K as well as many of the B complex vitamins. Friendly bacteria thrive on fermented milk products since these contain lactose, the natural food of the friendly bacteria. Yogurt is unique in that it contains bacteria that can actually help the friendly bacteria found in the healthy intestine because, unlike the bacteria in other fermented products, they are not killed at body temperature. Medical tests have shown that the yogurt bacillus remains active in the intestines even after the food has passed through, proving that the bacillus was alive and working throughout the entire digestive process.

The natural fermentation in a sourdough bread starter breaks down the phytin, releasing valuable minerals and trace elements. Again, lactic acid is formed, which aids digestion. Dr. Johannes Kuhl states that one of the reasons the Finns enjoy such robust health is because of the large quantities of sourdough rye bread they consume. This fermented natural grain bread is a superb source of vitamins, minerals, and trace elements. It is easily digested and tastes just marvelous.

THE GRAINS AND SEEDS

Grains, seeds, nuts, and legumes provide the bulk of calories and nutrients to most cultures. When these seeds are not refined, they contain all the nutrients necessary for the life of a new plant. Enzymes in all fruit, vegetables, meat, fish, and poultry begin the destruction of that food the moment the fruit is ripe, the vegetable is picked, or the meat is killed. Only in whole seeds, nuts, legumes, and grains is this reaction retarded.

Sprouted seeds have always been a favorite of many cultures. The Chinese have cultivated them for centuries, as have the Hunzakuts. The Marquesans eat a sprouted coconut whenever they find one, and the Tuareg love the tiny sprouts of desert seeds. These delicately flavored plants are becoming increasingly popular as people discover how easy it is to grow and harvest a crop at home. A sprouting seed is unique in being the only food that we can consume while its life force still reigns.

When a bean, grain, or seed is sprouted, its chemistry is changed. Its protein quality is improved, its carbohydrate content lowered, starch is changed to simple sugar, and chlorophyll appears. Sprouting increases the nutritional value of the seed, especially the B complex, sometimes an astonishing 100 percent. Vitamin C is introduced into the food where none existed before, Vitamin E increases about 20 percent, and the enzyme action soars as new enzyme systems are formed. Mung sprouts contain a factor that inhibits aging in cells. Horse trainers have fed these bean sprouts to burned-out race horses to get them back into racing trim. Many seeds can be sprouted at home. Rye seeds are wonderful and taste like wild rice. Radish sprouts really give a lift to salads; mung and alfalfa sprouts are delightful in soups, as a garnish, or in a sandwich. Sprouted seeds are soft and should be eaten raw. Wheat, when sprouted, becomes the most digestible protein known and sprouted wheat bread is unusually delicious.

EAT IT RAW

Meal preparation among the cultures examined is often a pretty complicated affair. Pits must be dug, fires built, stones heated, firewood obtained, and neither the Hunzakuts nor the Eskimos have any of the last to spare. Nomadic people usually eat on the run, so to speak, and elaborate meals are impossible to prepare. Farmers working in their fields certainly don't stop their sowing or plowing to go home for a hot meal and, as a result, eat much of their food raw.

The Marquesans like their fish raw, right out of the sea. The Hunzakuts love their vegetables raw, right out of the ground; immature corn and new potatoes are great favorites. Eskimos eat their frozen fish or meat uncooked and half-thawed. The Digueños were very fond of raw greens and berries. The Japanese and Chinese barely cook their foods, serving them still crunchy but hot. This method of half-cooking preserves most of the quality the raw food contained. In each of the cultures, milk is consumed raw. In the methods of cooking used by most isolated cultures, the heat does not penetrate to the very center of the food to destroy all of its enzymes.

Preference for raw foods, born of necessity, is an important factor in the health of these cultures for it has now been established that raw foods are a vital part of a healthy diet. Most meat should be eaten rare. Lightly cooked, it not only retains nearly all its protein value, but it is much easier to digest. It takes almost twenty-four hours for overcooked meat to be digested, but raw or rare-cooked meat begins the digestive process immediately. In the cooking process, amino acids, vitamins, and minerals are altered or destroyed.

The destruction of unknown elements, including the enzymes found in all raw foods, is perhaps the most disastrous result of cooking. Little is known about enzymes except that they disappear if the food is heated to 140 degrees. The human body contains almost a thousand types of enzymes. They are the catalysts that trigger all body functions. Each enzyme acts upon one substance. When its work is done, it is eliminated; thus countless enzymes are needed by our bodies in the course of our lives. Some nutritionists believe that if enzymes are not provided by the raw foods we eat, the enzyme-secreting organs and glands in the body must supply them. They feel the strain on these organs year after year contributes to the aging process.

All the elements built up by the sun and the nutrients found in the soil are retained in raw food. Certain legumes, brussels sprouts, peas, fish, and egg whites contain a Vitamin B inhibitor. These foods should be cooked, pickled, fermented, sprouted, or marinated in fermented food to destroy this inhibitor. The Marquesans dipped their raw fish into lime juice before eating them, the Eskimos dip theirs in seal oil and the Japanese use soy sauce, thus destroying this inhibitor.

The damage done to our bodies by the consumption of cooked food may not be immediately apparent because of the body's miraculous tolerance, but eventually it will catch up. A diet consisting only of cooked foods can sustain life, but it cannot regenerate the body-building elements needed for continued good health.

For instance, when milk is heated its biochemistry is altered. Its protein, essential fatty acids, carbohydrates, and minerals, including calcium, are made less available to the body. Enzymes, the Weizen (antistiffness) Factor, and up to 80 percent of its vitamins are destroyed.

Work done on the analysis of blood shows that cooked foods increase the number of white corpuscles the moment the food enters the stomach, while raw foods do not alter the blood composition in any way. The main function of white blood corpuscles is to fight infection and foreign substances in the body. Ideally, about half the food we consume should be raw and many foods that find their way into the pot can be eaten and enjoyed in their natural state. Spinach, zucchini, mushrooms, grated potatoes, beets, all fruits, and all sprouts can and should be eaten raw. Raw foods are easier to digest, provide needed bulk in the diet; during an illness additional raw foods should be eaten. They act as a cleansing agent in the intestine and help prevent constipation. Raw fibrous foods actually clean and exercise the teeth as you chew.

The Hunza diet, heavily dependent upon uncooked foods, is a perfect example of how these foods improve cell metabolism and increase the cells' resistance to aging. Many Hunzakuts live to be over 100.

When Dr. Bernard Jensen, D.C., visited centenarians around the world, to study their health, he found they all followed one dietary rule: They had eaten sparingly all their lives. None of them weighed much more than they had when they were 20 years old. In fact, an obese person is considered sick by primitive cultures. According to insurance statistics, people who are overweight are more apt to develop most of our degenerative diseases and die at an earlier age than those of normal weight. Studies now underway indicate that an excessive intake of food actually leads to premature aging of the cells.

BREAST FEEDING, A SUPERB START

Probably the biggest advantage these unsophisticated people enjoy is the marvelous start they get in life. They are all breast-fed. No matter how dissimilar their diets, their climate, or their living habits, one practice is common to all: Their children are not weaned from the breast until two or three years old. The infant is given supplemental food at about six months or so, but breast milk is the principal source of nutrition for the growing child. Along with abundant good health, there are a number of other benefits to nursing. For the mother, recovery from childbirth is faster as the uterus shrinks back to normal sooner. During nursing, the infant jaw develops properly. Because so many muscles are used, the dental arch is strengthened and shaped. But perhaps most important of all, the emotional well-being of the child is fostered as it is held and petted during nursing. A sense of security in infancy leads to a feeling of security and confidence in adulthood. In a society where this attitude is prevalent, hostility and antisocial behavior are often much less. The group is generally stress-free, able to meet the problems of living in a more rational and secure manner. Of course, there are exceptions, but the majority of these groups show little tendency to violence or aggression.

Another aspect of breast-feeding for up to two or three years is the general practice of avoiding pregnancy during lactation. The Eskimos have proven to be very vulnerable in this respect. Prior to adopting artificial feeding, the Eskimo family was fairly well spaced, with a child every three or four years; but urban Eskimo mothers now bottle-feed their children and many become pregnant every year, creating physical problems for the mother and social problems for the community.

In spite of all the evidence supporting the value of breast-feeding, the trend away from this natural method is worldwide. Even in tropical Africa, artificial feeding has become a status symbol. Since the mothers know nothing about nutrition, their babies are often bottle-fed a thin grain gruel until they can chew. The lack of sufficient nutrients in the children's diet is apparent in the rising mortality rates and chronically malnourished children found in developing areas of the world today. Only in England and the United States is there recent evidence that this trend is slowly being reversed as more and more women come to realize the importance of giving their children the proper start in life. Breast-fed babies receive natural immunities to help them resist infection, since human milk contains antibodies capable of fighting infection in humans. Cow's milk obviously does not contain antibodies to human disease.

Statistics support this evidence of natural immunity. An important study of infant development was conducted by Dr. C. G. Grulee of Northwestern University. Working through the Infant Welfare Society of Chicago, he followed the health of 20,000 children from birth to one year. Of those infants who died of respiratory infection during the survey period, 96.7 percent were wholly or partially bottle-fed and 3.3 percent were wholly breast-fed. The breakdown of all types of infection among the survey infants showed that of all those who became ill, 66.1 percent were bottle-fed, 27.2 percent partially bottle-fed, and 6.7 percent were wholly breast-fed. In addition, it was discovered that bottle-fed babies had 20 times more allergy problems than the breast-fed infants.

Analysis of colostrum, the milk secreted during the first five days after birth, shows that it is extremely rich in certain nutrients. It contains 6.8 percent protein, which later drops to 1.06 percent. It is five times richer in Vitamin A, twelve times richer in carotene; and the concentration of antibodies and antitoxins is four times higher than in the milk later produced by the mother. Later human milk contains forty times the Vitamin E of cow's milk, five times the Vitamin C, and twice the Vitamin A. Human milk contains lecithin; cow's milk does not.

Breast-fed babies are never constipated. Mother's milk forms soft, easily digested curds in the stomach and promotes the growth of desirable bacteria in the digestive system. Also, breast-fed babies are rarely fat. Plump and dimpled babies may be considered cute, but they may not be healthy. Cow's milk contains three-and-one-half times more protein and three times more sodium than breast milk. Energy from protein is used less efficiently by the body than energy from carbohydrates; thus the baby requires more cow's milk to meet his body's energy requirements. As the cow's milk intake increases, so does the calorie and sodium intake. According to Harriet Kohn of the University of Nebraska, excess calories actually build extra fat cells in an infant and cause an increased rate of growth while excess sodium causes water retention in the body, making the baby plump. The plump infant grows into a pudgy child, and later an overweight adult. There is no reason to believe that maximum weight gain in infancy is the optimal nutritional goal.

EAT IT ALL UP

After examining the eating habits of the various cultures, it is probably evident to the reader that very little food is wasted by these people and anything edible is consumed. Whether food is scarce or plentiful, every group makes a practice of eating the whole thing—the fish, vegetable, animal, even the fruit, pit and all. There are few food taboos; those that do exist usually have a religious or cultural origin. The Marquesan women are not allowed to eat wild pig; however, this meat is served so rarely it hardly constitutes a major sacrifice. Even the Moslems' taboo regarding alcohol is not practiced in Hunza. They make and enjoy a very fine wine.

Sophisticated food preferences have led most industrialized people into a dead end. They eat the muscle meat of an animal and overlook the brains and bones and organs. They eat the beet and throw away the tops that contain the most nutrients. Many Africans face such a staggering challenge just to sustain life that every edible part of the game they catch or the crops they grow is totally consumed. Even the Marquesans, with such an abundance of food, realize that there are limits to their island world, and that all the food should be eaten or returned to the earth to provide for their future. Western cultures that rely upon the market's seemingly endless supply of food blithely discard any portion of food that is either difficult to prepare or has an unusual flavor. We do ourselves a double disservice when this occurs.

First, the food itself is wasted, and second, the nutritional value is lost to the consumer. The liquids in which a food is cooked often contain nearly as many nutrients as the food itself. Analysis of nutrients found in one-half cup of canned peas and one-half cup of the liquid drained from them shows:

	Canned Peas, Drained	Liquid Drained from Peas
Calories	88.0	26.0
Protein	4.7	1.3
Calcium	26.0	10.0
Phosphorus	76.0	48.0
Sodium	236.0	236.0
Potassium	96.0	96.0
Iron	1.9	1.3
Vitamin B_1	.09	.10
Vitamin B_2	.06	.04
Niacin	.8	1.0
Vitamin C	8.0	10.0

When a potato is peeled, 20 percent of its nutrients are lost. A staggering 105 pounds of potato peelings for a family of four over the period of a year are thrown out. That represents a lot of money. In addition, the family will lose 500 milligrams of iron and nearly 10,000 milligrams of Vitamin C. Translated into other foods, that is equivalent to the iron in 500 eggs, the protein of 60 steaks and the Vitamin C of 95 eight-ounce glasses of orange juice. Beet and turnip tops have an extremely high nutritional value; actually, they are more nutritious than the root itself. If the family of four discarded these leafy tops and ate only the roots once a week for a year they would be throwing away nearly 6.5 million units of Vitamin A. Add to this nutritional waste the cooking liquids that are discarded, the carrot scrapings, asparagus ends and broccoli leaves that are thrown out and we are tossing away enough good food to ensure a healthy diet. What should you do with this so-called garbage?

Into the stock pot, just the way the Gandans do. Get a couple of pounds of bones from the butcher. If he's a friend, ask him to saw the bones into small pieces. Toss the bones; vegetable parings; slightly limp celery along with the leaves; the tough ends of asparagus; carrot, beet, or other green tops; leftover cooking liquids; anything and everything, into the pot. Fill with water, add a little acid like tomato, vinegar, or wine. The calcium from the bones will be leached into the stock. If it is an iron pot, all the better because the iron released during cooking can be used by the body very efficiently. Cook the mixture slowly for about 4 hours, strain and freeze the excess. Use this mineral-rich stock in soups, broth, gravies, sauces, whatever your pleasure. Bury the residue from the stock pot in your garden. It will enrich the soil and produce outstanding flowers and vegetables. The Indians buried a fish under the corn seeds they planted. This was a religious custom supposed to ensure a good crop and it certainly did. The world's best fertilizers are made from fish.

FORGET FOOD TABOOS AND PREJUDICES

Another serious disservice we do ourselves and our children is encouraging food taboos. No one is born with a strong like or dislike for certain foods; these attitudes are acquired. Scientists who have spent months in remote areas of the world, studying various cultures, have eaten the local food. Nothing else was available. Sometimes it took a little while actually to enjoy the native dishes, but without exception, they found the exotic and alien meals tasted better and better the oftener they tried them. Eventually these scientists discovered they really liked the raw fish, fermented breadfruit, gnat pies, and other foods that they would never have considered eating at home.

Many extremely nutritious foods are discarded or ignored because of these attitudes—the organ meats, leafy greens, fish, molasses, whole grain bread, and countless vegetables. A big improvement over a salad made with iceberg lettuce is one made with romaine lettuce or raw spinach. A comparison of the nutrients shows that 3½ ounces of each of the following greens contain:

	Vitamin A (IU)	Vitamin C (mg.)	Calcium (mg.)	Iron (mg.)
Iceberg lettuce	330	6	20.0	.5
Romaine	1,900	18	68.0	1.4
Beet greens	6,100	30	119.0	3.3
Mustard greens	7,000	97	184.0	3.0
Spinach	8,100	51	93.0	3.1
Dandelion	14,000	35	187.0	3.1

Some leafy vegetables are not too popular because of their texture. As the plant grows, the tender leaves become tougher and these leaves, although rich in nutrients, are often discarded. Don't toss them out. Chopped finely, they are pleasant to eat and often have a delicious flavor. Many greens develop an acid taste as they mature; this can be overcome by simmering them with a protein such as milk or meat broth. The protein neutralizes the acid and breaks it down. Not only that, but vegetables cooked in protein retain their color, suffer less vitamin loss, and gain in flavor. Chard is delicious and has a distinctive flavor; Chinese cabbage, kale, and mustard greens all rate high in nutritive value. Don't forget that sprig of parsley. One tablespoon of parsley contains 7 milligrams of Vitamin C, 290 units of Vitamin A and 7 milligrams of calcium. Parsley is a veritable vitamin pill and much less expensive than the bottled variety. Stop cursing the dandelion and try eating it. When the leaves are young, they are marvelous in a salad. They can be dried for future use in salads or soups; the tender greens are excellent when cooked like spinach. This is a spring treat, for the leaves become quite bitter as they mature.

There are literally hundreds of foods that we ignore because of phobias or taboos. Most primitive cultures wouldn't last long if they restricted their diets to a few specific foods or portions of those foods. Among the most valuable of meats are the organs—

the brains, kidneys, liver, and heart. These nutritious parts are the most overlooked. Brains are especially good. They are very tender and when properly prepared have a delicate flavor. In an experiment on the self-choice of foods by infants, Dr. Clara M. Davis discovered that the very favorite meat of all the children was calves' brains. They ate this meat in huge quantities, often more than a pound a day. Future research may show that brains are far more valuable a vitamin and mineral source than now believed. Almost every primitive culture considered the head of an animal the very best part. With the brain intact, the head was usually cooked whole, generally for special occasions, and portions of the brain carefully measured out for honored guests. Devoted parents saved the brain for their children and made do with other parts of the head for themselves. The fat behind the eyes was popular; this fat has an enormous concentration of Vitamin A. The gift of an animal head was considered the highest gesture of friendship or gratitude. All the evidence supports the theory that brain was the favorite part of the animal among many primitive cultures, probably because it tastes so good. Because the functions of organs in the living animal, including the brain, are to carry on vital life processes, they contain protein of superior quality and larger quantities of vitamins and minerals than do muscle meats.

To give a better idea of the relative merits of the raw organ meats, the following chart shows their nutritional value compared with 3½ ounces of raw beef.

	Protein (grams)	Calories (grams)	Iron (mg.)	Vitamin A (IU's)	Thiamine (mg.)	Vitamin B₂ (mg.)	Niacin (mg.)
Liver	19.9	140	6.5	43,900	.25	3.26	13.6
Heart	17.1	108	4.0	20	.53	.88	7.5
Kidney	15.4	130	7.4	690	.36	2.55	6.4
Brain	10.4	125	2.4	0	.23	.26	4.4
Melt (spleen)	18.1	104	10.6	*	*	.37	8.2
Sirloin steak	16.9	313	2.5	50	.07	.15	4.1

Bones of small fish and animals were often eaten along with the meat. The Digueños crushed the bones of small animals with a rock before putting them into the stew pot. The soft ends of large bones, a storehouse of excess calcium, were always chewed. The

* Unknown.

bones were then cracked and the marrow sucked out. This habit made mealtimes a noisy process in an Eskimo home.

Bone is an important mineral source. The calcium in bone is easily utilized by the body, the marrow is an excellent source of vitamins A and D, iron and other nutrients essential for the formation of red blood cells. Recent studies show that the gristle found on the bones and in the meat contains an important element which can lower blood cholesterol levels.

Why settle for ten or twelve common vegetables or meats when there are so many to choose from? Try them out. You have nothing to lose but your prejudices. And there may be little room in the world for these food prejudices in the not-too-distant future. The thought of eating locusts, termites, or gnats may be repellent, but these insects contain a high quality protein that may be needed to feed a hungry world. They're free, available, multiply fast—and they're nutritious.

FEAST ON FISH

Millions of people throughout the world live on a daily diet consisting of rice, a little fish, and a few wild greens. Day after day, this is all they eat, yet they remain healthy, fertile, and productive. Low in fat, high in protein, rich in phosphorus, and iodine, fish or shellfish provide sustenance for vast populations of the world. Most primitive cultures consume liberal amounts of seafood. They prefer it to other forms of meat. When Captain Cook brought goats to the Marquesans, the people allowed them to run wild and continued to eat their fish. This preference is another example of food selection that enhances health. For dieters, fish is a real blessing. Beef contains an average of 33 percent fat and pork about 50 percent, whereas fish is about 8 percent. This makes it the lowest in calories of all the major protein sources, while its protein is 13 percent more complete than that in meat.

Seafoods contain many minerals that are lacking in our depleted soils. They contain no preservatives, artificial flavorings, or coloring. They are not doped, chemicalized, or processed. There are no hormones or antibiotics found in fish. Because of contaminated lakes and streams, ocean fish is the safest to eat.

While canned foods should usually be avoided, fish canned with its bones is an exception. As long as the canned fish contains no chemical additives, the nutrients received from the bones outweigh the negative aspects of the can. A good source of lysine, the essential amino acid destroyed by high temperatures, should be eaten at the same meal. Good sources are greens, dairy products, and legumes that have not been heated above 212 degrees.

EAT NATURALLY

If no other single rule of good nutrition should be applied after studies of these healthy cultures, this one is beyond question the most important. Avoid processed and refined foods whenever possible. In most cases, the unsophisticated cultures enjoyed superb health on their native diet. It was only after the introduction of refined and manufactured foods that their health declined and disease began to take its devastating toll. The supermarket industry sees convenience foods as the wave of the future. Pop it in the toaster, shove it in the oven, drop it in boiling water. Soon everything will be precooked, preflavored, and preserved. Even the lowly potato, a fine and nourishing food, may disappear entirely from the vegetable section and reappear—leached, bleached, dehydrated, and chemically saturated—in boxes on the grocery shelf.

The dairy section is a trap for the unwary. Many people believe they are buying a dairy product because it is in a container like those holding a familiar dairy product such as milk, sour cream, or cottage cheese. It is displayed in the dairy section and is used for the same purposes. But read the label and compare it with the one on the natural dairy food. Then decide which product you would want to consume. The Council on Foods and Nutrition of the American Medical Association found there was a considerable increase of saturated fats in the imitation dairy product. They also found that the nutritional quality of the imitation milk varied from "good to shockingly bad." They issued a warning that this product should not be given to children. Most imitation dairy products are made with coconut oil, which is the only vegetable oil that is a saturated fat. Butterfat contains 57 percent saturated fat while coconut oil contains 86 percent. The advertisements for imitation milk state "no butterfat, no animal fat, only pure vegetable oil used." The vegetable oil is often coconut oil and this type of advertising patently deceives the public. To compound the problem, many processed foods are made with hydrogenated oils. There is reason to believe that high levels of hydrogenated fat in our diet contribute to cardiovascular diseases. In hydrogenation, nickel is added as a catalyst to the essential polyunsaturated natural oils and the oil is heated under high pressure. This hardened oil is used in most shortening, margarine, peanut butter, and nearly all baked goods. The result is a product that will not spoil, does not require refrigeration, and containing a fat that cannot be metabolized by the human cell. A favorite saying of many nutritionists, "Eat only foods that will spoil, but eat them before they do," is a good rule to follow.

SUGARS—SOME GOOD, MOSTLY BAD

The natural raw sugar in fruit, honey, or cane is easily assimilated by our bodies. It supplies quick energy, vitamins and enzymes needed for its digestion. But beyond question, the greatest culprit in modern civilized diet is refined sugar. Not only are all the valuable minerals and vitamins removed from the cane in processing, but the end product is actually harmful, and some nutritionists go so far as to say dangerous. In terms of damage done to the teeth, refined sugar can be dangerous indeed. Most dental caries are the direct result of sugar in the mouth forming bacteria colonies that attack tooth enamel. Vigorous brushing can break up these colonies and inhibit decay, but the whole point of brushing the teeth is not only futile but can actually be harmful if toothpaste is used. The American Pharmaceutical Association Handbook on Nonprescription Drugs (1973) lists the ingredients used in the manufacture of toothpaste. There among the various chemicals and additives found in several tooth-cleaning products is sugar. We could in fact be brushing our teeth with a product that causes tooth decay.

Many dentists recommend the dry-brush technique for cleaning the teeth. If this doesn't freshen the mouth enough to suit, dip the dampened toothbrush into a solution of baking soda or salt. This neutralizes the acids formed in the mouth and inhibits bacterial growth. It also polishes the teeth. Many primitive cultures dry-brush their teeth with blunt, fibrous twigs.

Once refined sugar has done its damage in the mouth, it continues on into the digestive system where it wreaks more havoc. An excessive sugar intake can lower the level of calcium in the blood. A deficiency of calcium can cause weak tooth development in young children that will make their teeth more prone to decay for a lifetime. It also causes a reduction in the protective alkaline balance of the saliva, thus creating hospitable conditions for the decay-causing bacteria to do their work.

Extensive work has been done on the analysis of saliva and it was found that when the body is in perfect mineral balance, saliva has defensive factors that control the growth of bacteria in the mouth. Successful new preventative measures are being taken by some dentists to adjust their patients' body mineral balance, and thus inhibit decay. Of course, sugar is prohibited in the diet.

Sugar robs the system of B vitamins necessary for its metabolism, and lowers the stomach's hydrochloric acid, needed for the proper and efficient digestion of protein. Furthermore, it discourages mineral metabolism, reduces our ability to fight infection, increases our rate of metabolism, and raises the cholesterol level in our blood. If that isn't enough to scare you to death, this should do the job. Some nutritionists maintain that fully 90 percent of present illness connected with heart, arteries, liver, skin, muscles, blood, kidneys, nerves, and ovaries—in other words, nearly every functioning system in our bodies—would vanish in ONE YEAR if refined sugar was totally eliminated from our diet.

Unfortunately, the consumption of sugar, far from declining, is increasing yearly. For the United States the figure now stands at about two pounds per person per week. The statistics for other countries are no more encouraging as sugar consumption increases throughout the world. This huge demand has led to higher prices for the product. The increase in price may be a blessing by forcing down sugar consumption, but this trend has so far failed to materialize.

For adults, a staggering 18 percent of all calories consumed are in the form of refined sugar added to food and drink. In the case of children, the figure is even more distressing—25 to 50 percent of their total caloric intake comes from sugar. No wonder they are "cavity-prone."

Sugar affects the diet in one of two ways: It is either taken in addition to a normal diet, causing weight gain, or is eaten in place of foods that contain essential nutrients.

Raw sugar still in the cane, raw honey in the comb, and raw fruit satisfy the natural craving for something sweet. They contain minerals, vitamins, fibers, and enzymes necessary for their metabolism. In the refining process, these important elements are not lost; they are removed. One by-product of refined sugar is brown or raw sugar, which does contain some nutrients, but the bulk of the food value removed from cane is found in the final residue, blackstrap molasses. It contains calcium, iron, potassium, and most of the B vitamins; but it will cause decay the same as sugar if left in the mouth. Control of sugar consumption rests with the consumer. There is hardly a processed or packaged food on the market today that doesn't contain sugar. How else could we consume two pounds a week? Certainly not from our sugar bowls. Even medicine is loaded with sugar. Most medication in syrup form—cough medicines, elixirs, liquid antibiotics, and vitamins—are so concentrated that a single teaspoonful of the medication may contain as much as a full teaspoon of sugar. While treating one problem, we're creating another. About the best way to avoid high levels of sugar in the diet is to prepare your own food, and substitute honey or blackstrap molasses for the offending product. This way you'll at least have some control over how much sugar you ingest.

The enviable health and boundless energy of the Orientals, the Hunzakuts, the Tuareg, the Marquesans, and all the other cultures described here are not limited to these people alone. Other primitive or isolated groups evolved diets that were correct for them in all elements. Their food was dictated by climate and geography, but the results are the well-balanced diets that account for their health and longevity. Given abundant food and nearly unlimited choice, there is little excuse for substandard nutrition in the wealthy and developed countries. But it does exist, in homes, schools, and even in hospitals. A little extra effort can produce meals of outstanding quality. Meals of outstanding quality can produce a life of outstanding health.

The Great Snack
Food Ripoff

The ubiquitous snack, that tasty bit of something we pop into our mouths so frequently, varies from culture to culture almost as widely as language. Less than a meal but more than a bite, snacks serve as a quick energy source during the hours between meals. They are a way to postpone the inevitable trip to bed for children all over the world, and they provide convenient excuses to relax with friends and co-workers for a few minutes during the day. Every culture and every civilization since time began has enjoyed a snack.

To primitive man, everything was a snack. If it was edible, he ate it. If it wasn't edible, he had a problem. Mealtime was any time food was available. As social groups formed and hunting and gathering gave way to planting and harvesting, regular mealtimes emerged, but the old ways died hard. The yen for a bite to eat at odd hours lives on in all of us.

MEXICO

From betel nut to doughnut, from fish and chips to raw fish, the quality of snacks varies infinitely with the infinite variety of foods. In Mexico, street vendors sell all sorts of seafoods, fruits, and vegetables as snacks: cucumbers, jicamas, pineapple, papaya, mango, and bits of fish sprinkled with lime juice and chile powder. Another popular snack item is corn on the cob roasted over a charcoal fire and sold on street corners. The tantalizing smell of charcoal and roasting corn is impossible to resist. At tiny shops along the street, steaming tamales stuffed with fruit or berries are a popular treat. Flan, a smooth and slithery egg custard, is sold in tiny cups and topped with fruit, making a light and delicious snack. Every market in Mexico has a great pile of sugar cane for sale and it is possible to see a stick of cane in the mouth of every child you meet at any given moment. The value of sugar cane as a sweet snack is twofold. First, it is an excellent energy source, containing the vitamins and minerals necessary for the absorption of its carbohydrates and, second, its fibers are a superb teeth cleaner. In fact, any raw, rough fruit or vegetable is a fine teeth cleaner.

In a Mexican home, the favorite snack is a leftover tortilla with a few beans from the eternally bubbling pot. Tortillas with cheese or chiles and a bit of meat will be wrapped in corn husks and carried off to the milpa for an afternoon snack by the farmers and everyone seems to carry a pocketful of sunflower seeds. Elaborate pastries are made for special occasions, sugar skulls for the day of the dead, and delicate lacy cookies for Christmas, but these are eaten infrequently in the villages. A study of dental health in several remote villages showed that 81 percent of the two-to-six-year-olds had perfect teeth, as well as 48 percent of the men and 39 percent of the women over sixteen. This is an enviable record compared with the rampant decay found in the more urbanized towns, where cola drinks and white flour bread have replaced fruit juices and tortillas.

Relaxing in the plaza with a beer or a pulque is a custom enjoyed by many Mexicans. If the beer is naturally fermented and contains no chemical additives, it is a nourishing drink, taken in moderation, of course.

Most American beer, however, is so laden with chemicals that it is a danger to drink, and not because of its alcohol content. Beer manufacturers in the United States need not list the ingredients in their product, so the public is totally ignorant about what is in their favorite brew. This is a dangerous situation.

JAPAN

In Japan, the snacks are as delightful and beautifully served as the meals. Dried seaweed, deep-fried, turns a clear transparent green. Crisp and crunchy, it is a favorite snack of the children. Steamed sweet potatoes sold from tiny stands are popular in winter, when they warm the hands and fill the stomach. All over Japan are tempura shops where bits of fish and vegetables are dipped in a light batter and deep-fried, a healthy and nutritious fast food item. Children trot off to school with *sushi,* a sweetened rice ball with tiny pieces of fish and vegetables mixed in and the whole thing tightly wrapped in edible seaweed—a sort of breadless sandwich.

Rice, plum, and cherry wines are enjoyed with or before meals, and these naturally fermented drinks are pleasant and nutritious. All these snacks, along with fresh fruit in season, are a healthy complement to the daily meals, but unfortunately the urban Japanese are discovering the dubious pleasures of french fries, doughnuts, soft drinks, and many other Western snack foods. Sugar-laden and high in useless calories, loaded with hydrogenated fats, these junk foods are beginning to cause serious health problems for city dwellers. A recent survey showed that 95.5 percent of the kindergartners in Tokyo had dental caries. This certainly qualifies that city as a modern, up-to-date metropolis. In the rural areas, more than 50 percent of the adults surveyed had perfect teeth. Meanwhile, Lt. Hiro Onoda, the Japanese soldier who hid out in the Philippines for thirty years, eating whatever he could gather, emerged with no cavities.

CHINA

Of course, the Chinese would have a charming name for snacks. They are called foods that "dot the heart." The varieties of dot heart are so numerous that an entire book could be written about these delicious and tantalizing morsels. The imagination and flair in their preparation and presentation typify all Chinese cuisine. In northern China, street corner vendors sell bowls of steaming noodles garnished with a bit of fish or pork to warm one on a winter day. Tiny shrimp in a delicate sauce, sautéed duck livers, pickled vegetables, fried wonton, and an almost limitless variety of foods are served as snacks in teahouses. In the old days, the elderly gentlemen would gather at the teahouses to gossip and tell their tales. Today the grandparents relax at home with a pot of tea and a platter laden with dot hearts—tidbits of fish, vegetables, and rice cookies. Again, most all of these snacks are healthful and nutritious, satisfying yet not fattening. Figures on dental health are not available from Mainland China, but the China Yearbook for 1974 gives the results of dental health exams in Taiwan for 1971. They show that among children under seven the cavity rate was 0.5 percent, and for persons twenty to twenty-four was 4 percent. In the United States, this last figure could be reversed: 4 percent of the children under six have perfect teeth while 96 percent do not.

THE MARQUESAS

Mealtimes in the Marquesas are so casual, it is a bit difficult to identify snacks; Marquesans really sort of snack all the time. Except for the rather elaborate feasts when an imu, or fire pit, is prepared, sit-down dinners are rare. When they travel from one village to another, the Marquesans will take some fermented breadfruit as a snack for their journey. Other than that, they pick whatever they feel like eating from the luxuriant supply of bananas, mangos, and coconuts found growing all over the islands. A great favorite is a sprouted coconut and a freshly caught raw fish marinated in lime juice. Nearly everything they prefer as a snack is eaten fresh and raw. The children all chew on sugar cane and carry a piece to school with them to supplement their school lunch. No dental records exist for modern Marquesans but during the 1930s, when most of the population still depended upon food from the stores, their dental health wasn't too good. Over 37 percent of their teeth showed serious decay. This is a sad comparison with the dental health of the Marquesans when Melville visited the islands. At that time it is believed they were completely free of dental caries.

HUNZA

Nuts are a popular snack in Hunza. A delicious sort of candy bar is made by mixing chopped almonds and walnuts, dried apricots and dried mulberries, all mashed together. Formed into balls and wrapped in leaves, they are ready to take along on a journey or just to eat for a little bite. This mixture, with any number of variations such as raisins or chopped dates, is so marvelous tasting it is hard to believe it is also good for you. It is also unparalleled as a quick energy source. The sugar in the fruit combines with the protein in the nuts to provide a filling and energizing lift. Mixtures of this sort are fast becoming popular with athletes and sportsmen in the West because they are light, easy to carry, and require no refrigeration.

Naturally, the enormous supply of dried fruit stored by Hunza families provides snacks all year round. In winter, a bit of fruit will be mashed up and combined with snow for a sort of ice cream treat for the kids. They have another snack idea that sounds great. They string almonds on a length of cord to wear around their necks. This edible lei may last for hours, and during the evening they restring it for the next day's snacks.

The grownups enjoy a rather potent mulberry wine. The astonishing health of the Hunzakuts is thoroughly detailed so it is unnecessary to tell again of their perfect teeth, their disease-free lives, and their longevity. They didn't get this way from drinking colas and eating Screaming Yellow Zonkers.

THE TUAREG

For the Tuareg, innumerable tea breaks, five or six a day, make snack time a major part of their lives. The only real meal of the day is in the evening when they make camp. Then the bread is made, the pot of stew or couscous is put on to simmer, and the family gathers to eat together. For their tea breaks, they drink herb tea, often served with fresh dates. A favorite snack of the Tuareg is dried date meal formed into balls and chased down with a sip of milk. While on the trail with their herds, they often have a bowl of millet cereal with clabbered milk, or they munch dried cheese as they walk along. As they cross the desert from oasis to oasis, especially in springtime, the females will gather young green leaves and sprouted seeds. These are a delightful snack and eaten right on the spot. Milk is drunk almost continuously as water is scarce and their need for fluids endless. With the enormous amount of calcium they get from the milk and the Vitamin D from the sun, it naturally follows that tooth development and dental health are superb.

THE ESKIMOS

There is usually a big supply of dried salmon available for an Eskimo snack. When the men go off to fish, they may put a few chunks into their pocket for a bite to eat later. Fermented fish heads buried during the summer run are a popular snack, rather like a strong Roquefort cheese. The children enjoy dried roe of salmon along with the livers and kidneys from various mammals. But the best treat of all is Eskimo ice cream, not to be confused with our commercial Eskimo pie. A quantity of grated caribou fat is placed into a large bowl. By slowly adding fermented seal oil and snow to the caribou fat while briskly beating it with the hand, a fluffy white meringue is formed to which berries and occasionally fish roe are added. This dish is saved for special occasions. A cocktail of fermented seal oil is a popular drink at the end of a hard day; its nutritional value is comparable to most naturally fermented drinks, with the advantage that it also supplies essential fatty acids and a large quantity of Vitamin A. Today's Eskimo parents, overindulgent to the point of poor judgment, love to buy special treats for their children. Chewing gum is very popular, along with soft drinks and store-bought cookies. A survey of dental health by Dr. Price showed that one group of seventy-two people living in isolation along the lower Kuskokwim River had such excellent teeth that they had only two cavities among them. In the same district was a group of eighty-one people who shopped in Bethel regularly and lived in part on store-bought food. Among this group, 394 teeth showed various degrees of decay and pyorrhea was a severe problem. Dr. Price found that people who lived mainly on marine foods have a high immunity to tooth decay, higher even than those who ate a primarily vegetarian diet.

THE GANDANS

Among the Gandans bananas are eaten so frequently, before, during, and after meals, they are hardly a treat for the children. What they really like is the swollen belly of a honey ant. They know just where to look for these tasty morsels and nothing is more fun than trotting off with a group of friends in search of a nest of honey ants. A Gandan mother makes high protein cookies from dried gnats as a special treat for her children. A small leather bag of roasted coffee beans is always carried by adults as a sort of combination hard candy and chewing gum. Sitting around visiting and chewing coffee beans is a pleasant way to spend an afternoon. In all Gandan homes, a great basket of peanuts is kept full, and a handful makes a filling snack. For trips, Gandans carry along manioc root which has been boiled and dried, or they'll munch on a raw sweet potato. Beer made from fermented bananas is the favorite drink. Strange and unfamiliar as these exotic foods sound, they are very commonplace to the Gandans. They also happen to be very nutritious, and probably account for the fact that Gandans eating their native foods have virtually no tooth decay. In one group of fifty-eight people, Dr. Price found only three decayed teeth.

THE DIGUEÑOS

No Digueño Indians live in the valleys and along the shoreline of Southern California today. All that remains of this flourishing culture are relics found in museums that tell the story of the tribe and its daily life. It isn't hard to piece together an accurate picture of the area, its food, and its people. For a snack they often ate piñon nuts gathered from the pine woods nearby, and leftover acorn mush was considered a delicacy. They also enjoyed a sort of chewing gum made from the sticky white juice of the milkweed. Chia seeds were a great favorite with the young men as they were believed to give them endurance and courage. Honey was gathered and the chewy comb shared among friends. The Digueños had a much more sophisticated diet than most Western tribes. They made delicious fruit drinks from crushed berries and water, although there is no evidence that they ever fermented this. They enjoyed a wide variety of nuts and fruits from cactus to blossoms to acorns, and nothing edible was overlooked. A study of pre-Columbian skulls shows that none of the children suffered from tooth decay, and only about 10 percent of the adults had one or more teeth pitted with cavities.

This is just a sampling of the sort of snacks enjoyed by the various cultures we've examined. Generally, they don't prepare something special as a snack, but they stick to things that are part of their regular daily diet. The main requirements are that the snack provide an energy lift and ease hunger pains by being filling. These requirements are met with nuts and fruits, vegetables, cheese, and bits of meat or fish which are also healthful foods. When refined or processed foods are introduced, the carbohydrate intake remains the same, but the form changes. Carbohydrates found in the fruits or grains are replaced by the useless and actually harmful sort found in sugar and refined flour.

AMERICAN SNACKS

While many American meals are hardly examples of outstanding nutrition, a leftover piece of meat loaf or cold vegetable would be infinitely superior to the prepared snacks now flooding the market. The caffeine-filled colas, the cavity-creating candy, and the cholesterol-causing cakes, crackers, and cookies contribute to our deteriorating health.

A recent flurry of charges, countercharges and cries of dismay was set off by the disclosure that all but three prepared breakfast cereals are worthless—and worse, totally misleading in their nutritional claims. In the presweetened variety the sugar content was often over 40 percent, and one ran as high as 50 percent. Among the rest the nutritional value was negligible, if not entirely missing. An attempt to have the FDA require the manufacturers to state the percentage of sugar in these cereals was rejected. They should not be given to children under any circumstances.

The importance of snack foods in the marketing of food products can hardly be overlooked. It is a multibillion-dollar-a-year business. The average American family spends somewhere around $950 a year on junk foods. Efforts to tempt and lure buyers involve huge advertising budgets and ever-increasing competition. The newest fad food is artificial potato chips. Several companies are now producing cookie-cutter-perfect pieces of potato product. Even cheese, a fine and nourishing food, has been artificially colored, flavored, and processed until the resulting product should hardly be called cheese. The tons of candy, the gallons of cola drinks, the mountains of cookies and cakes bought and consumed by Americans account for up to 50 percent of their total calorie intake. These are not foods that are part of a regular meal. They are especially created snacks and are about as nutritious as the container in which they are packaged. Most all snack foods produced in the United States are made with refined sugar and white flour along with hydrogenated oils, chemical preservatives, artificial flavoring and coloring, and they are often cooked in rancid fat. All these things have been proven to produce degenerative disease. None of them can promote or even maintain health.

Chocolate is the favorite of the school-age gang, but a disturbing fact has emerged. It interferes with the absorption of calcium, which is essential to growing and developing bones, yet 90 percent of the milk sold in school cafeterias is chocolate milk. Carbonated beverages and cola drinks now outsell coffee and milk. A *Boys' Life* survey revealed that the average Boy Scout drinks at least three bottles of cola a day, and one out of twelve drinks eight or more. Eight bottles of soda a day would cost about two dollars, which works out to about sixty dollars a month. The soft drink industry alone gobbles up several billion dollars a year of your food money. In addition, with a sugar content of up to six teaspoons per eight-ounce bottle, not to mention the caffeine and chemical additives, soft drinks can cause serious metabolic problems. Studies have shown that white cells have a significantly diminished capacity to cope with invading bacteria after ingestion of a single bottle of a cola drink. Moreover, this action lasts for several hours, certainly long enough for the next bottle to renew the effects. The amount of natural sugar a person can consume is self-limiting. The sugar in four one-inch squares of plain fudge is comparable to the sugar in fourteen medium-sized cantaloupes. While most anyone could eat four squares of fudge, it is very unlikely that he could consume fourteen cantaloupes during the course of a day. In this way, Nature protects us, but we bypass this safety factor when we ingest refined sugar because it is so concentrated.

Snacks are fun, and they're important in our lives socially and nutritionally. There's no need to give them up—just give up the bad ones. Real peanut butter, the kind that separates and turns oily, the kind that spoils and must be refrigerated, is a marvelous snack. Convenient and easy to prepare, peanut butter on whole wheat bread or spread on celery or a banana slice is so tasty. A crisp apple with a handful of nuts is a delightful and filling snack. So is just about any leftover vegetable. Cold eggplant Parmesan is a real surprise.

If you can't resist chocolate, and few people can, carob makes a perfect substitute, except that carob is very nutritious. Fresh fruit drinks, diluted half-and-half with water, are more refreshing than carbonated, artificially sweetened drinks, and at a fraction of the cost.

Snacks and desserts should contribute to good health. While sugar or some other sweetener may be necessary to make the food tasty, the amounts called for in any recipe can be reduced. With the addition of some other flavoring, an increased amount of vanilla, for example, the sweeteners can be further reduced. If blackstrap molasses can be substituted, the calcium and iron content is increased. Although brown sugar or honey do contribute a few nutrients, and white sugar none, they are not the ideal substitute. Curiously enough, raw sugar cannot be sold in the U.S. The sugar labeled raw is actually refined sugar to which molasses has been added for color and flavor. One brand doesn't even stop with this. They send the refined sugar through yet another process where it is crystallized to resemble raw sugar.

Raw honey is rare on the market. It is a thick, cloudy substance so heavy it will not pour. Commercial honey has been pasteurized to make it attractive and easy to pour. Even honey labeled "raw" may have been heated enough to kill valuable enzymes but not enough to be called pasteurized. True raw honey is by far the best sweetener to use when foods are not going to be cooked.

When cooking foods, however, blackstrap molasses should be used for at least part of the sweetener whenever possible. Both honey and blackstrap molasses are very concentrated sources of energy and, like any sweetener, should be used in moderation.

This chart compares the nutrients found in 100 grams of sweeteners.

	Calories	Iron (mg.)	Vitamin B_1 (mg.)	Vitamin B_2 (mg.)	Niacin (mg.)	Calcium (mg.)	Potassium (mg.)
White sugar	373	.1	0	0	0	0	3
Dark brown sugar	385	3.4	.01	.03	.2	85	344
Blackstrap molasses	213	16.1	.11	.19	2.0	684	2927
Honey	304	.5	trace	.04	.3	5	51

When substituting natural ingredients in your recipes, the results will be different. Whole grains are heavier, and honey is moister. The best difference, however, is a snack that is not only nutritionally superior, but tastes better too.

To replace refined foods with natural ingredients use the following proportions:

One cup white sugar equals ¾ cup honey. Reduce the liquid in the recipe by ¼ cup. If no liquid is called for, add 4 tablespoons flour. Lower oven temperature by 25°F.

If using molasses, reduce liquid by ⅓ the amount of molasses added.

In baking, one cup of white flour equals one cup whole wheat flour or ¾ cup coarsely ground wheat flour, or ⅞ cup whole wheat pastry flour. If the recipe calls for several cups of flour, as in bread, any of the following may replace one cup of wheat flour: ¾ cup buckwheat, ¾ cup coarse cornmeal, ¾ cup rye flour, ¾ cup soy flour, 1⅓ cups oatmeal.

Other equivalents are: 1 cup white rice equals one cup brown rice. 1 cup sour cream equals 1 cup yogurt, but as yogurt tends to liquefy rather easily it should be added very carefully and not stirred or heated much. 1 cup shortening or butter equals ⅔ cup oil, but count it as a liquid in the recipe. One ounce of chocolate equals three tablespoons carob plus one tablespoon water and 1 tablespoon oil. Carob is naturally sweet so other sweeteners may need to be reduced. Six teaspoons baking powder equals 3 teaspoons cream of tartar.

If you are adding wheat germ to a yeast dough it must be toasted. Enzymes in raw wheat germ will cause a runny dough.

THE SCHOOL CAFETERIA:
ROOM FOR IMPROVEMENT

Outside the supermarket, just about the greatest display of worthless (although very expensive) food can be found in schools. Great banks of vending machines selling every conceivable junk food tempt and lure the hurrying student. In the cafeteria things aren't much better. More varieties of cakes, pies, and frozen desserts are offered than vegetables. Salads are almost nonexistent. However, an interesting trend is becoming noticeable. Students are protesting. Why not vend apples and oranges instead of candy bars and ice cream cups? Why not dispense kefir and fresh fruit drinks instead of colas and chocolate milk? Why not packages of nuts and raisins instead of gum? Good, sound nutrition is becoming increasingly important to students all over the country. Recently, a group of high schoolers were called to the principal's office for disciplinary action because they left the school every day without permission. It finally came out, after prodding, that the food served in the cafeteria was inedible by their standards, and they were sneaking off to a health food store down the street for a lunch of kefir, yogurt, apples, carob cookies, and nuts. Many school cafeterias are now offering alternatives to the high fat and refined carbohydrate meals usually featured.

As long ago as 1932, Dr. Price established a school lunch program for Depression-age children. It featured an orange or tomato juice cocktail, and a rich and nutritious stew made with vegetables and bone marrow. The stew was similar to that prepared by many primitive cultures: whole fresh vegetables combined with lightly cooked meat and bone marrow. The stew was varied daily by using organ meats or fish in place of meat. It always contained bone marrow, finely chopped vegetables and plenty of carrots. Fresh milk and rolls made of freshly ground grain flour and spread with real butter were served with the stew. A dessert of fruit completed the meal. A supplement of cod liver oil was given each child.

For many of the children, this meal was about all the food they got all day, and it was designed with just that in mind. It contained all the nutrients necessary for their good health. Dr. Price carefully checked all the children at the beginning of the program and found that a majority of them suffered from undernutrition, or even malnutrition, and active tooth decay. The program ran for five months, and though no change was made in their diet at home or in their tooth care, during those five months the children's health showed dramatic improvement. Clinically, this program completely controlled the dental caries of each child. All the teachers remarked on the improvement of the children and one teacher could hardly believe that her worst student, a slow learner and serious troublemaker, had miraculously changed into her best student.

Pressure from the PTA and other parent groups can hasten these changes in schools all over the country. In the meantime the brown baggers can carry whole grain bread sandwiches, cheese, nuts, fruits, and carob cookies. If increasing awareness of good nutrition and the important part it plays in our lives leads to better eating habits in the future, in about ten years a comparison of dental health in the United States should be most enlightening. Things can only get better—how could a national tooth decay rate of 98 percent get much worse?

Tooth decay begins with the interaction of a type of bacteria that lives in the mouth with the sugar or starch particles in food. When these particles stay in the mouth for any length of time, they unite with the bacteria and produce acids that combine with the calcium in the tooth, causing the tooth to decay or erode. The faster these acids are formed, the greater their concentration is in the mouth and the greater the chance that the dentine will start to dissolve.

Dr. T. J. Belding, a member of the medical corps of the U.S. Navy, reported in 1938 that refined flour and refined sugar reacted with extreme rapidity, almost instantly, and the acids began their work at once. White bread seemed to be one of the worst offenders, while raw foods and whole grains fermented so slowly that little acid was produced.

Tooth decay affects more individuals throughout the modern industrial world than any other single affliction. Most tooth decay is caused by improper diet and is a forerunner of other degenerative diseases. This being the case, serious trouble lies ahead for modern man because the average seventeen-year-old now has nine decayed, missing, or filled teeth. In 1975, Americans spent almost $10 billion for dental care. Add this to the billions spent on the trash foods that caused the decay in the first place and it is obvious that an awful lot of money is being wasted, not to mention the pain and distress resulting from poor dental health.

The place to resolve this problem is in the kitchen of every home. It's much more pleasant than trying to salvage damaged teeth in the dentist's chair.

Science of Health

The art of eating for pleasure is very old but the science of eating for health is very new. The essentials for maintenance of life in every living cell in the human body are found in air, water, and food. It is from these elements that the body receives proteins, carbohydrates, fats, vitamins, minerals, and fibers. With these nutrients the body builds new tissue and obtains the energy necessary to carry on all of life's processes.

THE CALORIE

A calorie is a unit that measures the energy received from food. Excess food, that not needed for energy, is stored as fat (3500 calories equal one pound of body weight). In primitive cultures, obesity is so rare than an overweight person is considered ill. Figures from the Metropolitan Life Insurance Company reveal that in the United States 60 to 70 percent of adults over forty are overweight. While obesity is not in itself considered a cause of death, it is closely associated with other causes such as heart, circulatory, and digestive diseases, as well as diabetes. The people of cultures enjoying long and healthy lives eat sparingly.

For a rough estimate of your caloric needs per day, multiply your optimum body weight by sixteen. Extremely active people should multiply their weight by twenty to twenty-four. This is not a rigid rule and should be adjusted to the individual and his needs. For instance, middle-aged or elderly people should reduce the figure by five to ten percent, while children require more than the median.

All activities burn calories, even sleeping, which uses up about one calorie per minute. The calorie-burning rates of other activities are:

Activity	Calories Burned Per Minute
Eating	2.5
Normal moving	2.5
Serious walking	5
Bicycling	7
Swimming	11

PROTEINS

Obtaining protein mainly from aged, fattened, overcooked animal flesh is the custom of industrialized and sophisticated cultures. All primitive cultures receive their proteins from lean range animals, wild lean game, fish, milk products, or grains and beans. The milk products are nearly always consumed raw. The meat is often eaten raw or barely cooked. It is consumed freshly killed or it is immediately preserved for future use.

Protein is essential because it is the only nutrient that can build and repair the body. During a person's lifetime, this repair work goes on continuously so protein must be taken in constantly. In the digesting process, the body breaks up all types of proteins into amino acids, which it then uses to build body protein. Most foods contain the twenty-two known amino acids, but each in a different ratio. There are eight essential amino acids, ten for children, that must be present in the correct ratio and at the same time for the body to build new protein. If one of these amino acids is present in less than its optimum quantity, the effectiveness of all the other essential amino acids is reduced. The remaining amino acids are utilized as fuel for the body and are never converted to protein. Eggs contain the most perfect ratio and are used as a standard to rate the protein quality of all other foods.

The protein found in fish and dairy products is 80 percent usable, the protein in meat and poultry is 65 to 70 percent usable, as is the protein in brown rice, wheat germ, mushrooms, and fresh corn. The disadvantage of obtaining protein from rice, wheat germ, and mushrooms is that an enormous amount must be consumed to obtain the same quantity as meat provides. For instance, you'd have to eat three cups of cooked brown rice to get the usable protein found in three ounces of hamburger.

Most vegetables, seeds, legumes, nuts, and grains contain a limited essential amino acid, but when two complementary foods are eaten together the limited amino acid in one food is complemented by the large amount of that amino acid in the other food. Thus, a pattern is formed that may yield a higher utilization percentage than that of meat. Nature has made it easy to combine proteins. The basic complementary foods are:

1. Grains with beans
2. A small amount of meat, dairy products, poultry, or seafood with beans or grains
3. Beans and seeds. Sesame seeds are the only seeds that complement grains
4. Raw green vegetables combine well with all cooked protein foods

Some nutritious combinations are tortillas and beans, a bit of fish with rice, sesame seeds and rice, cereal and milk, baked beans and brown bread, macaroni and cheese, blackeyed peas and corn bread, potatoes with sour cream or cheese, garbanzo beans and sesame seeds, peanut butter on bread. However, in the case of peanut butter and whole grain bread, a little milk is necessary to make the protein complete. It also helps get the sandwich down.

When any of the above foods are eaten in the suggested combinations, the body obtains protein of the same quality as meat and more total usable protein than if any of these foods are eaten separately.

While sufficient protein is absolutely essential to life, an excess of protein is converted into carbohydrate or fat. The normal body can handle this conversion with no problem, but it does cause a strain on the liver and kidneys. Excess protein is used for energy, but the same energy can be obtained from fruits and vegetables or grains. These foods supply essential nutrients not generally found in meat protein and are available at a fraction of their cost. Protein not needed for body building or fuel is stored as fat. It can never be used as protein again.

To obtain maximum food value, the best way to consume protein foods is to eat a small amount at each meal rather than a large portion once a day. If such a food is eaten raw, rare, or cooked at a very low temperature, its protein can be more easily utilized by the body. The essential amino acid lysine is destroyed when protein is heated over 240 degrees. This means that protein found in most commercially canned or dried products, roasted cereals, seeds or nuts, or foods cooked in a pressure cooker may be deficient in this essential amino acid. When eating one of these foods, it's a good idea to include a food that contains a quantity of lysine such as raw or lightly cooked greens, legumes that have not been heated above boiling, raw-milk cheese, brewers' yeast, or raw wheat germ.

Proteins are digested in the stomach by hydrochloric acid. Most people over forty, or those who have had a low protein intake over a period of time, are apt to lack sufficient hydrochloric acid for the proper digestion of protein. It is a good idea to eat protein foods at the beginning of the meal because more hydrochloric acid is present in the stomach at that time. Often a little wine or apple cider vinegar will stimulate the flow of hydrochloric acid.

To establish the correct number of grams of protein you need each day, divide your ideal body weight by 2.2. This allowance is based upon the protein quality of meat. Children require more protein per pound than adults.

CARBOHYDRATES

Only in industrial countries are incomplete refined foods the chief source of carbohydrates. Healthy people in primitive cultures receive their carbohydrates from whole grains, beans, and seeds—foods that still have the ability to produce new life.

Carbohydrates are found in grains, seeds, nuts, fruits, and vegetables in the form of starch or sugar, and they furnish most of the body's energy. The body's demand for energy supersedes every other one of its needs. It will use protein for carbohydrate, ignoring the special functions of protein if it needs energy and lacks carbohydrates.

Starches are encased within plant cells and, for the body to utilize them, they must be broken down by cooking, liquefying, fermenting, or grinding before they are swallowed. The body changes all starch to sugar. Digestion of carbohydrates begins in the mouth during the chewing process. You may have noticed that bread chewed long enough begins to taste sweet.

Carbohydrates are essential to ensure the complete digestion and metabolism of fats and proteins. Some carbohydrate must be present before protein can be converted into carbohydrate. All flesh meats, poultry, and fish are the only foods which contain absolutely no carbohydrates.

A 128-pound woman requires 125 grams of carbohydrates per day for brain function alone, and 125 grams of carbohydrates is equal to 500 calories, or about half the amount of calories allowed in reducing diets. The popular low-carbohydrate reducing diets can be extremely dangerous when allowed for even short periods. Not only will the brain be severely deprived of glucose, but the drastic restriction of carbohydrate will prevent the conversion of protein into sugar, making it impossible to maintain a normal blood sugar level.

Obviously, refined sugar is a poor form of carbohydrate. It fills the energy requirements without providing the nutrients needed for its efficient use. In this manner it robs the body of nutrients necessary for digestion. It puts a strain on the body by causing an energy surge and it replaces the foods that do provide essential nutrients. As is well known, excess carbohydrates are stored as fat.

FATS

Healthy people in primitive or unsophisticated cultures obtained their needed fats from the oils found in seeds, grains or butterfat; raw animal fat was sometimes available. In most industrial countries today the main source of fat is unnaturally fattened animals, or vegetable oils that have been heated to high temperatures or otherwise processed.

Fat is so essential that the main cause of death among inland Eskimo populations is fat starvation. Fat is the energy storage bank of man and animal. Vital for the assimilation of Vitamins A, D, E, and K, it is also the source of essential fatty acids, and is needed to cushion vital organs as well. It is used in the production of bile, and regulates body temperature. Fats add satisfaction to a meal because of their slow rate of digestion. They also add flavor to foods. A deficiency of fat can cause dry lifeless hair, rough scaly skin, loss of sexual vitality, menstrual difficulties, and vitamin deficiencies.

Fats vary by degrees from saturated to unsaturated. Pecans and walnuts contain only 7 percent saturated fat. Percentages of saturated fat in some other foods are: eggs, 32 percent; beef, 48 percent; cow's milk, 55 percent; butter, 57 percent; and coconut oil, 86 percent. Coconut oil has a higher saturated fat content than any other food; it is used in most imitation dairy products such as nondairy creamers, margarines, artificial sour cream, and nearly all processed foods labeled as containing vegetable oil.

Three essential fatty acids, sometimes called Vitamin F, are found in unsaturated fat. They are needed for the proper utilization of cholesterol and saturated fats. The best sources of these essential fatty acids are nuts, seeds, grains and avocados.

Scientists agree that rancid fats are extremely detrimental to health. Not only do they cause digestive problems in humans but they cause cancer in laboratory animals. Fats become rancid when they are exposed to oxygen either in the cupboard or in a fryer. At the point when the fat begins to smoke it becomes rancid. The most stable fats are butter, sesame oil, and olive oil. Sesame oil smokes at 600 degrees, corn oil at 450, shortening and lard at 365.

Continuously heated fat used in deep-fryers becomes rancid. Deep-frying is fine; just make sure the fat is fresh and that it is not heated to a smoking temperature.

The natural oils in flour, wheat germ, shelled seeds, and shelled nuts soon become rancid, so these foods should be kept tightly sealed in a cool, dark place and used as quickly as possible. It is best to buy them in small quantities and only as needed. Commonly available polyunsaturated vegetable oils, unless specified on the label as "unrefined" or "cold-pressed" have undergone heat extraction, bleaching, and deodorization in which oils are usually held above 480°F for several hours.

Hydrogenation is another insult to oils. This solidifying process destroys the essential fatty acids and reduces the body's ability to metabolize the oil. Some physicians believe that it is the molecules of hydrogenated fat, absorbed by the cells in place of essential fatty acids, rather than foods containing cholesterol that cause high levels of cholesterol in the blood. Hydrogenated fats are found in nearly all processed foods that normally contain shortening. This includes margarine and most peanut butter.

Fats have two related constituents, sort of close cousins, cholesterol and lecithin. Cholesterol is found in saturated fats and is also produced by the liver. Studies show that a diet high in animal fat (2 eggs, 8 oz. beef, 2 cups whole milk, 1½ T. butter) includes about 800 milligrams of cholesterol a day, while the normal adult liver produces about 3,000 milligrams or more daily. (Liver biopsies show that when the dietary intake of cholesterol is extremely high, the production of cholesterol by the liver is almost suppressed. Conversely, when diets are very low in cholesterol, the liver overproduces, causing the amount of cholesterol in the blood to increase.) Cholesterol is essential because it creates the raw material from which Vitamin D, sex hormones, adrenal hormones, and bile salts are made.

In the early 1960s, J. D. Hunter studied the health of two Polynesian island groups, the Mitiaro and the Atiu. They live on a diet similar to the Marquesan diet, low in calories but rich in highly saturated coconut oil. While he found their serum cholesterol levels high, he was unable to discover by electrocardiographic readings any tendency to coronary heart disease.

These findings support the belief of Dr. Roger J. Williams and others that "the nutritional environment of the body cells involving minerals, amino acids and vitamins is crucial and that the amount of fat or cholesterol consumed is relatively inconsequential."

Lecithin appears to be a homogenizing agent capable of breaking up fat and cholesterol into tiny particles, which then readily pass into body tissue. Lecithin can be produced in the intestines, providing certain B vitamins and essential fatty acids are in the diet. Lecithin is found in egg yolk, liver, brains, soybeans, human milk (but not cow's milk), and all natural oils. When oils are hydrogenated, the lecithin is discarded. Similarly, the B vitamins essential in the body's production of lecithin are removed when grains are processed. When lecithin is destroyed in a blood sample from a healthy individual, within minutes large fat particles form in such quantities that the sample appears milky in color. These saturated fat particles are called triglycerides. The more triglycerides in the blood, the greater the clotting tendency.

While excess fat is stored in the body and causes weight gain, too little fat can do the same thing. When fatty acids are lacking in the diet, the body apparently changes sugar to fat more rapidly than normal. As this happens, the blood sugar level drops quickly producing the feeling of hunger. A deficiency in essential fatty acids is also responsible for water or fluid retention.

Ideally, everyone, whether on a reducing diet or not should consume at least 1 tablespoon of unsaturated oil a day in one of the following equivalents: 1½ tablespoons of mayonnaise, 6 tablespoons of avocado, 2 tablespoons of peanut butter, 2 tablespoons of seeds or nuts, 2 tablespoons of Thousand Island dressing, 9 tablespoons of wheat germ, 1 tablespoon of cold pressed or unrefined vegetable or seed oil. The very best sources of unsaturated oil are obtained directly from fresh raw seeds, nuts, and avocados.

The total fat in the normal diet should be restricted to 25 to 30 percent of the total calorie intake. To establish the maximum grams of fat required, divide 30 percent of your ideal calorie intake by 9.

FIBER

A favorite Eskimo recipe reads, roughly, kill bird, freeze, eat whole. The bird referred to is usually a nestling and it is eaten feathers and all, thus providing the Eskimo with much-needed fiber in a meat and fat diet.

Evidence is accumulating that low-fiber diets, those that mark the industrialized countries, are responsible for high blood cholesterol, heart disease, varicose veins, blood clots, obesity, and constipation—the universal disease of civilization. Worst of all, cancer of the colon is directly related to low-fiber diets. Fiber and bulk are absolutely essential for a healthy body. Although they have been almost completely ignored, probably because they contribute no calories and have little direct nutritional value, they do keep the digestive process active and functioning properly.

We get fiber and other bulk foods from the bran or outer coating of grains, fruits, and vegetables, especially the skins and cores. Good sources of fiber and bulk are legumes, nuts and seeds, whole grains, berries, cantaloupe, pears, figs, watermelon, eggplant, lima beans, wild greens, parsnips, yellow winter squash, and artichokes.

These high fiber foods produce larger stools, thus reducing the time that waste matter spends in the intestinal tract, and so shortening the stay of harmful bacteria in the body.

Sugar, refined flour, refined grains, meat, fat, dairy products, and most processed foods contain little or no bulk or fiber. The Tuareg of the Sahara desert balance their low-fiber milk diet with high-fiber dates and grains.

While Dr. Denis P. Burkitt found the daily intake of fiber of the Gandans of Lake Victoria to be 25 grams, it is believed that only about 15 grams a day provide enough fiber for proper elimination. With our refined foods and low residual diets, however, it is estimated that the average American is lucky to obtain as much as 5 grams daily.

LIQUID

No matter where one may wander in Hunza, there is some sort of water at hand, either in an irrigation ditch or a mountain stream. The water comes from melting glaciers, is pearly gray in color, and so full of minerals that it actually satisfies hunger.

About two-thirds of our total body weight consists of water. Next to oxygen it is the most important constituent for the maintenance of life. Dehydration kills far faster than starvation.

Water is the medium in which all the body's chemical reactions take place. It regulates the body temperature, acts as a transporting medium for nutrients, makes up a part of all tissue, and is essential for the excreting of waste from the intestinal tract as well as the kidneys.

A person's intake of water must equal his output. The normal body does not store water so what is lost must be replaced. On the average, a person loses about three quarts of fluid a day through lungs, kidneys, bowels, and sweat glands. Approximately one-and-a-half to two quarts must be replaced by liquids consumed during the day. The rest comes from the water content of foods and as the end product of food metabolism.

Hard water, that is, water with a high mineral content, can supply substantial amounts of the minerals needed by the body. In areas where water has a high mineral content, studies show that there is less heart disease, lower cholesterol levels, less high blood pressure, and less dental decay. Soft or distilled water can actually leach minerals from the body.

Rather than drink large amounts of liquid with a meal, it is better to drink it at other times. Too much liquid at mealtime may interfere with proper digestion and the utilization of nutrients.

VITAMINS AND MINERALS

During his travels, Dr. Price found that the healthy primitives he studied had a vitamin and mineral intake four to ten times greater than that recommended by most government experts. Most nutritionists believe that to maintain our vigor in this modern stress-filled world, today's healthy person needs many times more nutrients than our less sophisticated neighbors need to maintain their good health.

Vitamins are organic food substances that are essential in the body's utilization of proteins, fats, and carbohydrates. With the exception of a few which the body can partially synthesize, natural vitamins are manufactured only by plants. We must obtain our vitamins from the food we eat.

Vitamins, basic though they are, cannot function without minerals. These come from plants, which in turn receive them from the soil. If a mineral is lacking in the soil, it will be lacking in the plant and, eventually, in the body. An imbalance of minerals or the presence of harmful ones in the soil follows the same pattern.

Until recently vitamins and minerals have been thought important only as protection against the deficiency diseases that occur when they are missing in the diet. It was believed that vitamin and mineral intake only needed to be enough to prevent these diseases. Today we know that the functions of vitamins and minerals are closely interrelated, that individuals vary in the amounts they need for good health, and that when taken in amounts larger than previously thought essential, they enable the body to resist disease and infections. They promote the healing of wounds, maintain healthy nervous and cardiovascular systems; build strong bones, teeth, and blood; prevent premature aging; and help resist the effects of smog, toxic elements, and pollutants.

Vitamins build strong bodies, but they themselves are fragile. They are destroyed by air, light, heat, rancid fat, smoke, and chemicals. The normal processes of the body also destroy them. While minerals cannot be destroyed, they can be removed along with the vitamins when food is refined. Both minerals and vitamins are leached into the liquids used in cleaning, cooking, or rinsing of foods. They are also lost by excessive perspiration, urinating, diarrhea, or vomiting.

Greens contain varying amounts of oxalic acid, while phytic acid is found in grains and nuts. These acids occasionally interfere with the absorption of the minerals contained in these foods. However, it appears that the body tends to condition itself to these acids; so if they are eaten often enough, the undesirable effects are reduced.

New vitamins and minerals are still being discovered and many that are currently known to exist have still not been thoroughly researched. It is believed that when they are, each will prove to be as important to our good health as the following vitamins and minerals are known to be.

Vitamin A

The Eskimos, who never suffered from snow blindness, had a successful treatment for explorers who developed this affliction. They fed them animal eyes. The Vitamin A content in the eye of the animal was so high that it restored sight.

The chief dietary sources of Vitamin A are fish liver oils, liver, kidneys, egg yolk, cream, butter, fish roe, bone marrow, eel, and the flesh of fatty fish. The richest of all animal sources is found in the fatty tissues behind the eye. Carotene, the yellow pigment in many foods, is converted into Vitamin A by intestinal mucosa. This pigment is present in all yellow, red, or green vegetables. Outstanding sources of carotene are dark greens, carrots, red peppers, sweet potato, and cantaloupe.

Vitamin A is destroyed by nitrates and nitrites found in synthetic fertilizers and used as preservatives in many processed foods. It is also destroyed by oxygen and bright light. Rancid fat, smoke, smog, and baking soda—often used in cooking—also destroy it. Chronic diarrhea and certain laxatives containing mineral oil can also reduce the Vitamin A in the body. Diabetics probably cannot convert carotene into its usable form.

The prime importance of Vitamin A is in preventing infections of the skin, the eye, and the mucous membranes that line all body cavities. It also enables your eyes to adjust quickly when going from a light to a dark area. Research has established that a lack of Vitamin A will weaken resistance to an enormous range of diseases including tuberculosis, pneumonia, emphysema, salmonella, polio, impaired vision, and many types of cancer. Hay fever and other respiratory ailments are also more prevalent when the Vitamin A intake in the diet is low. It is a fat-soluble vitamin, and so not properly absorbed unless sufficient fat or oil is also ingested. Adequate protein as well as Vitamins D and E are also essential for its proper metabolism. Vitamin A is stored mainly in the liver, but a small amount is also found in the kidneys and lungs. Extra Vitamin A is stored as carotene in the fatty deposits of the body. The yellowish color of carotene is sometimes visible in the palm of the hand.

Excessive intake of vitamins is under constant discussion. How much is too much? Although a daily intake exceeding 50,000 international units (I.U.'s) may be toxic to an adult who does not have a deficiency of this important vitamin, no deaths have ever been reported from a Vitamin A overdose as they have from drugs as simple as aspirin. To ensure a sufficient quantity of Vitamin A in the diet, the government recommends a daily allowance for adult men of 5,000 I.U. and 4,000 for women. Nutritionists feel that an intake of 20,000 I.U.'s per day is not too much, and Dr. Price found that all healthy cultures ingested at least that amount.

Through the normal process of vision, Vitamin A is lost from the eye. The brighter the light or reflection of light, as from snow, the faster is Vitamin A lost from the body. Therefore, the requirements for Vitamin A are greater than normal for those who are exposed to bright light, either artificial or sunlight.

B complex

By and large, the more primitive cultures seem to be stress-free, and less prone to senseless violence. This is due in part to their isolation, but attention must also be given to their diet. The enormous amount of refined sugar consumed throughout the Western or industrialized nations, amounting now to more than two pounds per person per week, produces a serious Vitamin B deficiency. This causes nervous disorders, fatigue, and poor digestion, all of which can lead to antisocial behavior. It would be interesting to speculate whether the behavior of troublesome individuals could be modified if they were fed a highly nutritious and healthful diet. Most institutional food depends heavily upon refined, starchy, overcooked, and filling items rather than on nutritionally balanced meals. Can behavior be corrected by simply improving diet? It is an intriguing question.

The B complex vitamins are a group of closely related, water-soluble vitamins whose function is not clearly understood even today. Researchers have now isolated twenty-two members of the B-complex group; more will surely come to light in the future. There is such a close interrelation among these vitamins that a deficiency of one may impair the utilization of others. Likewise, a vitamin imbalance brought about by excessive intake of one of the group may create a deficiency of others in the family.

The major functions of the B complex center around the nervous system; they may be the single most important factor in the health of our nerves. They are also essential in the metabolism of protein and the digestion of carbohydrates.

Deficiency symptoms of this group are rather generalized. They may show up as a loss of appetite, lack of initiative, depression, irritability, fatigue, eczema, a sore mouth or tongue, a craving for sugar or alcohol, numerous digestive problems, constipation, or hypoglycemia.

Many or all of the B vitamins are destroyed, removed, or altered by the milling and refining of grains, as well as by unusual stress including gross physical activity or emotional trauma. Other substances that blight these vitamins are baking soda, high temperature cooking, sulfa drugs, oral contraceptives, antibiotics, barbiturates, sugar, caffeine, alcohol, and alkalizers. Hybrid crops are deficient in some of the B complex. Being soluble, the B vitamins can be dissolved into water and flushed from the body if an unusually large amount of liquid is consumed. It is plain to see that the B vitamins must be ingested daily to maintain their proper balance and quantity.

The complete B complex is generally found in organ meats, wheat germ, whole grains, brewers' yeast, legumes, seeds, and nuts. An incomplete form of the complex is found in blackstrap molasses, insects, muscle meat, fish, poultry, dairy products, eggs, and vegetables. A few members of the complex are synthesized in the body, mostly in the intestinal tract, but this only occurs if the proper bacteria are present. Fermented foods help sustain this type of bacteria so such foods are important assistants in nurturing the body's store of B vitamins. These friendly bacteria are destroyed by antibiotics and sulfa drugs so after an illness special attention must be given to proper diet.

As indicated above, B complex vitamins cannot be stored in the body, but must be supplied daily. Adelle Davis, the late famous nutritionist, based adult requirements for the various B vitamins upon the proportions in which they are found in human tissue.

Element	Amount in Human Tissue	RDA*
B_1	2 to 10 mg	.5 mg per 1,000 calories
B_2	same as B_1	.55 mg per 1,000 calories
Niacin	10 times B_1	6.6 mg per 1,000 calories
B_6	same as B_1	2 mg per 100 grams of protein
Pantothenic acid	10 times B_1	5 to 10
PABA†	20 times B_1	none
Inositol	500 times B_1	none
Choline	500 times B_1	none
Folic acid	same as B_1, with a good B_{12} source	0.4
B_{12}	3 mcg.	3 to 25 mcg.

The best way to ensure a complete intake of all the B vitamins your body must have is to eat several sources of the complete complex each day.

B_1, or *thiamine,* is essential for the digestion of carbohydrates. The more sugar and starches you consume, the greater your need for this vitamin. Thiamine has been effective in the treatment of alcoholism, diabetes, and some mental disorders. Some exceptionally good sources of Vitamin B_1 are pork, sunflower seeds, kidneys, rice polishings, liver, soybeans, and eggplant.

An enzyme in raw fish destroys Vitamin B_1 in the body, but fermented foods, acids like lemon or lime juice, and heat all destroy

* Recommended daily allowance.
† Para-aminobenzoic acid.

this enzyme. It is interesting to note that the Japanese, who are so dependent upon this vitamin because of their high intake of rice, have always consumed their raw fish in soy sauce, a fermented soybean product.

B_2, *riboflavin,* is important in cell respiration, good vision, and proper metabolism of all other nutrients. It has been found to have a role in preventing cataracts, and in some cases has even reversed their development if given in large quantities over a period of time. Good sources of riboflavin are organ meats, almonds, green leaves, and mushrooms. It is also found in cream but not in nonfat milk. Riboflavin is quite fragile and is destroyed by light. Glass jars and clear plastic wrap cause the loss of over half the riboflavin found in the food in as little as two hours. It is also destroyed by oral contraceptives.

Niacin, another of the B complex, helps "keep our heads in order." It is essential for mental health. In massive doses, niacin has been found to be an effective cure for many cases of schizophrenia. It has been estimated that 80 percent of the murders and other crimes of violence are committed by people with schizoid tendencies. Niacin has also been used in the treatment of alcoholism. Some fine sources of niacin are fish, poultry, and muscle meat.

B_6, *pyridoxine,* is essential for the digestion of protein. The more protein eaten, the more B_6 needed. It is also used in the formation of red blood cells, of antibodies so necessary for the fighting of infections, and for the proper metabolism of fat. B_6 has been effective in preventing edema and, during pregnancy, in relieving the symptoms of morning sickness; it also alleviates the nausea following radiation treatment. Certain kinds of rheumatism respond well to pyridoxine treatment. Bananas, avocados, milk, and egg yolk are all good sources of B_6. As with other B complex vitamins, oral contraceptives destroy B_6.

Following are some of the less well-known B vitamins which are also critical in maintaining our health.

Pantothenic acid promotes the production of cortisone, creates antibodies, and plays a large role in alleviating the tendency to allergic reactions. It has been used in place of ACTH or cortisone in the treatment of allergies, arthritis, and gout with some success, and without undesirable side effects. Good sources of this important B vitamin are egg yolk, organ meats, sesame seeds, turkey, and peanuts. It is found in many foods, but is very unstable when exposed to heat or freezing.

Para-aminobenzoic acid (PABA) is synthesized by healthy intestinal bacteria. It assists in the metabolism of protein and in the formation of red blood cells. Some doctors believe that PABA increases the efficiency of cortisone and insulin and helps raise estrogen activity. PABA ointment is considered a "wonder drug" in preventing skin damage from sunburn. Large quantities of PABA are found in liver, milk, and eggs.

Inositol is believed to be essential for the production of lecithin. It seems that men need more inositol than women because a deficiency appears to be responsible for baldness. Concentrations of inositol are found in organs that need a constant supply of energy such as the heart and the brain. It can be produced in a healthy body. Among the richest food sources are blackstrap molasses, wheat germ, brains, heart, citrus fruit, cantaloupe, and dried beans.

Choline, a constituent of lecithin, serves the body by metabolizing and transporting fat. It has been used successfully to lower blood cholesterol, reduce high blood pressure, and shield the body from the effects of some toxic drugs. It can be manufactured by the body, but it is an integral part of a team so folic acid, B_{12}, B_6, magnesium, and methionine (an amino acid) must also be present for choline to be produced. Good sources for this obscure but necessary B vitamin are egg yolks, soybeans, organ meats, milk, peanuts, and wheat germ.

Biotin seems to be essential in the synthesis and breakdown of fatty acids and amino acids. Researchers find that diabetics have a particularly high need for biotin, while a deficiency is also being linked with heart disease and lung problems. Biotin can be synthesized in healthy intestines, and the best food sources are liver, peanuts, cauliflower, mushrooms, dried beans, and halibut. It is, however, quite fragile, and caffeine is known to deplete the system of this B vitamin. It is also destroyed by avidin, an antagonist enzyme found in raw egg white. Eaten occasionally, raw egg white is not harmful, but over a period of time large amounts could cause a biotin deficiency. This harmful egg-white enzyme is destroyed when the albumen right under the shell is heated to 140 degrees.

B_{12} is vital in the formation of red blood cells and the production of bone marrow and nerve tissue. It is the only B vitamin that is stored in the body, where it is found in the liver. A deficiency of B_{12} causes pernicious anemia, which can be fatal if untreated. It is the only B vitamin that exists almost exclusively in food of animal origin, which means that vegetarians are apt to suffer a deficiency of Vitamin B_{12}. The only foods other than those of animal origin that contain appreciable traces of B_{12} are wheat germ, soybeans, garbanzo sprouts, seaweed, peanuts, and certain varieties of brewers' yeast. The best sources of B_{12} are liver; kidney; flesh meat of beef, pork, or lamb; fish; eggs; and milk. In an interesting symbiosis, Vitamin B_{12} is absorbed by an enzyme produced in the stomach. If a deficiency of B_{12} exists, the stomach cannot produce this enzyme. Even if sufficient B_{12} is added to the diet, it cannot be assimilated so it must be administered by injection until balance is restored. Like many other vitamins, B_{12} is destroyed by oral contraceptives.

Folic acid is important in the formation of red blood cells and nucleic acid; it must also be present for proteins to be properly utilized. Large doses of folic acid can disguise the symptoms of pernicious anemia, but they cannot cure it, so they must be obtained by prescription. Some of the best sources of folic acid are liver, dark green leaves, asparagus, and brewers' yeast. Again, oral contraceptives can destroy folic acid.

Vitamin B_{15}, pangamic acid, has the curative and protective powers of Vitamin E. Russian experimenters have used it successfully to reverse the effects of premature aging. They have also found it effective in improving athletic performances and in the treatment of circulatory problems, heart conditions, elevated blood cholesterol, diabetes, alcoholism, and drug addiction. B_{15} is found in fruit seed kernels, sunflower and pumpkin seeds, whole grains, and brewers' yeast. It is highly regarded in Russia, where it is considered a life-saving vitamin, but in the United States it is not considered an essential nutrient.

Nitrilosides, Vitamin B_{17}, is the most controversial vitamin ever discovered. Court battles are being waged over the importing and use of this vitamin because in many countries it is considered to be a successful cancer fighter. Doctors in the United States dispute this claim and, along with the FDA, have decided there is not enough evidence to support its alleged benefits. Laetrile, the drug made from B_{17}, is given to many terminal cancer patients in other countries, principally Mexico, and the pattern of improvement among patients receiving the drug has been encouraging to doctors and cancer victims. Despite these reports it is against the law to sell or dispense laetrile in the United States. The principal source of B_{17} is apricot pits. In fact, all seeds, legumes, maize, millet, buckwheat, cassava, sorghum, and flax contain some B_{17}. Sprouting seeds increase their B_{17} content fifty times or more. It is not found in brewers' yeast.

Vitamin C

For centuries man has suffered from scurvy. Until a source of Vitamin C was discovered, long sea voyages were virtually impossible because many crew members died or became incapacitated enroute. The early settlers of the United States were no exception. When scurvy struck the struggling band and threatened the future of the colony, the Indians showed them how to make a tea of pine needles that was guaranteed to help. Indeed it did; the Vitamin C content of the pine needles was enough to cure the existing cases and prevent future ones.

Vitamin C is present in most fresh fruits, vegetables, and flowers. Some of the best sources are citrus fruits, peppers, tomatoes, dark greens, raw berries, sprouts, raw seaweed, and wild rose hips—the bulbous part remaining after the petals have fallen. It is also found in raw liver; fresh, raw flesh meat; stomach contents of animals; and adrenal glands.

Because it is the most easily destroyed of all the vitamins, it is best to consume Vitamin C in fresh raw foods. With the exception of that found in some acid-based foods like oranges or tomatoes, heat, light and oxygen destroy it. Fright, worry, or other stress situations can also destroy Vitamin C. Drugs as innocent as aspirin or antihistamines can also damage it seriously. Nor are these the only menaces to this vital element of our diet. It is destroyed by baking soda, cyclamates, smog, and smoke. One cigarette uses up 30 milligrams of Vitamin C. It is also dissolved into rinsing and cooking liquids.

Having enumerated its weaknesses, let's look at its capabilities, which are many. Vitamin C stimulates the production of antibodies and white blood cells, thus strengthening our resistance to infection. It aids in tissue repair, helps form collagen which is needed to heal wounds, and promotes healthy blood vessels. When given in large amounts, it has been used successfully to kill viruses, to lower cholesterol levels, and to prevent colds. It has been used to help diabetics by lowering their insulin requirements, to heal poisonous insect bites, and to cure some childhood diseases. It can also prevent muscle cramps following exercise and, when teamed with antibiotics, helps them work more efficiently. Recent research indicates that Vitamin C may be a factor in reducing the risk of cancer. Its role in assisting other nutrients includes aiding folic acid, iron utilization, and helping Vitamin E protect unsaturated fatty acids from dangerous oxidation. The list of its benefits is almost endless.

Vitamin C is not stored in the body; it must be obtained daily. Because the body can absorb only a certain amount during any given period, it is better to take small doses often rather than one large dose. The government's recommended daily allowance is 45 milligrams. Most nutritionists feel that 500 milligrams should be the minimum daily dose of this valuable vitamin.

Bioflavonoids are found in most of the fruits and flowers rich in Vitamin C and help this vitamin work better. While Vitamin C is generally found in the juice and pulp of the fruit, the bioflavonoids are found in the fibrous white membranes and pulp of these foods. The richest source of them is the white membrane of citrus fruits and peppers. Bioflavonoid intake should equal about 2 to 20 percent of Vitamin C consumption.

Vitamin K

Vitamin K is synthesized in healthy intestines, but some of its best food sources are liver, greens, grains, egg yolk, and alfalfa sprouts. It is essential to the production of prothrombin, the substance that causes our blood to coagulate. Vitamin K is destroyed by freezing, rancidity, exposure to ultraviolet light, polluted air, irradiation, mineral oil, and some blood-thinning chemicals. The natural ability to synthesize this vitamin is destroyed by sulfa drugs and antibiotics. There is no recommended daily allowance.

Vitamin E

Before wheat was refined, every person in the United States received approximately 150 units of Vitamin E every day. It is estimated that most people now receive less than 5 units on their diet of refined and manufactured foods. Vitamin E prevents oil from oxidizing in the body, in the bottle, or in the whole grain. Found in whole grains, nuts, legumes, seeds, wheat germ, eggs, vegetables, and seed oils, Vitamin E is destroyed or removed when these foods are refined or exposed to oxygen, ultraviolet radiation, freezing, or bleaching agents used in making white flour. Iron salts, synthetic estrogens, rancid unsaturated fat, and oral contraceptives all destroy this vitamin in the body. Vitamin E is one of the most fragile, but also one of the most important discovered thus far.

Vitamin E has a profound effect in maintaining the tone and health of the cardiovascular system. It dilates blood vessels, strengthens heart action, lessens scarring of the heart after a coronary attack, and keeps unsaturated fatty acids from turning into toxic peroxides in the body or in the food. It promotes the health and long life of the red blood cells and is a natural anticlotting agent. A valuable aid in the healing of burns and skin grafts, it is also used successfully to treat gangrene. Vitamin E, along with Vitamin A, has been found to protect laboratory animals from some of the damage arising from air pollution. It is also beneficial in the treatment of phlebitis, emphysema, gallstones, varicose veins, and bedsores. Of particular importance for women is its role in regulating the menstrual cycle and preventing miscarriages.

Vitamin E combines with the circulating fatty acids that otherwise would merge with oxygen, thus keeping the oxygen pure and unbound so it can nourish tissues better. Even if blood flow is reduced as a result of narrowed arteries, the total amount of oxygen in the blood is kept high because the Vitamin E has kept it pure. This is particularly valuable to heart disease sufferers and people who engage in strenuous sports.

Vitamin E is fat soluble so, for the body to assimilate it, fat must be present. It is one of the few vitamins that the body can store.

The daily requirement established by the government is 10 to 15 units, but most nutritionists recommend 200 to 600 units a day.

It is vitally important to understand the need for Vitamin E. This need increases as the intake of unsaturated oil increases. A diet high in unsaturated oil which does not include a sufficient Vitamin E intake can lead to heart disease, cancer, and other degenerative problems. The proper ratio appears to be about ten units of Vitamin E for each tablespoon of unsaturated oil consumed.

Vitamin D

Rickets, a Vitamin D deficiency disease, is relatively rare today, except in some tropical countries where children are kept covered with clothes to shield them from the sun, or where women shield their faces as well as their bodies. The very best source of Vitamin D is sunlight.

Vitamin D is produced directly on the skin through a reaction of the ultraviolet rays of the sun and the natural oils of the body. The Vitamin D produced in this manner is absorbed directly into the bloodstream. The only food source of Vitamin D in quantities sufficient to promote health is fish liver oils. However, other sources are sunflower seeds, soybeans, flesh of oily fish such as mackerel or sardines, egg yolk (if the hen sat in the sun), cream, butter, roe, bone marrow, bones, mushrooms, guinea pigs, insects, and milk which is fortified with Vitamin D.

Paradoxically, sunlight on food destroys its Vitamin D and mineral oil removes it from the body. It is important to know that showering right after exposure to sunlight will wash off the Vitamin D before it has had a chance to penetrate. So it's a good idea to wait a couple of hours after sunbathing before hopping into the shower.

The utilization of calcium in the body is regulated by Vitamin D. Working in conjunction, they strengthen teeth and bones, so a Vitamin D deficiency is similar to a calcium deficiency.

Fat or oil is essential for the utilization of Vitamin D, either from the natural oils on the skin or in the food. It has been estimated that as little as half an hour's exposure to sunlight on the hands and face every day is sufficient to provide the Vitamin D needed by our systems. The weather should be clear, however, because ultraviolet rays cannot penetrate fog or smog, and it must be out-of-doors as the rays cannot penetrate window glass.

The daily requirement determined by the government is 400 units, but most nutritionists feel that up to 1,600 units give the best protection. Because it can be stored in the body, Vitamin D may be toxic if half a million units are taken daily over a period of several months.

Calcium and Phosphorus

Primitive people maintained a good calcium—phosphorus balance by eating the bones along with the meat. Many contemporary people are carnivores, but they remove the bones from the meat instead of eating them. By doing this, they very likely upset their mineral balance.

Calcium and phosphorus should be considered together because they are so closely related. A deficiency of calcium or an excess of phosphorus can cause a deficiency of the other. Ideally, calcium intake should equal or be up to two-and-a-half times that of phosphorus. A ratio of less than two parts calcium to three parts phosphorus, regardless of the absolute levels of intake, produces the same results as a simple calcium deficiency.

Foods containing a good calcium—phosphorus ratio are canned fish with bones soft enough to eat, milk products (except cottage cheese), sesame seeds, corn tortillas, bones, and bean curd.

The calcium in fermented milk is the easiest for the body to utilize. For the calcium to be assimilated, the phosphorus, magnesium, Vitamin D, unsaturated fatty acids, and hydrochloric acid must all be present in sufficient quantity. The primary functions of calcium are to build strong bones and teeth, help in blood clotting, maintain the acid/alkali balance in the body, and regulate the heartbeat. Best calcium sources are bones, milk and milk products, sesame seeds, blackstrap molasses, bean curd, pickled pigs' feet, fins and tails of fish, dark green leafy vegetables, stone ground grains, and certain kinds of clay.

Calcium deficiencies cause tooth decay; soft bones; muscle cramps, particularly in the legs; and the symptom often mistakenly called growing pains in children. It also leads to insomnia and premenstrual depression. Osteoporosis, the degeneration of bones usually associated with old age, is due to a calcium deficiency. The body maintains a certain level of calcium in the bloodstream at all times. When this supply falls below requirements, calcium is released from the bones, thus weakening them.

If calcium is consistently lacking in the diet, the skeleton will shrink and the bones become brittle or porous to the point where the slightest fall will result in a fracture. Sometimes the bone will simply give way and break even before a fall. In the United States, approximately every third person will develop osteoporosis.

The recommended daily allowance of calcium is 800 milligrams, but most nutritionists believe that one or more grams is preferable. Dr. Price found that primitive healthy cultures ingested an average of 3.4 grams of calcium a day.

Phosphorus is found in every human cell; thus it plays an important part in almost all the body's chemical reactions. It is essential for the body's production of lecithin. Foods high in phosphorus include all flesh meat, fish, poultry, organ meats, insects, grains, nuts and seeds, brewers' yeast, and legumes.

Nutritionists believe that phosphorus intake should be equal to or less than that of calcium. The daily requirement established by the government is 800 milligrams.

Magnesium

Magnesium is closely related to calcium and phosphorus. It is essential for the proper functioning of nerves and muscles, including that most marvelous muscle of all, the heart. Magnesium may also play an important part in preventing tooth decay. Indeed, it may be more valuable than calcium in this respect. Magnesium has been used successfully in the treatment of diseases of the prostate, heart disease, emotional disturbances, and alcoholism. It is found in seeds, nuts, legumes, wheat germ, greens, figs, apricots, blackstrap molasses, brewers' yeast, chile peppers, and curry powder. A high intake of protein, calcium, or phosphorus requires an increased intake of magnesium. Ideally, magnesium intake should be about half that of calcium. Stone ground and lime-softened corn tortillas contain the most perfect ratio of calcium, phosphorus, and magnesium of all foods.

Sodium and Potassium

Sodium and potassium are closely associated because an excess or deficiency of one affects the other. While most natural foods contain potassium, sodium, like water, must be obtained from sources other than food. It is believed by some scholars that great civilizations have developed in areas with an abundant supply of salt and collapsed when the salt became unobtainable. Early man required sodium to balance the high levels of potassium consumed in his daily diet. Ironically, the situation today is reversed. Processed foods are loaded with salt and additives containing it, while part of the potassium has been removed. Today, we need an additional source of potassium to balance this huge sodium intake. The best solution is to take the salt shaker off the table.

The wide variation in sodium content between natural and processed foods is shown by comparing the 40 milligrams of sodium in three ounces of roast pork and the 1,000 milligrams found in three ounces of ham. In 100 grams of fresh cooked peas there is one milligram of sodium, but in the same quantity of canned peas there are 236 milligrams of sodium, while their potassium content has been reduced from 196 milligrams to 96 milligrams.

The body loses sodium through sweating, vomiting, diarrhea, a high intake of potassium or pepper, or when the adrenal glands become exhausted. Sodium is essential for the formation and flow of saliva and gastric juices, as well as intestinal secretions. It is absolutely vital to the body because it maintains the fluidity of the blood and lymph systems and the water balance in cells. In this action it works in conjunction with potassium. Sodium also enables the nervous system to respond to stimulation and maintains the proper acid/alkali balance in the blood. Too much sodium, however, causes edema and high blood pressure. The general consensus is that we do not need more than 5 grams of sodium daily, but it appears that most people ingest 15 grams or more. Even lightly salting food at the table can add 3 grams per day.

While there is no recommended daily allowance for sodium intake, most nutritionists agree that it should nearly equal that of potassium.

Sources of potassium are blackstrap molasses, greens, potatoes, avocados, bananas, cantaloupe, whole grains, nuts, seeds, and legumes. Potassium is removed from the body by diuretics, digitalis, cortisone, vomiting, diarrhea, too much salt, or processing agents such as sodium nitrate or nitrite used as preservatives. All processing, including commercial freezing and canning, removes some potassium from food.

The interrelationship of minerals is again evidenced by the fact that potassium functions with calcium to regulate muscular activity. This includes maintaining a proper heart rhythm. Another function of potassium is to enable red blood cells to carry carbon dioxide to the lungs.

No specific requirement has been established for the quantity of potassium necessary for health, but again, potassium/sodium intake should be equal.

Iron

The ancient prescription for curing anemia sounds laughable. The patient was supposed to stick rusty nails into a sour apple, leave them overnight, remove the nails, and eat the apple. Curiously, this treatment had some sound basis in fact. Most inorganic iron, even iron rust, is easily utilized by the body. Because an iron deficiency produces anemia, this ancient treatment was probably fairly effective.

Iron available in most foods is not completely assimilated by the body. The iron found in liver, kidney, eggs, and apricots is the most fully absorbed of all sources. Other sources are wheat germ, blackstrap molasses, millet, legumes, greens, nuts, and seeds. A good nonfood source is cast iron cookware. A soup or stew simmered in a cast iron pot leaches iron right into the food. Food that is soft-textured usually contains iron that is more easily absorbed.

Iron is necessary for the formation of hemoglobin. Vitamin C enhances the assimilation of iron, and hydrochloric acid is necessary for proper absorption. Acid or fermented foods serve this function quite well. In a normal healthy person, only about 50 percent of the iron consumed is absorbed by the body, the rest is eliminated as waste. Women have a greater need for iron because they lose it during menstruation. Refined carbohydrates, alkaline preparations, as well as diarrhea all can decrease the amount of iron in the body.

Nutritionists agree that about 10 milligrams per day for an adult male and about twice that amount for an adult female will provide sufficient iron. However, Dr. Price found that healthy primitives often averaged more than five times that amount.

Iodine

Recent research into iodine and its effect on the body has produced some interesting conclusions. Along with preventing goiter, iodine was found to have a number of other important functions. It helps control the energy metabolism of the body and aids in healthy growth and development. It plays an important part in the proper development of the reproductive organs, while there are clear indications that women deficient in iodine are more prone to breast cancer. The best source of iodine is seafood. Kelp is an excellent source, but it isn't popular with most people. Iodized salt is considered acceptable, but its iodine is less easily assimilated than that found in seafood. Fruits and vegetables grown in iodine-rich soil also provide this necessary mineral. Synthetic estrogens, however, can rob the body of iodine.

Trace Minerals

Though little is known of the various functions of most of the trace minerals found in the body, they are essential to life. Needed in only minute quantities, they nevertheless play a role in maintaining vigor and fighting disease.

The trace mineral *zinc* is a constituent of insulin and sperm. It helps in the synthesis of nucleic acid and the metabolism of Vitamin A. Little known and often overlooked, zinc plays an important role in maintaining health. It has been used successfully to speed the healing of wounds, prolong the effects of insulin for diabetics, and help overcome impotency and prostate problems.

Fragile and elusive, zinc can be removed from the body in any number of ways. A large intake of phosphorus such as in a diet too rich in flesh meats, consumption of alcohol, profuse sweating from physical activity, and synthetic estrogens are just some of the enemies of zinc. Furthermore, at one time it was plentiful in all fruits and vegetables, but extensive use of chemical fertilizers and pesticides has leached zinc out of much of our farming land. The best sources of zinc are now bones, liver, kidney, pancreas, oysters and other shellfish, seeds with points, barley, and kelp.

Selenium helps Vitamin E work more effectively both in preventing cancer and heart disease. Because it is stored in the testes in men and lost in semen, males have a greater need for selenium than females. Good sources are brewers' yeast, eggs, and tuna.

Sulphur, essential for the secretion of bile and an important fighter of bacterial infection, is found in vegetables of the cabbage family and most protein foods.

Silicon helps build strong tooth enamel and sturdy bones. Good sources are mushrooms, carrots, liver, buckwheat, oatmeal, and lentils.

Fluorine, found in nature, protects teeth by discouraging the growth of acid-forming bacteria. It also strengthens tooth enamel. Natural fluorine is found in bones, shrimp, and spinach.

Chlorine is a constituent of hydrochloric acid and is needed to help the liver remove toxic waste from the body. The best sources are seaweed, greens, rye, ripe olives, salt, and seafood.

Manganese promotes lactation in nursing mothers and builds up resistance to disease. This trace element can be found in the bran of unmilled grains, greens, beets, egg yolks, legumes, and nuts.

Cobalt plays a role in blood formation. It is a component of Vitamin B_{12} and also promotes iron absorption. It is found in liver and all greens.

Chromium helps the body utilize carbohydrates. The organ meats, brewers' yeast, and cream provide this important element. It is removed in the process of producing nonfat milk.

Molybdenum deficiency can lead to uric acid formation and tooth decay. Fortunately, there is no need to suffer a deficiency, because it is found in legumes, whole grains, greens, organ meats, and whole milk, although it too is removed in making skim milk.

Copper assists in the formation of red blood cells, and the metabolism of amino acids. Organ meats, nuts, legumes, whole grains, brewers' yeast, seafood, kelp, and greens all contain copper.

TIPS ON FOOD STORAGE AND PREPARATION

The following tips can help save many of the nutrients found in food. Foods that are not protected by a thick skin should be stored in a dark place at a temperature of about 45 degrees. When washing foods before cooking, do so quickly and dry them as fast as possible. Dried beans that are soaked overnight should be cooked in the same water.

Many foods do not require salt at all, but those that do should be salted just before serving. Salt added during cooking leaches many nutrients from the foods.

Avoid using a knife to peel foods; it carves off too much of the food value found just beneath the skin. Use a vegetable peeler instead. In many cases, a good scrubbing instead of peeling is all that is necessary to make the skin edible. If foods are to be chopped or cut up before cooking, coating them lightly with oil or an acid liquid like lemon juice or vinegar and returning them covered to the refrigerator will preserve much of their nutritional value.

In cooking fruits or vegetables, it is best to drop them into rapidly boiling water. This will quickly kill the enzymes that destroy vitamins. The heat should then be reduced to a simmer to continue cooking. Protein foods should always be cooked at a low temperature so they remain tender and retain their nutrients and protein quality.

Clear glass cooking utensils let in so much light that considerable vitamin loss results. A cast iron pot with a tight fitting lid is ideal. Whatever kind of pot you use, the food should be covered whenever possible while cooking.

Foods lose all their identity, along with their nutrients, when they are overcooked. If they must be cooked, do it gently and quickly.

Foods cooked until all liquids are gone have suffered terrible vitamin loss. Stuck to the bottom of the pan is where these nutrients will be found. Foods should never be rinsed after cooking.

Always save the liquids from cooked food. Into the stock pot they go or into the freezer for future use in stews, soups, or gravies.

While fresh tomatoes are preferred, canned tomatoes appear to retain more nutrients than other canned vegetables. As a convenience food to use as a base for cooking other fresh foods such as in soup or stew they are acceptable.

Frozen vegetables often contain more nutrients than fresh vegetables bought at the supermarket. They are quickly processed almost immediately after they are picked so that most of their nutrients are preserved. Vegetables and meat at the market may sit a week or more in heat, light and air, all of which destroy vitamins.

Seeds, nuts, sprouts, and fruit are superior raw food sources and whenever possible should be eaten uncooked. Many people have trouble chewing nuts, seeds, and dried fruit thoroughly enough for their proper digestion. Soaking these foods for a few hours or overnight in a liquid or juice such as apple juice, pineapple juice, or even water will make them easier to digest. Be sure to consume the soaking liquid with the food. There is an advantage to occasionally eating cooked greens. Since cooking reduces their volume considerably a person can eat a much larger serving and thus obtain more nutrients than from a raw green salad. Some vegetables, for instance raw carrots, are very tough. It is almost impossible to chew them well enough to obtain all the vitamins they contain. While the unchewed cells do not cause digestive problems, vitamins are lost to the body. It is a good idea to eat these vegetables half cooked, as the Chinese and Japanese do.

TIPS FOR HEALTHFUL EATING

Our body is a fantastic machine, incredible in its complexity, yet simple and functional. Even when mistreated and neglected, it can keep going. Bad fuel may not have an immediate and discernible effect, but over the long run things will begin to malfunction. Degenerative disease will set in and few will suspect poor nutrition, begun long ago, as the initial cause. The problem is that modern civilization and industrialization have caught us in a double squeeze. With the stresses and the pollution we endure plus acquired deficiencies, our nutritional requirements are higher than ever before; but the processed and refined foods we eat result in severe nutritional loss. Many needed elements are missing in the soil, and therefore lacking in our food, making the chances of getting enough of these essential nutrients pretty slim.

All the foods we eat should contribute to our health, not detract from it. Even with the wide array of supplemental vitamins and minerals available, food is still our best source of nutrients. Ideally, a person should obtain one-third of his required protein; a minimum of one-third of desirable body weight in grams of carbohydrate; and one teaspoon of unsaturated fat or its equivalent at each of three meals. Most of the calories needed should be consumed during the day, when the body needs energy most. The lightest meal should be in the evening. At least one raw food should be consumed at each meal. By eating all parts of a plant at one meal, a root, a green, a seed, and a fruit, a good balance of nutrients —known and unknown—can be obtained. If supplements are necessary, the following are some of the best natural concentrated sources.

VITAMINS A AND D	fish liver oil, by spoon or capsule
B COMPLEX VITAMINS	brewers' yeast, rice polishings, wheat germ, and desiccated liver
VITAMIN C COMPLEX	rose hips or acerola cherries
VITAMIN E	wheat germ oil
CALCIUM	bone meal, calcium lactate, or non-instant powdered milk
IRON	desiccated liver or blackstrap molasses
MAGNESIUM	epsom salts, dolomite, or magnesium oxide

Many of these can be found in tablet or powder form. Most other minerals can be found in bone meal, alfalfa seeds, and kelp.

Powdered supplements can be mixed in the blender to make a drink, rather than taking them by the spoonful. Some powdered supplements can be added to cooked foods. When using brewers' yeast, wheat germ, or desiccated liver concentrates, their high phosphorous content must be balanced by additional calcium and magnesium.

Protein chelated mineral tablets, recently introduced, are the most easily assimilated mineral supplements. In taking mineral supplements, it is important that they be taken before a meal because the concentration of hydrochloric acid, essential for the proper metabolism of these minerals, is greatest in the stomach at that time. Acid foods such as citrus fruits, yogurt, wine, or apple cider vinegar help in the absorption of minerals. Oil-based Vitamins A, D, and E should only be taken with meals that contain a good oil or fat source, since fat is necessary for their proper absorption. All the other vitamins can be taken at any time, providing large amounts of liquid are not going to be consumed along with them. It is better to take Vitamins C and B complex in small amounts throughout the day rather than in one large dose.

To enhance the nutritive value of any meal, it should be eaten in a relaxed and happy manner. Good conversation, laughter, and companionship while leisurely enjoying the meal will bring out the best in the food, aid digestion, and reduce the possibility of stomach distress. The family dinner table is no place to discuss controversial matters, air grievances, or relate unpleasant events. All efforts should be made to have it the happiest time of the day.

IMPACT OF GOOD NUTRITION

In 1971, a joint task group made up of representatives of the U.S. Department of Agriculture and the state universities along with land grant colleges, prepared a report entitled "An Evaluation of Research in the United States on Human Nutrition." This report states that if nutrition were improved, it would have a dramatic impact on total health. Most of the leading causes of death in the United States could be reduced by improved diets.

The report goes on to state that the following number of people could be spared death or disease in the course of one year through proper nutrition:

Heart and vascular disease—over 1.2 million fewer cases.
Cancer—64,000 fewer deaths and 120,000 fewer cases.
Respiratory and infectious diseases—49.2 million fewer cases.
Infant health and congenital birth defects—37,500 fewer deaths and 3 million fewer cases.
Arthritis—8 million fewer cases.
Diabetes—2 million cases avoided or improved.
Osteoporosis—3 million fewer cases.
Blindness—16,200 fewer cases.
Corrective lenses—over 17 million fewer lenses required.
Duodenal ulcers—3.5 million fewer acute conditions.
Hay fever and asthma—over 3 million sufferers relieved.
Alcoholism—825,000 fewer addicts.
Mental health—2.5 million fewer disabilities.

This is an incredible list of suffering that could be relieved or prevented by diet alone. The report further stated that in every age group and at every socioeconomic level in the United States, approximately 50 percent of that group is suffering from some form of malnourishment.

Examination of the health of many primitive or isolated cultures still following their ethnic diets shows that they do not suffer extensively from any of these diseases. When they adopt the foods of industrial society, these diseases become rampant.

Have a Care

Man, the relentless survivor, persists in spite of all odds. Inferior to animals in most of the senses, with no fangs or claws to aid in hunting food, his one outstanding advantage is his ability to protect himself.

From tree to cave to house, over the centuries man has continued to improve his defenses. The walled castle, the mountain-top fortress, are examples of protection against other human beings. But human life was constantly threatened by other dangers. Among these were the thousands of poisonous plants that grew everywhere and must have accounted for many deaths among the primitive human groups. Before language and social organization developed, before tribal dietary laws dictated what foods were edible, man could easily have been wiped out by eating the poisonous roots, berries, and fungus plants that grew in such abundance. Over and over again he must have accidentally poisoned himself, not knowing which of the many plants he ate was responsible for his ensuing illness. That he survived these experiences seems to indicate some sort of natural protection, very likely a result of the wide variety of nutritious foods he ate along with the toxic ones. Man's ability to survive natural organic poisons increased over the centuries. Survivors passed on this ability and, as long as their diet retained all the nutritional requirements, the species struggled on, growing in numbers and size.

Modern man doesn't have to protect himself from poisonous plants; he knows which ones they are and successfully avoids them but another and even greater threat is facing him today—how to cope with the enormous quantities of poisons in our industrialized world.

SOME NEW POISONS

Tolerance to certain toxic substances developed over the centuries, but within the last two generations poisons never before encountered are finding their way into our food and water. We are ingesting these alien chemicals at a rate of five pounds per person per year. They are chemical additives in prepared foods, residuals from fertilizers and insecticides, and particulates in the air that make their way into the gullet.

To compound the problem, the natural protection that would come from a nutritionally sufficient diet is decreasing at a time when it is most needed because of the poor quality of commercially grown foods and our consumption of refined foods. When we need more protection, we are getting less. Detoxifying the chemicals that we ingest puts an enormous strain on the body. Organs, blood, and enzyme systems are overworked and, unless they are nourished, degeneration begins and disease eventually follows.

All the requirements for the maintenance of life in every cell in the body are obtained from the air we breathe, the water we drink, and food we eat. What is happening to these three essentials? The food is being treated with heavy doses of chemicals to preserve or enhance it; the water is loaded with more chemicals to "purify" it; and the air is laden with smoke, smog, gas, and dust.

Every cell from blood to brain to nerve needs oxygen to survive. This vital oxygen is in the air we breathe but in some areas there are a few other things in the air: nitrogen dioxide, hydrocarbons, lead, sulphur dioxide, carbon monoxide, all with varying degrees of toxicity.

Our bodies were never built to cope with these pollutants. The respiratory system is equipped to protect us against certain amounts of certain kinds of pollutants. Nose hairs and cilia which line our breathing tubes filter out a considerable amount of dust and dirt. In the past most organic pollutants, such as smoke from burning wood, dirt particles, and animal hair, were eliminated by a highly effective system of cilia to trap the pollutant, sneezing to blast it out, and mucous lining to cough up whatever irritant entered the lungs. In just the last twenty-five years this system has been rendered obsolete. It is simply not equipped to handle industrial pollution being belched into the air in droplets so minute they easily bypass the cilia and make their way into the lungs and even into the bloodstream.

That these pollutants are dangerous indeed is borne out by some frightening figures. Auto emissions killed 4,000 Americans last year and caused nearly four million sick days. Damage to crops and property from air pollution comes to more than $12.3 billion annually, according to Environmental Protection Agency (EPA) estimates. Smog in high concentrations, enough to cause problems to health and to food crops, has been measured more than fifty miles from urban areas in the eastern third of the country.

Air pollution is dangerous for more than the obvious reasons of lung cancer, emphysema, and heart disease. In a normal, healthy body, breathing impure air depletes the body of Vitamin A necessary for the formation of the mucous membranes that line our body cavities, including the lungs. When these mucous membranes fail to develop properly, the ability to resist disease is reduced. Fortunately, Vitamin E helps protect Vitamin A from being destroyed by pollution—perfect example of nutritional symbiosis.

Lab tests on rats living in an atmosphere simulating heavy smog concentrations, showed that those fortified with extra Vitamin E lived twice as long as those without the supplemental E. Protecting Vitamin A, which E can do, is the best safeguard against the effects of air pollution.

In many cases polluted air is an occupational hazard. Miners, and workers in asbestos and certain other industries subject to high levels of pollution, might be expected to show degeneration, but living beside a busy highway can also be hazardous to health. Dr. Walter Blumer of Netstal, Switzerland, reported that over a twelve-year period, seventy-five of his patients died of cancer and seventy-two of them lived within fifty yards of a heavily traveled highway. In addition, patients who lived within fifty yards of the road suffered twice as much from headaches, depression, fatigue, digestive disorders, and nervousness as those living beyond that range. Suspecting that lead and other pollutants from auto emissions might be the cause, Dr. Blumer treated the patients with calcium edetate, plus Vitamins B and C. Nearly 70 percent of his patients recovered from their headaches and other disorders and 20 percent showed improvement.

AN OLD POISON

While much of the air pollution we are forced to live with is beyond our ability to control, one extremely toxic pollutant is ingested by choice—that is, tobacco. Of all the self-destructive follies man pursues, smoking is probably the worst. It is widely known that smoking causes lung cancer, but, it is also directly responsible for a number of other fatal diseases—heart disease, high blood pressure, and emphysema. It also interferes with the proper function of the brain, the eyes, and the nervous system. Most of these symptoms are related to the constriction of the small blood capillaries which occurs as a result of smoking. In addition, most tobacco is heavily sprayed with poisonous insecticides, thus intensifying the toxic effect.

Tobacco tar is more dangerous than the nicotine, but not much. If the nicotine from less than three cigarettes were injected into the bloodstream, it would prove fatal. Fortunately, most of the nicotine is exhaled into the air. However, nonsmokers are then subject to this pollution because second-hand smoke is just as noxious as the original. Tar, however, goes straight into the lungs. One pack of cigarettes a day provides the smoker with 27 fluid ounces of tar in the course of a year. A single cigarette robs the body of 30 milligrams of Vitamin C. According to Dr. Bertram W. Carnow, Director of Occupational and Environmental Medicine at the University of Illinois School of Public Health, one cigarette can paralyze the body's defense mechanism whereby foreign materials are expelled from the lungs for up to fifteen minutes. Cigarette smoke causes oxidation of unsaturated fats in the tissues and, according to the *American Journal of Public Health,* the arsenic content of the tobacco leaf is thirty times more than the amount permissible by federal law in marketed foods. Lecithin is destroyed by tobacco smoke and loss of lecithin in the lungs can cause emphysema. To protect themselves, smokers should take large amounts of supplemental vitamins, particularly C, A, and E.

OUR TREACHEROUS WATER

Water covers two-thirds of the earth. It comprises up to 68 percent of our body; it nurtures plant life that sustains human life. Most creatures will die much sooner from lack of water than lack of food. It is, in short, vital to life on earth. As recently as the last century, no one gave a thought to water unless it was to curse a flood. The quality of the water was never questioned. But things change rapidly. In 1974 alone, over 26,000 permits were issued to various industries allowing them to dump limited waste into the nation's waterways. An EPA check showed that two out of three industries have violated these permits by dumping illegal and poisonous waste. New pollutants never before encountered are now being detected in our water supply. In 1974, the EPA stated: "The assumption that our water is safe is subject to question." Their study found minute quantities of cancer-causing organisms in all eighty of the water systems tested.

In an effort to control these pollutants—the results of run-off from farm fertilizers, the leaching of pesticides into streams and lakes, the residue of mining and oil field operations, as well as industrial waste—enormous amounts of additional chemicals are dumped into reservoirs. The public water engineer has forty-eight chemicals he uses regularly, at his own discretion. As an example, the chemicals added to the drinking water of Columbus, Ohio, in one year included: 500 tons of aluminum ore; 8,000 tons of lime; 8 tons of liquid chlorine.

Among the most serious contaminants in our water supply are the nitrates leached from fields treated with inorganic nitrogen fertilizers. These nitrates are antagonists of Vitamin A and, when combined with secondary amines in the stomach, can cause cancer.

Chemically softened water is extremely dangerous. Calcium and magnesium are removed in a chemical reaction and sodium is introduced into the water in huge amounts. When installing a water softener, have a separate drinking water tap that bypasses the softener system.

In a somewhat misguided effort to reduce tooth decay among children, many communities have introduced fluoride into their water systems. Removing soft drinks from the school cafeteria would bring better results but credit must be given for recognition of a problem and the attempt to correct it. It has not proven successful, however; any decrease in tooth decay has been shown to be only temporary; in fact, the teeth later become brittle and cause more problems. But there may be further far-reaching consequences to the use of fluoride. It is a highly toxic chemical and its protracted use over a period of years could cause a cumulative effect and endanger various organs of the body such as the heart, liver, and kidneys. More than 7 ppm (parts per million) damages the calcification process of the secondary teeth during the first six years and it is known to accumulate in the placenta. Authorities by no means agree as to the benefits of fluoride in the water either. Tooth decay has sometimes actually increased after fluoridation. Newburgh, New York, Baltimore, Maryland, and Puerto Rico have all reported increases in tooth caries, while in Puerto Rico 64 percent of the adolescent boys have permanently mottled teeth as a result of fluoridated water.

Actually, little is known about fluorides and, as with any unknown element, caution is advised until the years show the results. In any case, if water is fluoridated, increased quantities of Vitamins B and C, as well as calcium and iodine, will help give protection.

COFFEE, COLA, ALCOHOL

If worry over drinking polluted water results in an increased consumption of alternative liquids, a word or two about coffee, soft drinks, and alcohol is in order.

In the first place, if the coffee is made with local water, however bad it may be, converting it into coffee does not improve the situation. As any coffee hound knows, caffeine is a strong heart stimulant. It dilates the coronary arteries and the effect is cumulative. One hour after drinking a cup of coffee, a subject will show a 10 percent increase in the basic metabolic rate. Overindulgence in caffeine prevents iron utilization and is suspected of being responsible for deficiencies in biotin and inositol, both B vitamins related to choline, necessary for the control of fatty acids and cholesterol, in the body. Adding sugar to the coffee increases the destruction of the B vitamins. The abromine and theophylline in tea and cocoa have the same effect as caffeine. One cup of coffee contains about 100 milligrams of caffeine. Ten grams is fatal to humans. As little as one-fifth of a gram can cause nervousness, muscle twitching, insomnia, and poor circulation. It is absolute poison to an ulcer victim. An intake of more than five cups of coffee per day doubles the risk of heart attack. About three cups should be the upper limit for any coffee drinker; this is a little over the 250 milligrams considered tolerable. The destructive results of overindulgence in coffee, tea, or cocoa don't generally appear until late in life so caution in drinking these is advised.

Americans can take all the credit for a worldwide epidemic whose ultimate consequence may be the total destruction of teeth. Carbonated, supersweetened, chemically colored and chemically flavored soft drinks—these bottled beverages can be found everywhere. No country is too remote, no village too small. Cola drinks and decayed teeth are now the common denominator in human life. In developing countries, money that should be spent on nourishing food is wasted on cola drinks. In poverty areas soft drinks have replaced milk among people with the greatest need for good nutrition.

Cola drinks are made from phosphoric acid, which has an acidity of about 2.6 percent, the same as vinegar; enough sugar to mask the acid (usually about three tablespoons per cup); artificial coal tar flavoring and coloring; and caffeine. If caffeine is not added, the FDA considers the drink is mislabeled.

Cola drinks do not contain one bit of food value. They do contain empty calories and artificial stimulants, which no one needs.

Naturally fermented beverages are an important part of life to many cultures. These drinks are enjoyed at festivals and religious holidays and they mark a special occasion, but such occasions are infrequent and drinking at those times doesn't pose a social or health problem. Indiscriminate drinking is warping lives all over the world. Russian officials, who conceal any unfavorable aspect of their controlled existence, are readily admitting alcoholism is responsible for reduced factory output, poor agricultural production, and serious health problems in the People's Republics. Alcoholism is self-induced. It is caused by the body's inability to handle the carbohydrate intake, resulting in too much insulin's being released into the system. This causes low blood sugar and fatigue. A drink will raise the blood sugar and temporarily relieve the symptoms of jitters and nervousness and so the cycle is self-perpetuating. Individuals who overindulge as adolescents permanently damage the function of glands that control their insulin flow. In addition, alcohol destroys magnesium and flushes zinc from the system. This may account for the destructive effect that drinking has on male sexuality. An editorial in the *New England Journal of Medicine* (1 August 1974) states:

> Alcohol inhibits the conversion of Vitamin A into a form required for the production of sperm. The mechanism is analogous to the one causing night blindness in alcoholics. Simultaneously, the toxic effect of alcohol and the nutritional deficiencies induced by it combine to interfere with breakdown of estrogen (female hormone) by the liver. The high levels of estrogen tend to feminize the male alcoholic, diminish his libido, and contribute to impotence. By two different pathways, then, the nutritional deficiencies of the alcoholic may deprive him of a normal sex life and the ability to father children. The Vitamin B complex and protein are the keys to restoring liver function if treatment is instituted before the process reaches the point of no return.

To counteract the effect of alcohol on the system, large amounts of B vitamins should be taken and all refined carbohydrates should be avoided.

The best bet of course, is to drink milk, fruit drinks, and bottled water and try to avoid the risk of too many chemicals.

The effects of air and water pollution can be minimized with the intake of additional vitamins and minerals, so naturally one would turn to foods rich in these elements to achieve protection. An exercise in futility. Not only are the foods laden with more alien chemicals, but their nutritional quality has also deteriorated.

CHEMICALS IN OUR SOIL,
CHEMICALS IN OUR FOOD

In a cycle of self-destruction that must baffle more unsophisticated cultures, American farmers load their fields with chemical fertilizers which fail to maintain a good soil balance. Because of this the plants are subject to insect infestations, so widespread use of pesticides follows. Damaged plants and trees are stunted and produce fewer and poorer quality crops. To raise productivity the farmer will again load his fields with chemicals.

The produce from these farms puts the consumer in a double bind. Processed and refined foods, which take up fully 75 percent of the grocery store shelf space, offer little in the way of vitamins, minerals, fibers, and trace elements that would help detoxify the chemicals we ingest. Turning to fresh fruits and vegetables increases the amount of poisons we consume, for there is hardly a food in the market that hasn't been sprayed or treated with some sort of toxic material before it reaches the consumer. The safest, of course, are the foods that must be peeled, although it means loss of nutrients as a result. Always use a vegetable peeler to peel foods because the nutrients are concentrated right under the skin. The ripe and glowing apple has been subject to more poisonous sprays in its short lifetime than anyone would believe possible. Because leafy green vegetables are quick to absorb poisons, the outside leaves should be discarded. A rinse in vinegar water, about one-fourth cup in a couple of gallons of water, will neutralize up to 85 percent of the chemicals on the food. Ample protein and Vitamins A, C, E, the B complex and the essential fatty acids help to protect the body from pesticides. There are alternatives to nitrate and nitrite fertilizers and they should be in general use. An enormous amount of fossil fuels is used in the production of chemical fertilizers, fuels that cannot be replaced and that will become exorbitantly expensive as the world supplies dwindle.

THE ORGANIC FERTILIZERS

One fertilizer that can be found in ever-increasing amounts is "night soil," the time-honored and time-tested method of enriching the land. Human excrement produces bountiful harvests of nutritious crops. The Japanese have used it for centuries, as have the Chinese and nearly every other agricultural society. Currently Japanese scientists are working on ways to disinfect and make better use of night soil, for there is a danger of spreading disease if it is used undecomposed and the resulting foods are eaten raw. Light cooking or pickling eliminates this danger.

Fields fed with natural organisms stay fertile for centuries. Chinese agriculture, based on the use of natural manures, has endured for over forty centuries without exhaustion of soil fertility. While United States farmers produce enormous crops and high acreage yields, soil depletion is a grave problem. In less than two centuries something like 100 million acres of America's land have been exhausted and barren fields are increasing yearly.

One of the serious results of improper soil care is the loss of trace elements. Zinc, in minute amounts, is vital to human health; so are magnesium and a number of other elements. Soil cannot manufacture these minerals and the plant won't have them unless the soil contains them. These minerals and elements must be returned to the land so the land can return them to man. The farmers of Hunza, China, Japan, Latin America, and many other areas know that they must return to the soil that which the soil needs to sustain life and that the cycle must not be broken.

There are some peripheral advantages to using natural fertilizers. In a study conducted by Dr. Barry Commoner, thirty-two farms, ranging in size from 171 to 875 acres, were surveyed. Sixteen of the farms used natural fertilizers and sixteen farmed the conventional way with commercial fertilizers. All the farms were equally and fully mechanized but the farmer using natural fertilizer saved an average of sixteen dollars an acre because of the enormous cost of petroleum-based fertilizers and insecticides. The results of the study showed that the two types of farming had virtually identical yields of soybeans and wheat and comparable yields in oats. One of the farmers in the survey related how his whole family had been sick for years. The skin rashes, allergies, fevers were finally traced to the chemical spray he used on his farm. He switched to natural fertilizers fourteen years ago and his family has had no health problems since. For pest control he uses ladybugs and crop rotation, for weed control he maintains a well-balanced soil whose healthy plants choke out weeds. Fertilizer from compost costs $3.25 per acre as opposed to $20 to $50 per acre, the constantly fluctuating price of petrochemical fertilizers. And the quality of the food? The organically fertilized corn was tested at Iowa State University and showed 12.3 percent protein. Commercially fed corn runs about 4 to 8 percent protein.

THE GENTLE INSECTICIDES:
ANIMALS AND PLANTS

Man has many friends on this beautiful planet. Animals that help us far outnumber our competitors in the animal world. There are more birds that eat insects than there are rats that attack grain. There are more insects that prey on plant-eating bugs than animals that destroy crops. Given half a chance these birds, bugs, and animals will save more food than they consume. Salt Lake City boasts a handsome statue of seagulls in flight. It is to commemorate the occasion when a swarm of invading locusts was destroyed by a huge flock of seagulls, thus saving the first harvest of the tiny Mormon settlement. The ranchers in Humboldt County, California, have erected a monument to the tiny chrysolina beetle. This insignificant bug has saved them over $12 million in lost grazing land by destroying the Klamath weed that nearly took over the area. Animals that ate this weed suffered sore mouths, skin scale, and blisters. No one has yet erected a monument to a cobalt-60 gamma ray device, but it would be appropriate. Gamma rays were used to sterilize screwworms that were devastating animal life throughout the South and West. Cattle, sheep, goats, and wild life were all being viciously attacked by this parasite. Spraying was hopeless, insecticides useless, and damage kept increasing. Finally the particular habits of the screwworm were turned against it. The females mate only once but the males mate many times. Introducing males sterilized by gamma rays into the infected areas could reduce larvae growth. The best test came with an opportunity to try the plan on an isolated offshore island. Within thirteen weeks screwworm was eliminated. A massive program in the United States has reduced the annual $120 million loss by 96 percent, and not a drop of chemical or poison was used.

The botanical world is an endless source of natural pesticides. Probably the most effective all round pesticide ever discovered is pyrethrum. It is an herbaceous perennial chrysanthemum and legend has it that the Chinese used it nearly 2,000 years ago. This is probably true. Because it breaks down readily in sunlight and has no residual effect, it is an ideal preharvest spray. The USDA terms pyrethrum the safest of all insecticides for use on plant food.

Other plants that are effective insecticides are tobacco; the South American quassia tree; derris or tuba root; rotenone from the roots of several South American trees; ryania, a shrub native to Latin America and the Caribbean; and sabadilla, known since the sixteenth century to be an effective and versatile insecticide for the control of corn borer, army worm, webworm, aphid, cabbage looper, squash bug, and several other pests.

All these plant insecticides have low residual quality and do not accumulate in the human body.

Many animals keep fat and healthy eating garden pests and farmers use them to good advantage. Frequently an "orchard flock" of chickens will be found pecking around the fruit trees, happily keeping down the insect population. Farmers have built structures for bats to use so these hungry predators will stay near their fields. Intelligent cooperation between man and the creatures he lives with can be beneficial to both. A chemical spray doesn't select its victims; it kills everything within its range, the good with the bad. We can't afford to lose our animal friends while trying to save our food.

DINING TABLE OR CHEMISTRY LAB?

Now, the food has been harvested and it awaits the buyer. What has happened to it from farm to market? In the case of fresh foods, it has been trimmed, sorted, and packaged. To prevent spoilage, some foods are gassed, some are covered with wax, and some are dipped in a chemical bath. By the time they are trucked to market, several days may have elapsed and valuable nutrients have been lost. With frozen foods the situation is different. The foods are left to ripen longer before picking, and frequently the freezing plant is close at hand. Often the foods are frozen and packaged the very day they are picked. Of course, there is nutritional and enzyme loss in freezing but there are advantages too. Either way, the supermarket isn't your best source of good, nutritious food. It is hoped a farm stand isn't too far away.

If the food has gone through any refining or manufacturing process, it is virtually worthless. Not only have the vitamins and minerals been destroyed but any one of more than 700 chemical substances, singly or in groups, are routinely added.

In the course of one day, the average person will consume great quantities of these chemicals. For instance, there is benzoic acid (a preservative used in nearly everything), polysiloxane (antifoaming agent used in juices, jellies, soups), butylated hydroxyanisole (antioxidant used in cereals, margarines, soups, crackers, candy, fruit pies), sodium acetate monoglyceride, calcium propionate, and a whole rainbow of artificial colors from Red Dye 2, which has finally come under some well-deserved suspicion, to FD&C 3 (yellow) and FD&C 1 (blue). This chemistry lab is found in bread, butter, meat, milk, soups, candies, sodas, lunch meat, hot dogs, ice cream, canned vegetables, and cheese. Those chemicals that are presumed safe need not be listed on the food container, which leads to an incredible problem for the parents of hyperactive children. Dr. Ben F. Feingold of Kaiser Permanente Medical Care Program has established a link between food additives and hyperactive children. The only way to control the problem is to eliminate the additives in the diet, and the parents must assume that all prepared foods contain the offending products.

Unhappily, the human body has no natural defense against synthetic additives. Every time an adulterant is added to food or a natural substance removed, the balance of nature is disturbed. It took thousands of years for our bodies to adjust to environmental changes; they are incapable of instant adjustment to the whims of chemists. Sadly enough, so many of the additives are entirely unnecessary. Dumping suspicious chemicals into food for cosmetic effect is insane. Some preservatives are necessary because of our food marketing system, but tampering with the natural flavors or colors of the food by adding chemicals is totally irresponsible.

The law is pretty lax when it comes to food additives. No testing is required for carcinogenicity, so we have no idea how many of the so-called "safe" chemicals are cancer producers. In addition, an agent that may be harmless in a single product may react violently when consumed with another product containing a different agent or when combined with other compounds that may be antagonistic to it. Claims that these agents are not toxic in such minute quantities are not borne out by the facts. In truth, our health is declining with each tiny dose.

Few items in the American diet are tampered with quite as much as meat. Beef, pork, and fowl contain twice as many parts per million of pesticides as any other food. In addition, indiscriminate use of antibiotics in animals and fowl provides the eater with a constant dosage, thus increasing his tolerance of these drugs. Doctors are alarmed at the rate with which many life-saving antibiotics are becoming useless and ineffective.

The long-range effect of synthetic chemicals was sadly demonstrated in the case of stilbestrol, an artificial female sex hormone. It is given to beef and fowl and can increase their weight 15 percent with 12 percent less food. Stilbestrol is said to be responsible for a 675 million-pound increase in beef weight annually; however, the weight is all fat. But stilbestrol has a tragic history of pain and grief. In the 1950s many women were given the drug to prevent miscarriage. It was effective and seemed safe for the user, but it has proven a time bomb for the female fetus. Many of these girls, now grown up, developed vaginal cancer during their adolescence, a type of cancer previously unknown in young women. About 85 percent of all beef cattle are fed stilbestrol; in 1970, the FDA doubled the amount growers were permitted to use.

When meat is processed, all sorts of things are done to it. Ham, lunch meat, bacon, and hot dogs have a chemical pedigree that is truly impressive. An additive-free hot dog cannot be called a hot dog, according to the FDA. To qualify for that label, it must contain nitrates. The problem with nitrates is that they change to nitrites which can combine with secondary amines in the stomach and create nitrosamines which are known to be powerful cancer-causing chemicals. Some sources of amines are beer, cigarettes, wine, cereals, and other common food. Vitamin C can block this transformation.

At the University of California at Davis, experiments are underway to test the effectiveness of formaldehyde as a means of making beef fat polyunsaturated. The cholesterol levels were lowered significantly in test subjects who ate beef that had been fed small amounts of formaldehyde. Granted that high cholesterol is suspected of being the cause of many heart attacks, there is a better way to control it than introducing even *more* chemicals into our food.

With the fat of meat and poultry already showing .281 parts per million pesticide residue (as compared with grain, with only .008) combined with the five pounds per year of pollutants we ingest, we just don't need any more toxic substances in our diet. All efforts should be made to reduce these levels or deal with them effectively.

YOU *CAN* PROTECT YOURSELF

What is the best defense? A healthy body, of course, a well-balanced diet, and a very careful scrutiny of grocery store labels. If it is at all possible, a backyard garden is the best solution, concentrating on the leafy vegetables which absorb more of the poisons in sprays and are harder to wash off. Cabbage is a lovely crop, zucchinis are so popular that many backyard gardeners grow nothing else. Just about any vegetable sold in the market is easily grown at home. A compost heap will ensure a large and delicious crop and mail order ladybug beetles will keep it healthy.

Many apartment dwellers have grown a limited variety of vegetables in tubs on their terraces and everyone can grow one of the finest foods known, sprouted seeds.

If home-grown isn't for you, careful selection and treatment of foods can reduce their toxicity. The best meats are lamb and range beef; they are not fattened at the feed lots where most of the damage is done. Ocean fish is additive-free, but in some cases it may be subject to pollutants leached from the land. Meat from Argentina is excellent and desiccated Argentine beef liver is best because chemical sprays are forbidden there. Reducing meat consumption and substituting grains and legumes can reduce pesticide ingestion up to 1800 percent.

Watercress, parsley, and endive are usually not sprayed. Beef liver is an outstanding food but the catch is that the very function of the liver may make it suspect. The liver is the detoxifier in the body and over the years it may become saturated with waste. Animals are subject to the same pollutants humans are. The best bet is the liver of a young animal, one that hasn't had to work so long keeping its body healthy.

Whole grains and fibers that get waste material out of the body quickly are essential in protecting ourselves. If highly toxic material consistently stays in the intestines for many hours, damage can be devastating and irreversible. Legumes, fresh fruit, fermented foods, and nuts are also excellent for regulating elimination.

Trace elements are vital to the maintenance of good health. Little is known of the part they play, but a deficiency of some obscure element found in our body in the tiniest quantity can cause a host of ills and problems. However, there are some trace elements that we do not need, cannot use, and have little ability to eliminate. They get into our food through additives and chemicals. They accumulate in our bodies. These are the culprits and they can cause all sorts of trouble.

WHEN ELEMENTS ARE OUT OF BALANCE

Cadmium is an element that is increasing in our environment due to industrial processing. It is released into the air when steel scrap is melted down. It finds its way into soil fertilized with phosphates, and it is in the residue of burned motor oil. There is reason to believe that cadmium contributes to emphysema, high blood pressure, and heart and circulatory diseases. Studies have shown that there is no system or function of the human organism that has not been subject to, and damaged by, concentrations of environmental cadmium. Zinc is an effective antagonist of cadmium. It is the best protection possible but the fact is that zinc is being depleted from our soil at a rapid rate and is not being replaced. Our soil used to contain sufficient zinc, but this important trace mineral has dropped below the danger level in thirty-two states. In another example of harmony in Nature, cadmium is found in the starchy part of the grain, the endosperm, and zinc is in the bran. The whole grain creates a perfect balance. When grain is refined however, the zinc is removed with the bran while cadmium is left in the endosperm.

The grotesque period of paintings of Goya hold a repellent fascination for the art lover. Weird shapes and colors make the observer wonder about this Spanish artist's state of mind. The fact is, his state of mind was terrible and so was his physical condition. It is believed he suffered and nearly died from lead poisoning contracted from the lead-based paints he used. For over a year he quit painting entirely, hoping to recover from his near-fatal illness and, except for becoming permanently deaf, he did recover sufficiently to resume his work.

Some highly respected experts make a good case for lead poisoning's being responsible for the fall of the Roman Empire. Debilitating and crippling diseases, the result of storing wine, water and food in lead containers, rendered the Romans incapable of defending their empire.

Of course, lead is carefully controlled now. No more than .5 percent is allowed in paint and many paints contain none at all. But, for instance, every day about eighteen tons of the stuff are deposited on Los Angeles. Except for the 4.3 tons that are blown into adjacent towns, all that lead settles to the ground and accumulates. Most of it comes from auto emissions; about 75 percent of the lead in gasoline finds its way into the atmosphere. Vegetables from farms along the freeways were found to contain fifty times more lead than the amount considered tolerable in food. Toothpaste from the end of the lead-lined tube shows seventy-two times more lead than that at the beginning of the tube. Lead waterpipes leach into drinking water, while burning newspapers cause lead from the ink to float into the air. Improperly glazed pottery leaches lead into food and lead found in some hair dyes is absorbed into the system. The blood of hyperactive children showed an elevation of lead and tests indicated high lead levels led to hyperactivity in mice. In areas where there is heavy traffic, it is safe to assume higher amounts of lead exist. Inasmuch as it appears to be impossible to avoid ingesting lead, some protection from poisoning is found in Vitamin C. Tests on mice have shown that the trace mineral chromium also protects against lead poisoning. Chromium is found in the bran and germ of grains.

Mercury becomes toxic when it settles to the ocean floor and by bacterial action is converted to methyl mercury. The bacteria then become part of the food chain through plankton. The plankton-eating fish consume the tainted food and the dangers start. Marine biologists were stunned to find seals that lived a hundred miles offshore in the Bering Sea had heavy concentrations of mercury in their livers. Obviously, mercury is found in the food chain from the smallest organisms to the largest marine mammals. How did it get there? How was it introduced into this vitally important food source? Over 5,000 tons of mercury are dumped into the sea every year, the residue of industrial manufacturing. In addition, 90 percent of all commercial seeds are treated with a mercury compound to inhibit fungus growth. Check the seeds you buy for sprouting. Some golf courses use a mercury-based spray to protect their greens. Even a small hospital can actually drop and lose up to 150 pounds of mercury a year. It is essential to protect oneself against mercury poison, and fortunately the trace mineral selenium detoxifies it successfully. Selenium is found in eggs, whole grains, nuts, and brewers' yeast. Interestingly, tuna has always had a high level of mercury in its flesh but it balances this by having a high level of selenium too.

Aluminum, like many trace minerals, normally appears in the body. It has been found in minute amounts in the bodies of animals which are never exposed to aluminum. However, the natural aluminum found in fresh foods is not metallic. The introduction of metallic aluminum in our diet through the use of metal foil, storage containers, and cooking pots can result in phosphate and calcium deficiencies, stomach disorders leading to ulcers, obesity, and problems of the nervous system.

Aluminum is a soft metal that food acid can dissolve quite easily. For instance, orange juice stored in an aluminum container can dissolve 37 parts per million of the metal, stewed tomatoes show an increase of 15.5 percent aluminum after only twenty minutes and lemon pie filling a surprising 118 percent when cooked in an aluminum pan. There is some confusion as to whether aluminum pots and pans pose a problem. It is felt that toxicity from cooking utensils isn't too likely. But why wonder if aluminum pots are harmful when it is well established that iron pots are beneficial? Food cooked in iron pots absorbs an easily assimilated iron that our bodies can use. The Seventh-day Adventists do not allow cooking in aluminum; they recommend stainless steel, glass or iron. Enamel pans are also considered safe as long as they are not chipped.

Aluminum is so much a part of our daily lives we hardly realize how often we come in contact with it. Many prepared frozen foods are stored in aluminum containers and they must be cooked in these containers too. Millions of yards of metal foil are used by housewives yearly for freezing, cooking, and storing food. Aluminum storage containers of every shape and size are in constant use, each making its tiny contribution of metallic aluminum. The convenience of metal foil makes it difficult to abandon. It is an effective wrapper for food preservation, but if the cooled food is first wrapped in wax paper and then in metal foil, preservation is just as efficient and the food is protected. Glass jars are ideal storage containers. It is easy to see the contents; it is also possible to freeze foods in glass jars if some precautions are taken. Leave room for expansion and wait until the food is thoroughly chilled before putting it in the freezer. Butchers paper can be used to wrap food for freezing and special parchment paper can be obtained for use in cooking food.

Arsenic, the fabled poison of mystery stories and Sunday supplement writers, is not limited to use by mass murderers. It is used by manufacturers of rodent poisons and pesticides and is also found in wood preservatives and some phosphate-high detergent cleaners. Curiously, pigs and chickens grow faster if just a bit of arsenic is added to their food. However, it does have a tendency to accumulate in the liver.

Because such small quantities of these elements find their way into our bodies, the symptoms of poisoning are not acute and identifiable. Capable of combining with the enzymes and inhibiting their normal function, these pollutants cause a host of complaints and lead to vague illnesses with no specific origin. Digestive problems, constipation, a feeling of nausea from time to time, skin rashes, loss of vitality, all easily confused with organic or bacterial infections. Without taking the trouble to identify and analyze all toxic elements in our system, it is certainly safe to assume that we are ingesting too much of some or all of the above. The logical conclusion would be to protect ourselves against all of them. Additional Vitamin C, fiber, chromium, and selenium offer vital protection; whole grains are a good source of these minerals.

SOME NEW MENACES

An interesting type of pollution, that is to say, an unnatural environmental change, has been getting a lot of attention these days. It is light pollution and it is treated with the seriousness it deserves. It has been shown that extended exposure to fluorescent light causes behavioral problems for children and adults. People working under these lights become nervous, irritable, and hyperactive. A 1970 article in the *New England Journal of Medicine* stated that calcium absorption, endocrine function, and other physiological activities were adversely affected by exposure to fluorescent light. It has a short light wave and a restricted spectrum. A new light has been developed that gives 92 percent of the light spectrum of the sun at noon and will eliminate that aspect of light pollution.

Research indicates that light affects your physical and mental health by glandular reaction through your eyes. The use of inadequately balanced light for long periods of time can cause adverse effects. Artificial light, window glass, spectacles, sunglasses, and contaminated air all limit our absorption of the full range of natural sunlight. Arthritis, acne, bursitis, hay fever, and even ulcers have all been reported to have improved when the full spectrum of sunlight is allowed to enter the eye. Natural sunlight is essential to all life. It is important to spend some of your daylight hours out-of-doors. An effort should be made to see that invalids, small children, and the elderly are also exposed to the natural sun rays.

A new complaint that symbolizes modern man is jet lag, disturbance of the diurnal rhythms. This leads to nervous tension, indigestion, fatigue, and poor judgment. The daily routine of rising, eating, working, and sleeping determines our biological clock; forcing it into new patterns causes considerable stress. Countless light/dark experiments with cockroaches, small mammals, and birds have shown how easy it is to drive them mad by consistent tampering with their diurnal rhythms. Good nutrition with emphasis on the B vitamins, Vitamin C and protein can help the body in times of stress. Allowing an extra day or two for adjusting to jet lag is worth the extra time. Better yet, go by boat.

Another risk our ancestors never faced is radiation poisoning. The only real protection from absorbed radiation discovered so far is through diet. Studies have shown that radioactive substances, like all other toxic material, can to some extent be removed from the body or rendered neutral by certain elements. These are Vitamins E and C in large doses, calcium, bone meal, the B complex (especially B_6 and pantothenic acid), brewers' yeast, kelp, unsaturated oil, and cod liver oil. In addition, it would help to eat foods that contain pectin: apples, lemons, and sunflower seeds are rich in this nutrient.

Low level radiation in extremely small amounts may come from the television (never sit close), x-rays and other radiation treatments, even the slow release of radioactivity from a nearby nuclear plant. Fallout has been found in leaves of plants and pond water as far as 2,300 miles from an explosion site. This is a very slow and cumulative danger and simple precautions following known procedures can help prevent future problems. Just take the supplemental vitamins and minerals.

Plastics are a new material so long-term studies on their toxicity are only now appearing. One rather frightening development is the incidence of a rare type of liver cancer showing up among workers exposed to vinyl chloride, used in the production of plastics. The symptoms only appear after prolonged and constant exposure, but they do demonstrate the potential toxicity of plastics.

There is proof that formaldehyde is released into hot foods served in plastic containers. In one study up to 28 parts per million were detected. Formaldehyde reacts with chlorine and a hot beverage made with tap water and served in a plastic cup could contain up to 62.7 milligrams of formaldehyde. A group of volunteers agreed to eat from 100 to 200 milligrams of formaldehyde a day with their normal food; at the end of ten days they all began to show the symptoms of metal poisoning. Formaldehyde inhibits the metabolism of oxygen in the cells and is definitely one of the chemicals to avoid.

OXYGEN, THE BASIC NUTRIENT

The most important of all nutrients is oxygen and one of the major benefits of prudent exercise is the increase of oxygen intake. To get the greatest benefit, one should exercise in a smog-free area. Avoid jogging alongside a busy highway. If smog levels are high, that is over .10 parts per million, avoid outdoor exercise and take extra Vitamins E and A. Working in a garden raising naturally fertilized plants is a marvelous form of exercise. Growing plants are the very best source of oxygen. House plants, lately so popular, not only add natural beauty to any room but also make a positive contribution by supplying additional oxygen.

Our beautiful blue planet has its problems and pollution is certainly one of them. No one can isolate himself to avoid contamination as, indeed, no one would want to. It's our world and we live in it. But just as we use seat belts, carry insurance, and learn to swim, so can we protect ourselves and help our miraculous bodies overcome these pollutants. Well-balanced soil inhibits weed growth and discourages insects and the well-balanced human organism can isolate and reject most of the toxic chemicals we encounter. The higher the pollution level, the greater the amount of help in the form of supplemental vitamins and minerals we need. The human body can rid itself of the alien matter but the toll may be devastating. Vitamins and minerals will be depleted and various functions hampered while the body struggles with the invaders. Heavy artillery in the form of protective nutrients and a well-balanced diet will guarantee victory.

A diet that is high in protective nutrients is one that is rich in the B vitamins, Vitamins A, C, and E, calcium, iodine, fibers, pectin, essential fatty acids, zinc and other trace minerals. To help these along and allow them to do their work, avoid processed and refined foods. Increase fish consumption, cut down on meats, and trim away all the fat on the meat you do eat. Keep coffee drinking down to three cups a day and never drink it from plastic cups. Use moderation in drinking fermented beverages and, if you do, take some extra B vitamins. If you smoke be sure to include Vitamins A, C, and E in your diet and be considerate of your family and friends who do not want to inhale your smoke.

All these rules are designed to help the body rid itself of toxic chemicals, but they seem to be the same rules recommended for reducing heart attack risk, increasing vitality, and guaranteeing a long, healthy life. In truth, there are no special rules for protecting yourself from pollutants: good sensible eating protects you and prevents other illness at the same time.

The following charts compare the nutrients found in the meals described for the nine cultures and the United States.

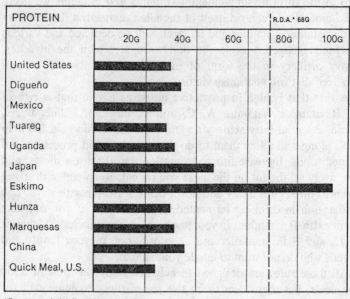

PROTEIN   R.D.A.* 68G

	20G	40G	60G	80G	100G
United States					
Digueño					
Mexico					
Tuareg					
Uganda					
Japan					
Eskimo					
Hunza					
Marquesas					
China					
Quick Meal, U.S.					

*Recommended daily allowance

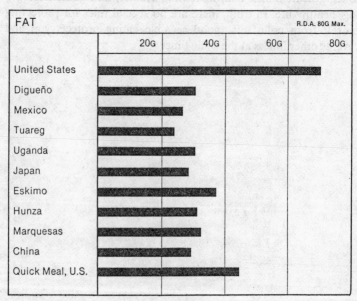

FAT   R.D.A. 80G Max.

	20G	40G	60G	80G
United States				
Digueño				
Mexico				
Tuareg				
Uganda				
Japan				
Eskimo				
Hunza				
Marquesas				
China				
Quick Meal, U.S.				

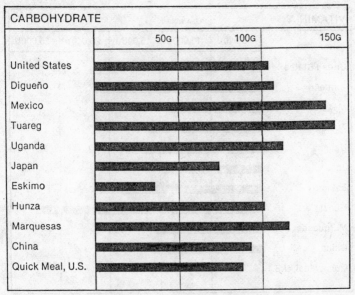

CARBOHYDRATE

	50G	100G	150G
United States			
Digueño			
Mexico			
Tuareg			
Uganda			
Japan			
Eskimo			
Hunza			
Marquesas			
China			
Quick Meal, U.S.			

Note: Since excess protein is used as carbohydrate no deficiency will exist as long as the calorie intake is adequate. However, it is essential for some carbohydrate to be present before protein can be metabolized.

CALORIES

R.D.A. 2,400 G.

	500G	1000G	1500G	2000G	2500G
United States		WITHOUT PIE →			
Digueño					
Mexico					
Tuareg					
Uganda					
Japan					
Eskimo					
Hunza					
Marquesas					
China					
Quick Meal, U.S.					

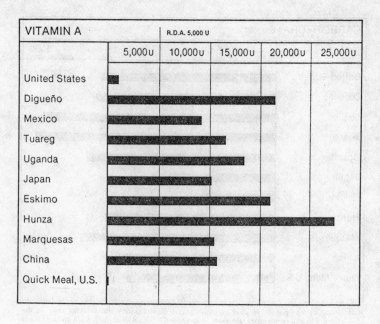

VITAMIN A   R.D.A. 5,000 U

	5,000u	10,000u	15,000u	20,000u	25,000u
United States					
Digueño					
Mexico					
Tuareg					
Uganda					
Japan					
Eskimo					
Hunza					
Marquesas					
China					
Quick Meal, U.S.					

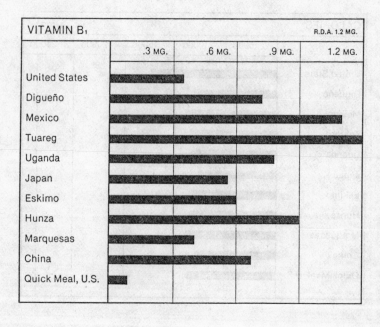

VITAMIN B₁   R.D.A. 1.2 MG.

	.3 MG.	.6 MG.	.9 MG.	1.2 MG.
United States				
Digueño				
Mexico				
Tuareg				
Uganda				
Japan				
Eskimo				
Hunza				
Marquesas				
China				
Quick Meal, U.S.				

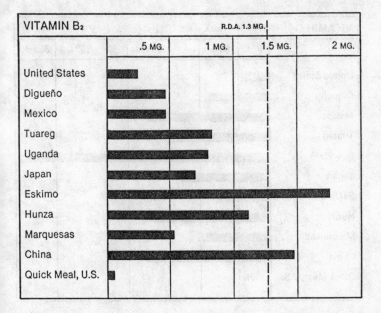

VITAMIN B₂

	.5 MG.	1 MG.	1.5 MG.	2 MG.

R.D.A. 1.3 MG.

United States
Digueño
Mexico
Tuareg
Uganda
Japan
Eskimo
Hunza
Marquesas
China
Quick Meal, U.S.

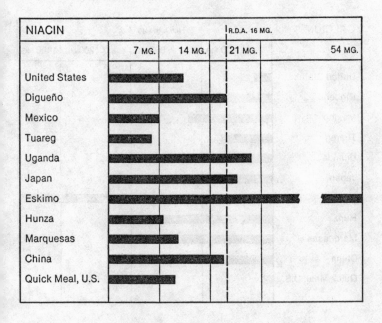

NIACIN

	7 MG.	14 MG.	21 MG.	54 MG.

R.D.A. 16 MG.

United States
Digueño
Mexico
Tuareg
Uganda
Japan
Eskimo
Hunza
Marquesas
China
Quick Meal, U.S.

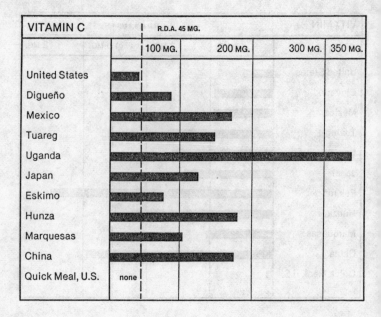

VITAMIN C — R.D.A. 45 MG.

	100 MG.	200 MG.	300 MG.	350 MG.
United States				
Digueño				
Mexico				
Tuareg				
Uganda				
Japan				
Eskimo				
Hunza				
Marquesas				
China				
Quick Meal, U.S.	none			

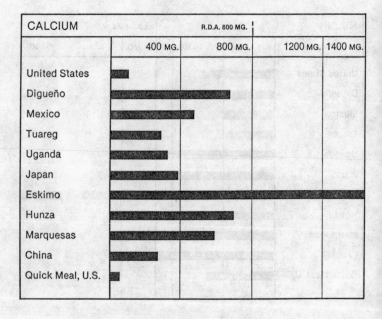

CALCIUM — R.D.A. 800 MG.

	400 MG.	800 MG.	1200 MG.	1400 MG.
United States				
Digueño				
Mexico				
Tuareg				
Uganda				
Japan				
Eskimo				
Hunza				
Marquesas				
China				
Quick Meal, U.S.				

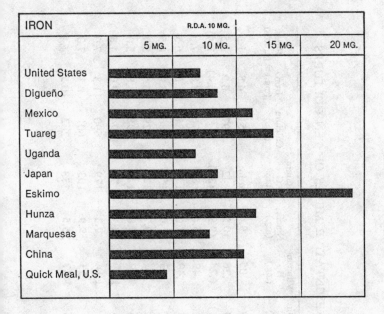

IRON	R.D.A. 10 MG.			
	5 MG.	10 MG.	15 MG.	20 MG.
United States				
Digueño				
Mexico				
Tuareg				
Uganda				
Japan				
Eskimo				
Hunza				
Marquesas				
China				
Quick Meal, U.S.				

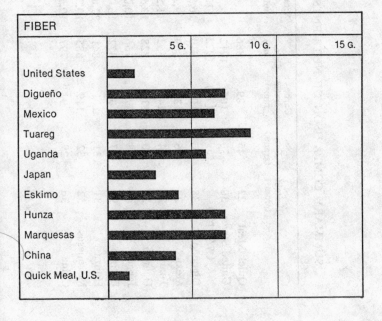

FIBER			
	5 G.	10 G.	15 G.
United States			
Digueño			
Mexico			
Tuareg			
Uganda			
Japan			
Eskimo			
Hunza			
Marquesas			
China			
Quick Meal, U.S.			

SUMMARY COMPARISON OF NUTRIENTS IN REPRESENTATIVE MEALS OF TEN CULTURES

	Protein (grams)	Fat (grams)	Carbo-hydrates (grams)	Calories (units)	Vitamin A (units)	Vitamin B₁ (mg.)	Vitamin B₂ (mg.)	Niacin (mg.)	Vitamin C (mg.)	Calcium (mg.)	Iron (mg.)	Fiber (grams)
Quick Meal	23	45	89	886	40	.08	.05	9.4	none	51	4.8	1.3
United States	30	70	105	1212	1224	.33	.26	10.2	42	97	6.9	1.5
(w/o pie)		(59)	(74)	(972)	(1216)	(.31)	(.24)	(9.9)	(39)		(6.4)	(1.4)
Digueño	35	30	109	810	16,550	.72	.49	16.4	88	676	8.8	7.0
Mexico	27	26	135	889	9,240	1.14	.49	7.0	177	481	11.0	6.5
Tuareg	29	24	142	852	11,535	1.2	.83	6.0	153	286	13.0	8.5
Uganda	32	30	114	828	13,510	.8	.8	19.7	322	329	6.5	5.9
Japan	47	28	77	766	10,021	.56	.69	17.8	129	395	8.8	3.0
Eskimo	94	37	38	872	16,095	.6	1.7	54.1	77	1494	19.0	4.6
Hunza	31	31	101	841	22,885	.9	1.14	7.3	179	690	11.3	7.0
Marquesas	32	32	119	885	10,316	.4	.53	9.9	103	601	8.1	7.0
China	36	29	93	797	10,671	.66	1.47	15.5	178	262	10.5	4.4

Index

Abalone, 86–87, 100
Abromine, 332
Acerola cherries, 324
Acid-alkali balance, 316, 318
Acid foods (*see also* Fermentation; specific foods): and minerals, 324
Acne, 345
Acorns (flour; mush), 84–85, 89 ff., 102, 104, 288; Recipe for Mush, 107
Additives, 265–66, 337–39
Adrenals, 146, 301, 312, 318
Africa(ns), 41, 113, 117–18, 170, 271, 273. *See also* specific peoples
Agar, 205
Agave (mescal), 85–86, 94–95. *See also* Pulque
Aging, 65, 268, 270, 311. *See also* Degenerative disease; Longevity
Agriculture, Department of, 325
Aguamiel, 236
Agutuk. *See* Ice cream: Eskimo
Airola, Paavo, 143
Air pollution, 313, 314, 327–29, 342, 345, 346–47. *See also* Smog
Alaska. *See* Eskimos
Alcohol (fermented beverages), 258, 259, 307 ff., 311, 317, 320, 325, 332, 347. *See also* Beer; Wine
Aleurone layer, 263, 264
Alfalfa seeds, 324; sprouts, 81, 268, 313
Algae, 205, 234
Algonquin Indians, 135
Alkalizers, 307, 319
Allergies, 309, 335
All Souls' Night, 230
Almond Cookies, 194–95
Almonds, 309; Chinese use, 180–81, 185, 189, 194–95; Fruit and Nut Snack, 80; Digueños use, 108, 109; Granola with, 108; Hunza Breakfast with, 79; Hunza use, 70, 73, 79, 80, 285, 286
Aluminum, 343–44; in water, 330
Amedama, 29–30
American Journal of Clinical Nutrition, 118
American Journal of Public Health, 329

American Medical Association, 278
American Pharmaceutical Association Handbook . . . , 279
Amines, 330, 339
Amino acids, 184, 269, 296 ff., 310, 321
Amoebic dysentery, 137
Anemia, 98, 117–18, 121, 311, 319
Antelope, 42
Antibiotics, 307, 308, 313, 339
Antibodies, 309, 312
Antihistamines, 312
Ants, honey, 287–88
Aphid, 337
Apoplexy, Digueños and, 91
Appendicitis, Gandans and, 117
Appetite, loss of, 307
Apples, 290, 345 (*see also* Vinegar); Chinese use, 179, 196; Cranberry Relish on Greens with, 154; custard, 243; Hunza use, 57, 63, 69, 70, 79
Applesauce, Raw, 79
Apricot Jam, Recipe for, 76
Apricots (oil; pits), 179, 312, 317, 319; Fruit and Nut Snack, 80; Hunza Breakfast with, 79; Hunza use, 57, 58, 63, 64, 69–70, 73, 75, 76, 79, 80, 285
Argentina, meat from, 340
Arhant's Fast, 195–96
Army worm, 337
Arrowhead, 98
Arrowroot, 16, 21
Arsenic, 329, 344
Arteries, 169, 280, 331. *See also* Atherosclerosis; Cardiovascular system; Cholesterol
Arthritis, 141, 203, 205, 239, 309, 325, 345
Artichokes, 44, 242, 302
Asbestos workers, 328
Ascorbic acid. *See* Vitamin C
Asparagus, 311; Summer Soup with, 78
Aspirin, Vitamin C and, 312
Asthma, 325
Atherosclerosis, 70, 203. *See also* Cholesterol
Athletics (sports), 311, 314
Atiu, the, 301

Atole, 91, 100, 101–2, 238 (*see also* Acorns); Recipe for Acorn Mush, 107
Atomic Energy Commission, 140
Auklets, 148
Auto emissions, 328, 342
Avidin, 310
Avocados, 300, 302, 309, 318; Mexican use, 227, 232, 235, 242, 247, 250, 257
Avocado Sauce, 247; Recipe for, 250
Aztec culture, 227, 228

Bacon, 339
Baldness, 310
Baja California, 83, 90–91
Baked goods, hydrogenated fat in, 279
Baking, flour substitution in, 292
Baking powder, 292
Baking soda, 279, 305, 307, 312
Baleen whale, 147
Baltimore, Md., 331
Bamboo shoots, 178, 199, 210, 221
Banana and Vegetable Stodge, 132
Banana beer (mwenge), 114, 116, 125, 288
Banana poi, 28–29
Bananas, 309, 318; in Fruit Cocktail, 25; Gandan (Ugandan) use, 4, 111, 113–14, 116, 119–20, 125, 126, 128, 129, 132, 134, 287 (*see also* Banana beer); Marquesan use, 11, 12, 17, 20, 23, 25, 28–29, 285; Mexican use, 235, 243; Steamed, Recipe for, 129
Bantu(s), 110–11
Barbiturates, 307
Barley, 40, 68, 209, 320; and Garbanzo Curry, 78; Hunza Breakfast with, 79; Hunza use, 67, 68, 78, 79
Bass, 112
Bathhouses, Eskimo, 142–43
Bathing (showering), 206–7, 315
Bats, 337
B complex. *See* Vitamin B
Bean(s), 3, 4, 68, 267–68, 297, 310, 321 (*see also* Legumes; Sprouts, specific types); and Carrots in Tofu Sauce, Kidney, 225; Fish Soup with Green, 131; Chinese use, 169, 174–76; in Couscous Dinner (green), 51; Gandan use, 131, 133; Hunza use, 67–68; Japanese use, 201, 210–11, 222, 225, 226; Mexican use, 7, 227, 228, 232, 233, 235, 236, 238–39, 240, 245 ff., 253, 254, 257, 283; Paste, 226; Refried, Recipe for, 249; Stodge, Peanut and, 133; in Stuffed Squash Blossom Omelet, 253; Tamales with, 254; in Tempura (green), 222

Bean curd, 316; Chinese use, 166, 168, 175, 192–93, 195, 196; Fried Puffy,

196; Japanese use (tofu), 202, 209–10, 216, 218, 221, 222, 225, 226, 266; skin of, 195, 196; Szechwan, Recipe for, 192–93
Beavertail cactus, 97, 104
Bedsores, 314
Beef, 300, 311, 338–39, 340 (*see also* Hamburger); compared with algae, 234; compared with cornmeal, kidney beans, 240; compared with insects, 100–1; compared with organ meats, 276; fat vs. pork and fish, 277; formaldehyde and fat, 339; Japanese use, 202, 205, 211, 221; Jerky, 107–8; Mexicans and, 235; Sukiyaki, Recipe for, 221
Bee larvae, 100
Beer, 230, 283, 339. *See also* Banana beer
Beets and greens, 126, 129, 242, 270, 273 ff.
Begert (anthropologist), 91
Belding, T. J., 294
Benzoic acid, 338
Beriberi, 161
Bering Sea, 342
Berries, 302, 312 (*see also* specific kinds); Diegueños and, 84, 87, 102, 108, 288; Eskimos and, 140, 142, 145 ff., 151, 154, 160, 266, 268, 287; Pemmican with, 108; for Relish on Greens, 154
Bethel, Alaska, 136, 287
Bicycling, 296
Bieler, Henry, 87
Bile; bile salts, 301, 320
Bioflavonoids, 37, 43, 69, 235, 239, 313
Biotin, 310, 331
Birds (wildfowl), 336, 345 (*see also* Eggs); Diegueños and, 87, 99; Eskimos and, 140, 142, 146, 148, 302
Bird's nest soup, 183
Birth defects, 325
Bitter melon, 179
Black beans, 174, 210, 232
Blackberries, 148
Blackfish, 138, 141, 142, 144, 146, 152
Blackstrap molasses, 281, 291, 307, 310
Bleaching agents, 314
Bleu cheese, 266; and Butter Spread, 156
Blindness, 90, 325; snow, 305
Blood, 269, 277, 280, 301, 309 ff., 318, 321 (*see also* Anemia; Arteries; Blood pressure; Capillaries; Circulation; specific constituents); clotting, 301, 302, 316; in Eskimo diet, 141, 142, 160, 266; seawater as, 205
Blood pressure, 60, 121, 167, 203, 232, 310, 313–14, 318, 329, 341

Blood sugar, 167, 299, 302, 332–33. *See also* Hypoglycemia
Blossoms. *See* Flowers
Blubber, 139
Blueberries, 147, 154
Blumer, Walter, 328
Bok toy, 177
Bone marrow, 277, 305, 310, 315; Eskimos and, 140, 141, 146, 149; Paste, 107; in school lunch program, 293
Bone meal, 92, 93, 100, 102, 104, 276, 324, 345
Bones, 2, 65, 274, 276–77, 278, 315, 316–17, 320, 321 (*see also* Bone marrow; Bone meal); Gandans and, 122; Eskimos and, 146, 152, 277; fractures, kelp and, 206; Hunzas and, 61; Marquesans and, 17, 25; Tuareg and, 37
Bonito, 209, 214
Botulism, 144
Boy Scouts, 290
Brain, the, 299, 210, 329
Brains (as food), 276, 301, 310; in Ground Nut Sauce, 132
Bran, 200–1, 262 ff., 302, 321, 342; Granola with, 108
Bread, 134, 152, 157, 266, 267, 268, 293, 294, 297, 299 (*see also* specific forms); Chinese, 170, 176; Diegueños, 92, 109; Mexican, 283; Seventh-day Adventists and, 258; Sourdough Rye Recipe, 155; Tuareg, 41, 286
Breadfruit, 9, 11, 13, 15 ff., 23, 25, 266, 285
Breakfast, Hunza, 79; Recipe for, 82
Breast cancer, 201, 259, 320
Breast feeding (lactation), 16, 113, 136, 230, 270–72, 321
Brewers' yeast, 307, 311, 317, 320, 321, 324, 345
Britain (England), 169, 271
Broccoli, 177, 178, 185, 187; Braised, Recipe for, 190
Brussels sprouts, 269
Buckwheat (groats), 68, 312, 321; Chinese use, 176; Diegueños and, 103, 105; with Pumpkin Seeds, 105; Hunza use, 67, 68; Japanese use, 209; substituting in baking, 292
Buffalo, 113
Bulgur: Lentil and Wheat Stew, 53; Salad, 53
Bulk, 302–3. *See also* Fiber
Buns, 6; Lotus, 191
Burkitt, Denis P., 117, 262, 303
Burning (*see also* Smoke): newspapers, 342
Burns, 314. *See also* Sunburn
Bursitis, 345
Butchers paper, 344

Butter (butterfat), 4, 42, 46, 63, 71, 278, 292, 300, 305, 315
Buttermilk, 41, 63, 70, 72, 73, 75, 266
Butylated hydroxyanisole, 338
Buwei Yang Chao, 195 n

Cabbage, 99, 196, 210, 275, 320, 340; Chinese use, 163–64, 177–78, 196; Japanese and, 210, 224; in Pickled Mixed Vegetables, 224; Mexican use, 242
Cabbage looper, 337
Cacao, 119
Cacti, 85, 97, 239, 243. *See also* types
Cactus worms, 234
Cadmium, 341
Caffeine, 290, 307, 310, 331
Caillas, Alen, 98
Cake, Nut, 256
Calcium, 3 ff., 62, 206, 264, 269, 273 ff., 280, 281, 290, 291, 315, 316–17, 324, 343 ff., 347, 352, 354; Chinese and, 169, 174, 175, 177, 178, 180, 181, 186, 187; Diegueños and, 92, 93, 97, 99, 100, 103, 104; Eskimos and, 140, 141, 146, 149–50, 152, 153; Gandans and, 113, 115, 120 ff., 127, 128; grains vs. legumes, 68; Hunzas and, 66, 67, 69 ff., 74, 75; Japanese and, 209, 212, 213, 217, 218; Marquesans and, 17 ff., 21, 24, 25; Mexicans and, 231, 233, 237, 247, 248; milks vs. bean curd, 175; sesame seeds vs. milk, 213; Tuareg and, 36, 40, 48, 49, 286
Calcium edetate, 328
Calcium lactate, 324
Calcium propionate, 338
Calcium sulfate, 175
California, 259. *See also* Diegueños
California, University of, at Davis, 339
California holly, 96
Calories, 3 ff., 65, 264, 272, 273, 280, 291, 295–96, 349, 354; Chinese and, 174, 186, 187; cornmeal, kidney beans, beef compared, 240; Diegueños and, 93, 101, 103, 104; Eskimos and, 146, 153, 154; Gandans and, 120, 124, 127, 128; grains vs. legumes, 68; Hunzas and, 65, 66, 68, 70, 74, 75; insects vs. beef, 101; Japanese and, 209, 213; Marquesans and, 17, 24, 25; Mexicans and, 240, 247, 248; milks vs. bean curd, 175; organ meats vs. beef, 276; sesame seeds vs. milk, 213; Tuareg and, 40, 48, 49
Camels and camel milk, 32, 35 ff., 41–42, 266
Camembert cheese, 266
Cancer, 259, 262, 300, 302, 306, 311–12 ff., 320, 325, 328 ff., 338, 339, 346; Diegueños and, 91; Eskimos and, 141;

Gandans and, 117; Japanese and, 201, 203; Mexicans and, 232
Candy, 15, 204, 285–86; Coconut, 29–30; Peanut Butter, 133
Cannibalism, 8
Canning, 264, 265 (see also specific foods); and potassium, 318
Cantaloupe, 290, 302, 305, 310, 318
Cantonese cuisine, 165, 166
Capillaries, 329
Carbohydrates (starches), 3 ff., 5, 65, 267, 269, 289, 297 ff., 307, 308, 319, 321, 323, 332, 349, 354 (see also Starches); Chinese and, 174, 186, 187; Digueños and, 93, 97, 103, 104; Eskimos and, 140, 141, 146, 152, 153; Gandans and, 115, 120, 122, 127, 128; Hunzas and, 65, 66, 70, 74, 75; Japanese, 209, 217, 218; Marquesans and, 17, 19, 24, 25; Mexicans and, 238, 247, 248; Tuareg and, 40, 48, 49
Carbonated beverages. See Soft drinks
Carbon dioxide, 319
Carbon monoxide, 327
Cardiovascular system, 62, 279, 314, 325. See also Circulation; Heart and heart disease
Caribou, 138, 140, 142, 149, 287
Carnitas, 247; Recipe for, 250
Carnow, Bertram W., 329
Carob, 291, 292
Carotene, 305, 306. See also Vitamin A
Carp, 162, 166, 168, 180
Carrots, 305, 321, 323; Chinese use, 185, 188; Hunza use, 61, 69, 73, 77; Japanese use, 201, 210, 218, 222, 224, 225; and Kidney Beans in Tofu Sauce, 225; Mexican use, 242; Pickled Mixed Vegetables with, 224; Tuareg use, 44, 47, 49, 51; Winter Stew with, 77
Cashews, 180, 181
Cassava (manioc), 114 ff., 118, 120, 121, 126, 288
Cataracts, 309
Cattail, 97–98; Pollen Flour, 109
Cattle. See Cows
Cauliflower, 177, 310
Cavanaugh, and kelp, 206
Celery, 148, 210, 211, 242; Chinese use, 177, 185, 189, 191
Celery cabbage. See Cabbage
Cell respiration, 309
Cellulose, 67, 121, 262
Century plant (mescal), 85–86, 94–95. See also Pulque
Cereal, 289, 298 (see also specific grains); Granola, 108–9; Hunza Breakfast, 79, 82; Japanese and, 204
Cesium, 137, 140

Chapattis, 7, 62–63, 66, 72, 73, 75; Recipe for, 76
Chard, 23, 120, 242, 275; in Coconut Cream, Baked, 26–27
Chard cabbage, 177
Chawan-Mushi, 224–25
Cheese, 6–7, 266, 289 (see also Bean curd); and Butter Spread, Bleu, 156; Chiles and, 256; Curd Curry, 55; Date Balls, 54; Hunzas and, 63, 70; Mexican use, 232, 235, 244, 253, 256, 257; Squash Blossom Omelet with, 253; Tuareg use, 35, 37, 42, 46, 54, 55, 286
Chemicals. See Additives; Pollution
Cherimoya, 243
Cherries, 179; acerola, 324
Cherry, holly-leaved, 96
Cherry wine, 284
Chestnuts (see also Water chestnuts): Japanese and, 212
Cheung, T. K., 173
Chewing, and digestion, 299
Chewing gum, 287, 288
Chia (and seeds), 86, 89, 94, 100, 288
Chicken(s), 337, 344 (see also Eggs); Almond, Recipe for, 189; Chinese use, 162, 167, 183, 187 ff.; Couscous Dinner with, 51; Custard, Main-Dish, 224–25; Digueños-style (including recipe), 103, 105; Gandan, 123, 130; Giblet Soup, Recipe for, 188; Hunzas and, 71; Japanese use, 204, 211, 216, 218, 224–25; Mexican use, 232, 235, 246, 255–56; and Rice Soup, 255–56; Thick-Curried, 130
Chick peas. See Garbanzos
Chicory, Salad with, 104
Children, 265, 289 ff., 295; and amino acids, 296; Chinese, 167–68, 170 ff., 285; Digueño, 87–89, 90, 288; Eskimo, 136–37, 140, 144, 271, 287; and fluoride in water, 330–31; Gandan, 113, 123, 128, 287–88; growing pains, 316; Hunza, 59, 60, 64; hyperactive, 338, 342, 344; and imitation milk, 278; Japanese, 202–3, 284; Marquesan, 9–10, 14, 15–16, 285; Mexican, 230, 233, 236; in Michigan suburb, 233; and organ meats, 276; protein requirements, 298; Seventh-day Adventist, 259; Tuareg, 34, 38, 46
Chiles (and sauce), 227, 228, 232 ff., 238, 241–42, 245, 246, 248, 249, 251, 253, 256, 283; and Cheese, 256; and magnesium, 317; to skin, 249 n
China (Chinese), 13–14, 161–97, 204, 266, 268, 284–85, 334–35, 336, 348 ff.
Chinese cabbage. See Cabbage
Chisso Chemical plant, 207

Chlorine, 206, 321, 330
Chlorophyll, 267–68
Chocolate, 290, 291; for Mole Poblano, 251–52
Cholesterol, 60, 70, 139, 231, 262, 280, 300 ff., 310, 311, 313, 339
Choline, 308, 310, 331
Chopsticks, 185, 187, 200
Chorizos, 232
Chow Haak Look, 185; Recipe, 188–89
Chromium, 321, 342, 344
Chrysolina beetle, 336
Ch'u Yuan, 161
Cider (see also Vinegar): toyon, 96
Cigarettes. See Tobacco and smoking
Cilantro, 182, 239
Cilia, 327
Circulation, 234, 311, 332, 341. See also Cardiovascular system
Citrus fruit, 212, 310, 312, 313, 324
Clams, 141; Fish Soup with, 154
Clay, 92, 102, 316
Clothing, 10, 33–34, 36
Coal tar additives, 332
Cobalt, 321
Cobalt-60 gamma rays, 336
Cockroaches, 345
Cocoa, 228, 236, 245, 331. See also Chocolate
Coconut (see also Coconut cream; Coconut oil): Candy, 29–30; Granola with, 108; Marquesans and, 12–13, 16, 17, 19, 25–26, 29–30, 267, 285; Pudding, 29; Toasted, 25–26
Coconut crabs, 13
Coconut cream, 12–13, 23, 25; Recipe for, 26
Coconut oil, 278–79, 300, 301; Marquesans and, 10, 17, 19
Cod, 146; liver oil, 293, 345
Coffee, 116, 119, 125, 245, 259, 288, 331–32, 347; Dandelion, 109
Colache, 246 ff.; Recipe for, 248
Cola drinks, 6, 290, 332; Japanese and, 204; Mexicans and, 236, 237, 283
Colds, 91, 205, 234, 313
Collagen, 312
Collard greens, 126; Recipe for, 129
Colon, 266; cancer, 203, 262, 302
Coloring, artificial, 265, 290, 338
Colostrum, 272
Columbus, Ohio, 330
Comal, 227, 246
Comino, 245
Commoner, Barry, 335
Compost heap, 340
Condiment sauces, Chinese, 191
Confucius, 162, 177
Congee, 168, 177, 185, 193

Constipation, 70, 98, 206, 239, 262, 270, 272, 302, 307, 344
Convenience foods, 278
Cook, Captain James, 277
Cookies, 204, 283, 287, 288; Chinese Almond, 194–95
Cooking. See Preparation, food
Copper, 321
Copra traders, 13, 14
Coriander, 182, 239
Cormorants, 148
Corn (cornmeal), 68, 274, 296, 300, 335 (see also Corn oil; Maize); Cakes, 250; Chinese use, 176; Hunza use, 61, 62, 67, 68, 72, 78, 268; kidney beans, beef compared to, 240; Mexican use, 227, 228, 230–31 ff., 235–36 ff., 240, 246, 248, 250, 254, 282; Mush, 107; Pumpkin Pudding with, 106; substitution in baking, 292; Summer Soup with, 78; Sweet Tamales, 254; tortillas (see Tortillas)
Corn borer, 337
Corn oil, 300
Coronary problems. See Heart and heart disease
Cortés, Hernando, 234
Cortisone, 309, 310, 318
Cottage cheese, 41, 70, 82, 85; Curd Curry, 55
Coughing, 327
Couscous, 35, 36, 46, 51, 286; Recipe for, 52
Cows (cattle), 59, 336. See also Milk
Crabs, 13, 100
Cramps, muscle, 313, 316
Cranberries, 148, 152, 159; Ice, Ice Cream, 159; Relish, 154
Cream, 40, 63, 305, 309, 315, 321; sour, 292, 300
Cream cheese: Date Balls, 54; Snacks, Tuareg-style, 55
Creamers, nondairy, 300
Cream of tartar, 292
Crime, Mexicans and, 232
Crock pot, 12
Cucumber(s), 201, 209, 210, 216, 218, 257, 282; Fish, 216, 218–19; in Gazpacho, 252; Summer Soup with, 78
Cucurbocitrin, 121
Cuero, Delfina, 90–91
Cumin, 245
Currants, red, 148
Curry, 317; Barley and Garbanzo, 78; Cheese Curd, 55; Hunzas and, 73, 75, 77, 78; Lamb, 77; Sauce, Tuareg-style, 55; Spinach, 75; Tuareg and, 43, 46, 47, 50, 55
Custard, 244, 283; Main-Dish, 224–25
Custard apple, 243

Cuttlefish, 166
Cyclamates, 312

Daikon (radish), 201, 210, 212
Dairy products, 66, 278, 296, 297, 303, 307 (*see also* specific products); imitation, 278–79, 300
Dandelion, 275; Coffee, 109; Digueños and, 99, 102, 104, 109; Hunzas and, 69, 73; Mixed Greens with, 155; Salad with, 104
Dashi, 211, 214. *See also* specific dishes
Date(s), 285; Balls, 54; Chinese and, 179; Tuareg and, 35–36, 39–40, 41, 46, 54, 286, 303
Davis, Adelle, 308
Davis, Clara M., 276
Day Lily Blossom Omelets, Stuffed, 252
Death, 137, 325. *See also* Longevity
Deep-frying, 300
Deer, 89, 99
Degenerative disease, 203, 270, 290, 314–15, 323. *See also* Longevity
Dental arch, 270. *See also* Teeth
Depression, 307, 328
Derris, 337
Detergents, 344
Diabetes and diabetics, 117, 203, 259, 305, 308, 310, 311, 313, 325
Diarrhea, 137, 305, 318, 319
Digestion, 44, 70, 122, 235, 239, 242, 266, 267, 280, 296, 298 ff., 304, 306–7, 328, 344. *See also* Hydrochloric acid; Intestines; Stomach
Digitalis, 318
Digueños, 83–109, 262, 276, 288–89, 348 ff.
Diphtheria, 13
Dipping gravy, Gandan, 125, 126
Dirt, 327
Disease. *See* Health and disease
Diuretics, 318
Diurnal rhythms, 345
Diverticulitis, 262
Dock, 99
Doctors, Chinese, 171–72
Dogs, Eskimo, 137, 151
Dolomite, 324
Donkeys, Hunza, 59
Doong gwah, 179
Dot hearts, 183, 284
Doughnuts, Japanese and, 284
Dried foods, 263. *See also* specific foods
Dropsy, 91
Dr. Siegal's Natural Fiber . . . Diet, 200
Drugs, 258, 259, 307, 310 ff., 339. *See also* specific items
Ducks, 148, 164, 165; eggs, 182; livers, 284; Peking, 190–91

Duke University, 98
Dumplings, Chinese, 165, 176
Duodenal ulcers, 201, 325
Dye, mesquite, 95
Dysentery, amoebic, 137

Eating, and calorie-burning, 296
Eczema, 307
Edema, 309, 318
Edible pod peas. *See* Snow peas
Eel, 21, 200, 214, 305
Eggplant, 178, 290, 302, 308; Grilled, Recipe for, 219; Japanese use, 201, 210, 216, 219, 222; Stew, 52; Tempura with, 222
Eggs, 42, 269, 296, 300, 301, 305, 307, 309 ff., 313 ff., 319 ff.; Chinese and, 182–83, 196; Digueños and, 87, 99, 109; Eskimos and, 140, 142, 149; Hunzas and, 71; Japanese and, 209, 212, 220; Mexicans and, 241, 244, 245, 252; and minerals, 319 ff., 343; Stuffed Squash Blossom Omelets, 252; Tuareg and ostrich, 43
Egg wrapper, 220
Elephant, 113
Emotional disturbance, 307, 317. *See also* Mental health
Emphysema, 259, 306, 314, 328, 329, 341
Emulsifiers, 265
Enamel pans, 343
Endive, 340
Endocrines, 344. *See also* Hormones
Endosperm, 263, 264, 341
Energy. *See* Metabolism
England (Britain), 169, 271
Entebbe, 116
Environmental Protection Agency (EPA), 328, 330
Enzymes, 265, 266, 268 ff.
Epsom salts, 324
Eskimos, 135–59, 263, 265–66, 268, 269, 287, 299, 302, 305, 348 ff.
Estrogens, 310, 314, 320, 333. *See also* Oral contraceptives
Estrom, James E., 259
Exercise (activity), 172–73, 296, 307, 346 (*see also* Sports); sweating, 318, 320
Eyes (*see also* Eyesight): eating, 100, 123, 146, 276, 305
Eyesight (eyes; vision), 60, 90, 203, 305, 306, 309, 325, 329, 345

Fairbanks, 135
Fallout, radioactive, 345–46
False Bay, 83
Fasting, 37
Fast meal. *See* Quick meal
Fatigue, 306–7, 328, 332, 345

Fats, 3 ff., 65, 263, 264, 277, 290, 297, 299–302, 303, 305, 306, 309, 310, 314, 315, 323, 324, 329, 339, 347, 348, 354 (*see also* specific fats); Chinese and, 174, 181, 186, 187; cornmeal, kidney beans, beef compared, 240; Digueños and, 89, 93, 100, 101, 103, 104; Eskimos and, 138–39, 146, 147, 153, 154, 287, 299; Gandans and, 120, 124, 127, 128; Hunzas and, 63, 65, 66, 69, 74, 75; in imitation dairy products, 278–79; insects vs. beef, 101; Japanese and, 203, 206, 209, 212 ff., 217, 218; Marquesans and, 17, 19, 21, 24, 25; Mexicans and, 238, 240, 244, 245, 247, 248; sesame seeds vs. milk, 213; Tuareg and, 36, 40, 43, 44, 48, 49

Fatty acids, 67, 213, 269, 299 ff., 310, 313 ff., 347; Chinese and, 175; Digueños and, 93, 94; Eskimos and, 287; Gandans and, 124; Hunzas and, 70; Japanese and, 212, 213; Mexicans and, 242

FDA, 289, 311, 332, 339

FD&C, 338

Feathers, 146, 148, 302

Feingold, Ben F., 338

Fermentation, 266–67, 308–9, 312, 332, 340. *See also* Alcohol; specific foods

Fertilizers, 62, 305, 320, 330, 333, 334–35, 341. *See also* Night soil

Fiber, 3 ff., 262, 264, 270, 302–3, 340, 344, 347, 353, 354; Chinese and, 174, 186, 187; cornmeal, kidney beans, beef compared, 240; Digueños and, 93, 103, 104; Eskimos and, 146, 148, 152, 153; Gandans and, 117, 120, 127, 128, 303; Hunzas and, 66, 74, 75; Japanese and, 201, 209, 217, 218; Marquesans and, 17, 24, 25; Mexicans and, 231, 238 ff., 245, 247, 248; Tuareg and, 39 ff., 48, 49

Field beans, 116

Figs, 179, 302, 317

Finns, 267

Fire (*see also* Burning): ash, 92

Fire pit (imu), 11–12, 15, 22–23, 285

Fish, 274, 277–78, 293, 296, 299, 305, 307 ff., 311, 315 ff., 340, 342, 347 (*see also* specific fish); Chinese and, 164, 165–66, 168, 174, 176, 180, 183, 196, 284; with Coconut Cream, 27; Cucumber, 218; Digueños and, 86, 87, 89, 100; drying, 263 (*see also* Fish: Eskimos and); Eskimos and, 136 ff., 150–51 ff., 158, 266, 268–69, 287; Fried, 28; Gandans and, 112 ff., 120, 123, 125, 126, 128, 131, 134; Japanese and, 200, 202, 205, 207–8 ff., 214, 216, 218, 219, 222, 284, 309; liver oil, 315, 324 (*see also* Cod: liver oil); Marinated, 28; Marquesans and, 11, 12, 21, 23, 25, 27, 28, 268, 269, 277, 285; and mercury, 207–8, 342; Mexicans and, 282; Soup (Eskimo), Recipe for, 154; Soup (Ugandan), Recipe for, 131; Steamed, 128; Steamed Dried, 158; Stock, 131; Sun-Dried, 158; Tempura with, 222; Teriyaki with, 219

Five-spice, 182

Flan, 244, 283

Flavorings, artificial, 265, 290

Flax, 312

Flounder, 146

Flour, 44, 237, 289, 290, 292, 294, 300, 303, 314 (*see also* Bread; specific kinds of flour); gluten of, 195–96

Flowers (blossoms), 93, 94–95, 234, 239, 312, 313 (*see also* specific plants); dried tiger lilies, 195; Omelets, Stuffed Blossom, 252

Fluorescent light, 344

Fluoride, 330–31

Fluorine, 321

Foil, metal, 343

Folic acid, 310, 311, 313

Foo gwah, 179

Formaldehyde, 339, 346

Fowl. *See* Birds; Poultry

Fractures, 206

Freezing and frozen foods, 262, 265–66, 313, 314, 318, 322, 337, 344

French, the, 10, 14, 32

French fried, 284

Fright, 312

Fruit, 160, 263, 270, 281, 291, 293, 297, 298, 302, 312, 313, 320, 322–23, 334, 340 (*see also* specific fruits); canning, 264; Chinese, 179; Cocktail, Tropical, 23, 25; Digueños and, 93, 102, 108, 109, 288; Hunzas and, 7, 61, 62, 63–64, 66, 69–70, 79, 80, 82, 263, 285–86; Japanese and, 210, 213, 284; Leather, 80; Mexicans and, 232, 235, 242–43; and Nut Snack, 80; Pemmican with, 108

Fudge, 290

Fungi, 98

Fuzzy melon, 179

Gai choy, 177–78

Gallstones, 314

Gambia, 119

Game (hunting), 37, 42–43, 87, 88, 99–100, 113

Gamma rays, 236

Gandans (Uganda), 4, 110–34, 287–88, 303, 348 ff.

Gangrene, 314

Garbanzos, 68, 311; in Couscous Dinner, 51; Curry, Barley and, 78; how to sprout, 81; Hunzas and, 64, 67, 68, 78, 81; Mexicans and, 235; Sesame Dip, 52–53; Tuareg and, 41, 51 ff.
Gardening, 340, 346
Garlic, 43, 44, 166, 167, 182
Gasoline, 342
Gastric juices, 318. See also Hydrochloric acid
Gastrointestinal problems. See Digestion; Intestines
Gazelle, 42
Gazpacho, 252
Geese, 148; eggs, 182
Gerard (herbalist), 239
Germ (grain), 262 ff., 342. See also Wheat germ
Ghee, 35, 36, 42, 70
Ginger, 43, 46, 73, 166, 167, 182
Ginkgo, 195
Ginseng, 167
Giraffe, 42
Gizzard, chicken, 185, 188
Glass, 322, 343–44; window, 345
Glasses (lenses; spectacles), 325, 345
Glucose, 299
Gluten of flour, 195–96
Gnats, 115, 116, 119, 124, 288
Goats (cheese, milk), 336; Gandan, 123; Hunza, 58, 59, 63, 65, 70, 71; Marquesan, 11, 22, 277; Mexican, 244; Tuareg, 32, 35, 37, 41–42, 47
Goiter, 121, 319
Goldfish, 180
Golf courses, 342
Gourds, 209, 210
Gout, 91, 309
Goya, Francisco de, 341
Grains, 5, 258, 259, 262–63, 267–68, 292, 297, 298, 300, 302, 303, 305, 307, 311, 313, 314, 316 ff., 321, 340 ff. (see also Bran; Bread; specific grains); Chinese and, 169, 176; Digueños and, 262; Gandans and, 116, 117; Hunza Breakfast, 79; Hunzas and, 62, 63, 66–67, 79, 262; Japanese and, 208–10; Mexicans and, 232, 237–38; Tuareg and, 36, 40–41, 46, 303
Granola, 108–9
Grapefruit, 243
Grapes, 179
Grasses. See Seeds; Sorrel; Sprouts
Grasshoppers, 100
Grayling, 146
Greeks, 56–57
Green beans. See Beans
Greens, 5, 17, 263, 275, 277, 278, 302, 305, 309, 311 ff., 316 ff., 321, 323, 334 (see also specific greens); Chinese and, 174, 177–78; Digueños and, 87, 93, 99, 102, 104; Eskimos and, 140, 142, 145, 146, 151, 155, 266, 268; Gandans and, 114, 120–21, 122, 126, 129; Hitachimono, Recipe for, 219; Hunzas and, 66, 69; Japanese and, 201, 209, 210, 216, 218 ff.; Mexicans and, 232, 235; Mixed, Recipe for, 155; Steamed, Recipe for, 129; Tuareg and, 286
Gristle, 277
Ground nuts. See Peanuts
Groundnuts, Eskimo, 140, 147, 152
Growing pains, 316
Grulee, C. G., 271
Grunion, 86, 100
Guacamole, 247; Recipe for, 250
Guadalajara, 237
Guavas, 235, 243
Guinea pigs, 315
Gum (see also Chewing gum): mesquite, 95
Gums, seaweed and, 205
Guy Gon Tong, 185, 188
Gypsum, 175

Hair: animal, 327; baldness, 310; dyes, 342; fat deficiency and, 300
Hair vegetable, 195
Halibut, 138, 216, 219, 310
Ham, 318, 339
Hamburger (beef patty), 3, 4, 6
Hamites, 111
Hanford Laboratory, 140
Harris, Robert S., 233
Haupia, 29
Hay fever, 306, 325, 345
Hazel nuts, 212
Headaches, 234, 328
Health and disease (illness; infection), 271–72, 280, 304, 305–6, 312, 320, 325 (see also Drugs; Pollution; Viruses; specific illnesses, nutrients); Chinese and, 163, 170–72; Chinese Restaurant Syndrome, 182; Digueños and, 87, 90, 91; Eskimos and, 135, 137, 139, 141–42; Gandans and, 116, 117–18; Hunzas and, 59, 60; immunities, breast feeding and, 271; Japanese and, 201, 203; Marquesans and, 10, 13; Mexicans and, 232–33; Seventh-day Adventists and, 259–60; sugar in medicine, 281
Heart (as food), 134, 276, 310; Barbecued, 52; in Chinese soup, 188
Heart and heart disease (coronary problems), 65, 67, 167, 169, 259, 262, 280, 301 ff., 310, 311, 314, 316 ff., 325, 329, 331, 332, 341 (see also Cardiovascular system); and air

pollution, 328; Eskimos and, 139; Gandans and, 117; Hunzas and, 60; Japanese and, 201; Mexicans and, 232

Heat, 308–9, 312 (*see also* Preparation, food; specific foods; substances); prostration, 35–36

Hemoglobin, 319

Hemorrhoids, 262

Herbs. *See* Spices and herbs

Herb tea, 62, 286 (*see also* Mint); Digueños and toyon, 96

Herring, 146

Heung New Fun, 182

High blood pressure. *See* Blood pressure

Highways, living near, 328

Hilton, James, 72

Himalayas. *See* Hunzas

Hippopotami, 113

Hitashimono, 216, 220

Hoggar, 31

Hokkaido, 199

Holly, 96

Holly-leaved cherry, 96

Homes (houses): Chinese, 183–85; Digueño, 101–2; Eskimo, 144, 150–51; Hunza, 58, 72–73; Japanese, 206, 214–15; Marquesan, 22; Mexican, 228–29; Tuareg, 45–46

Honey, 16, 63, 87, 102, 281, 288, 291, 292

Honey ants, 287–88

Honshu, 199

Hormones, 201, 209, 339. *See also* Endocrines; Estrogen

Horses, 32, 59, 166, 268

Hospitals, 342–43

Hot Cakes, Sourdough, 156

Hot dogs, 338, 339

House plants, 346

Houston, Robert, 118

How to Cook and Eat in Chinese, 195 n

Huacamotes, 239

Humas, 52–53

Humboldt County, Calif., 336

Hunter, J. D., 301

Hunting. *See* Game

Hunzas, 7, 56–82, 262, 263, 266, 268, 270, 273, 285–86, 348 ff.

Hybrid crops, 307

Hydrocarbons, 327

Hydrochloric acid, 235, 280, 298, 316, 319, 321, 324. *See also* Gastric juices; Stomach

Hydrogenated fats, 279, 284, 290, 300–1

Hypoglycemia, 307. *See also* Blood sugar

Hyperactivity, 338, 342, 344

Ice, Cranberry, 159

Iceberg lettuce, 275

Ice cream: Cranberry, 159; Eskimo, 139, 147, 159, 287; Hunza, 64, 286

Iguana, 234

Illness. *See* Health and disease

Imjudara, 53

Immunities, breast feeding and, 271

Impotency, 320

Imu. *See* Fire pit

India, opium in, 169

Indian fig. *See* Tuna cactus

Indian potato, 148

Indians, 274, 312. *See also* Digueños; Mexicans

Infants, 325. *See also* Children

Infection. *See* Health and disease

Initiative, lack of, 307

Ink, lead in, 342

Inositol, 308, 310, 331

Insanity, 232; schizophrenia, 309

Insect bites, 312

Insecticides. *See* Pesticides

Insects, 277, 307, 315, 317, 336 (*see also* specific kinds); Digueños and, 100–1; Gandans and, 114–15, 119, 124, 287–88; Mexicans and, 243–44; nutrients compared to beef, 101; Tuareg and, 45

Insomnia, 316, 332

Insulin, 310, 320, 332, 333. *See also* Diabetes and diabetics

Intestines (and gastrointestinal problems), 44, 123, 141, 167, 262, 266–67, 270, 301, 303, 305, 308, 310, 313, 318, 340 (*see also* Colon); in Eskimo diet, 147; Gandans and, 117, 122

Iodine, 277, 319–20, 331, 347; Digueños and, 98, 99; Eskimos and, 140; Gandans and, 121; Japanese and, 201, 205, 206; Marquesans and, 19

Irish moss, 205

Iron, 3 ff., 97, 206, 263, 264, 273, 275, 277, 281, 291, 313, 314, 319, 321, 324, 331, 353, 354; Chinese and, 169, 174, 175, 177, 178, 181, 186, 187; in cornmeal, kidney beans, beef, 240; Digueños and, 92 ff., 97, 100, 101, 103, 104; Eskimos and, 140, 141, 146, 149, 152, 153; Gandans and, 120, 123, 124, 127, 128; grains vs. legumes, 68; Hunzas and, 64, 66 ff., 74, 75; insects vs. beef, 101; Japanese and, 209, 212, 213, 217, 218; Marquesans and, 16 ff., 24, 25; Mexicans and, 231, 233, 238 ff., 242, 244, 245, 247, 248; milks vs. bean curd, 175; organ meats vs. beef, 276; pots, 274,

322; Tuareg and, 39 ff., 44, 45, 48, 49
Irradiation, 313
Irritability, 307, 344
Islay, 96

Japanese, 1, 177, 198–226, 266, 268, 269, 283–84, 309, 334, 348 ff.
Jellyfish, 214
Jensen, Bernard, 270
Jerky, 107–8, 109
Jet lag, 345
Jicama, 241, 257, 282
Jimson weed, 87–88
Judgment, poor, 345
Junk foods, 289–90 ff.; Japanese, 284

Kai choy kou, 181–82
Kale, 177, 275
Kamabako, 214
Kampala, 116
Kanten, 211
Karam, 73, 75
Kasha. See Buckwheat
Kefir, 266
Kelp, 99, 140, 146, 149–50, 152, 166, 205, 206, 320, 321, 324, 345
Kidney bean(s), 116, 232, 240; and Carrots in Tofu Sauce, 225; cornmeal, beef compared with, 240; how to sprout, 81; Paste, 226; Refried, 249; Stodge, Peanut and, 133
Kidney(s), 121, 134, 147, 276, 280, 287, 297, 305, 306, 308, 311, 319, 331; Stew, 157
Kinton, 226
Klamath weed, 336
Kobe, 202
Kohn, Harriet, 272
Kombu, 211
Kuhl, Johannes, 267
Kuskokwim R., 136, 138, 145, 149, 287
Kweifei chicken, 162
Kyushu Island, 207–8

Lactase, 113
Lactation, 321. See also Breast feeding
Lactic acid, 141, 266, 267
Lactose, 71, 267
Ladybugs, 335, 340
Laetrile, 311–12
La Jolla, 83
Lake Chapala, 237
Lake Victoria. See Gandans
Lamb, 311, 340; Couscous Dinner with, 51; Curry, 77; Spinach Curry with, 73; with Vegetable Curry, 50
Lamb's quarters, 99
Language, Marquesan, 15
Lard, 181, 238, 248; stability of, 300
Laxatives, 305

Lead, 327, 341–42
Lecithin, 169, 175, 272, 301, 310, 329
Leek, Tempura with, 222
Legumes, 67–68, 269, 278, 297, 302, 307, 312, 314, 317 ff., 321, 340. See also specific kinds
Lemon juice, 308
Lemon pie, 343
Lemons, 345
Lent, 230
Lentils, 41, 47, 49, 64, 67, 68, 73, 321; how to sprout, 81; and Wheat Stew, 53; Winter Stew with, 77
Leprosy, 13
Lettuce, 3, 232, 275. See also Romaine
Leukemia, 259
Lichen, 140
Light, 312, 344–45 (see also Sunlight; Ultraviolet); and Vitamin A, 305, 306
Lima bean(s), 174, 210, 232, 302; Paste, 226
Lime, 330
Lime juice, 235, 243, 269, 308
Lin Yutang, 161, 165
Ling cod, 146
Liquid, 303–4, 312. See also Water; specific uses
Liver (including use as food), 276, 280, 297, 301, 305, 306, 308, 310 ff., 319 ff., 324, 331, 333, 340, 342, 344, 346; Chinese and, 185, 187, 188, 192, 284; Eskimos and, 137, 140, 141, 146, 147, 152, 157–58, 159, 287; Gandans and, 123, 134; oil (see Fish liver oil; Seal oil); Paste, Recipe for, 157–58; Stir-Fry, 192
Lizards, 99; iguana, 234
Lobster, Tempura with, 222
Locusts, 45, 115, 119, 124, 336
Lok baak, 178
Loma Linda, Calif., 259
Long beans, 210
Longevity (life expectancy), 37, 59, 270; Chinese, 163, 169–70, 171
Loquats, 179
Los Angeles, Calif., 342
Lotus, 181, 210; Buns, 191
Lunch meat, 339
Lungs, 65, 259, 306, 310, 327 ff.; in Eskimo diet, 140–41
Lymph system, 318
Lysine, 41, 278, 298

Mackerel, 315; Fish Soup with, 154
Magnesium, 67, 69, 71, 264, 310, 316, 317, 324, 332, 335
Magnesium oxide, 324
Maguey (agave), 85–86, 94–95. See also Pulque
Maguey worms, 243–44

Maize, 165, 312
Malaria, 117
Malva (mallow), 233–34, 235, 241
Mammals (see also Sea mammals): light/dark experiments with, 345
Mandarin oranges, 213
Manganese, 321
Mangos, 12, 17, 20, 23, 25, 235, 282, 285; in Fruit Cocktail, 25
Manure, 335
Manzanita, 96
Mare's tail, 148
Margarine, 279, 300, 301
Market day, Mexican, 229–30
Marquesans, 1, 8–30, 266, 268, 269, 272, 273, 277, 285, 348 ff.
Marriage. See Sex and marriage
Marrow. See Bone marrow
Matoke (stew), 113, 116, 120, 125; Recipe, 130
Mayan culture, 228
Mayonnaise, 6, 302
Measles, 91, 135
Meat, 258, 259, 263, 268–69, 273, 293, 296, 297, 299, 303, 307, 309, 311, 312, 320, 321, 338–40, 347 (see also Organ meats; specific dishes, meats); Chinese use, 165, 169, 174, 177, 180, 193, 196; Diguéños and, 99–100, 107–8; Eskimos and, 149; Gandans and, 113, 116, 123, 125; Hunzas and, 58, 62, 64–65, 71, 266; Japanese and, 202, 203, 211, 214; Jerky Recipe, 107–8; Mexicans and, 229, 232, 235, 244, 253, 254, 283; Mormons and, 259; Pemmican, 108; in Squash Blossom Omelet, 253; Szechwan Bean Curd with, 193; Tamales with, 254; Tuareg and, 35, 37, 42–43, 46
Medicine (see also Drugs; Health and disease): sugar in, 281
Melon (see also specific kinds); Chinese and, 179; Gandans and, 121; Japanese and, 210; Tuareg and seeds, 44
Melt, 276
Melville, Herman, 9
Meningitis, 16
Menstruation, 300, 314, 316, 319
Mental health, 325 (see also Emotional disturbance; Insanity); depression, 307, 328
Mercury, 207–8, 342–43
Mescal, 85–86, 94–95. See also Pulque
Mesquite, 95
Metabolism, 37, 280, 290, 309, 320, 331. See also specific substances
Metate, 227, 231, 246
Methionine, 310
Methyl mercury, 342

Metropolitan Life Insurance Company, 295
Mexicans (Mexico), 7, 227–57, 282–83, 348 ff.; and laetrile, 311
Mice, 99
Michigan, 233
Milk (and products), 268, 269, 293, 296, 300, 301, 309 ff., 315, 316, 321, 324 (see also Breast feeding; Dairy products; specific products); almond, 181; chocolate, 290; and early sexual maturity, 203; fermented, 267 (see also Yogurt); Hunzas and, 62, 63, 66, 70–71, 75; imitation, 278; Mexicans and, 244; mungo bean, 176; sesame seeds vs., 213; soy, 175; Tuareg and, 35, 36–37, 40, 41–42, 46, 266, 286, 303
Milk sugar. See Lactose
Milkweed, 288
Millet, 68, 118, 312, 319; Chinese and, 165, 170; for Couscous Dinner, 51; Gandans and, 111, 113 ff., 123; in Hunza Breakfast, 79; Hunzas and, 61, 63, 67, 68, 79; Recipe, 49–50; Tuareg and, 35, 37, 40–41, 47, 49–50, 51, 286
Mineral oil, 305, 313
Minerals, 99, 233, 266, 269, 280, 303–4, 305, 316–21, 323–24, 342, 347 (see also specific minerals); Hunzas and, 62, 65, 71, 72
Miners, 328
Minimatu Bay, 207–8
Mining residue, 330
Mink, 136, 138
Minnows, 200
Mint, 43, 44, 46, 62, 73; Recipe for Tea, 80
Miscarriage, 314, 339
Miso, 209, 266
Mission Bay, 83
Missionaries, 14, 83, 89–90
Mission Valley, 83
Mitiaro, the, 301
Mok gwah, 179
Molasses (see also Blackstrap molasses): substituting in cooking, 292
Mole poblano, 236, 244; Recipe, 251–52
Molybdenum, 321
Mongols, 162
Monosodium glutamate, 182
Monroe County, Fla., 62
Montezuma, 234
Mortar and pestle, 246
Mormons, 259–60
Morning sickness, 309
Moslems, 272–73. See also Hunzas; Tuareg
Mosquito larva paste, 234

Motor oil, burned, 341
Mountain sorrel, 148
Mousenuts, 149
Mouth, sore, 307
MSG, 182
Mucous membrane, 306, 327, 328
Mulberries, 57, 63, 81, 213, 285
Mulberry Wine, 286
Mungo beans (sprouts), 176, 268
Murder, 309
Muscles, 67, 280, 313, 316, 317, 332
Mushrooms, 270, 296–97, 309, 310, 315, 321; Buckwheat Groats with, 105; Chinese use, 185, 189, 195; Digueño use, 84, 98, 102, 105, 109; Japanese use, 201, 210, 216, 218 ff., 224, 225; Pickled, 224; Summer Soup with, 78
Mustard, 87, 94, 102; greens, 216, 218
Mustard cabbage, 177–78
Mwenge. See Banana beer

Nails, rusty, 319
Nameko, 210
Nanking, 163
Napalitos, 104
Napaskiak, 136, 138, 142, 145
Nausea, 309, 344
Navy beans, 174
Needlefish, 138, 141, 146
Nerves (nerve tissue; nervous system), 280, 306–7, 310, 317, 329, 343. See also Nervousness
Nervousness, 308, 332, 344, 345
Newburgh, N.Y., 331
New England Journal of Medicine, 323, 344
Newspapers, burning, 342
Niacin, 3 ff., 264, 273, 291, 308, 309, 351, 354; Chinese and, 174, 186, 187; in cornmeal, kidney beans, beef, 240; Digueños and, 93, 94, 97, 101, 103, 104; Eskimos and, 146, 152, 153; Gandans and, 120, 124, 127, 128; grains vs. legumes, 68; Hunzas and, 66, 68, 70, 74, 75; insects vs. beef, 101; Japanese and, 209, 213, 217, 218; Marquesans and, 16, 17, 24, 25; Mexicans and, 236, 238, 240, 242, 244, 247, 248; organ meats vs. beef, 276; sesame seeds vs. milk, 213; Tuareg and, 35, 39, 40, 48, 49
Nickel, 279
Nicotine, 329
Niger area, 31
Night soil, 170, 203–4, 334
Nitrates, 305, 330, 334, 335, 339
Nitrilosides. See Vitamin B₁₇
Nitrites, 305, 334, 335, 339
Nitrogen dioxide, 327
Nitrosamines, 339

Nome, 136
Noodles, 41, 42, 44, 165, 176, 185, 196, 197, 209, 221, 284; peastarch, 195; Recipes, 194
Nopales, 239, 243
Nori, 211, 216, 219
Nose hairs, 327
Nucleic acids, 98, 311, 320
Nut Cake, 256
Nuts, 290, 297, 298, 300, 302, 305, 307, 314, 317 ff., 321, 340, 343 (see also specific kinds): Chinese and, 180–81; Digueños and, 87, 91 ff., 109, 288; Hunzas and, 7, 63, 64, 70, 80, 285–86; Japanese and, 212; Pemmican with, 108; soaking, 322–23; Toasted, 26
Nut Snack, Fruit and, 80

Oats (and oatmeal), 63, 67, 68, 321; Granola with, 108–9; Hunza Breakfast with, 79; substituting in baking, 292
Obesity (overweight; reducing), 117, 201, 206, 262, 270, 295, 299, 302, 343
Ocotillo, 85
Octopus, 100, 166, 200, 209, 214
Oil fields, 330
Oils, 262, 299, 300, 302, 314, 315, 324, 345 (see also specific kinds); Chinese and, 174, 181; in imitation dairy products, 278–79; Japanese and, 209, 212; substituting in cooking, 292
Okra, 44, 122, 126, 129 ff.
Olive oil, 300
Olives, ripe, 321
Ollas, 227
Olmec culture, 228
Omelets, Stuffed Squash Blossom, 252
Onions, 97; Chinese use, 185, 188 ff.; Digueño use, 87, 96–97, 102, 104; Eskimo use, 148, 152; Gandan use, 122, 126, 129 ff.; Hunza use, 61, 69, 73, 78; Japanese use, 216, 218, 221, 222, 224; Mexican use, 235, 242, 246, 248, 249, 252; Pickled Mixed Vegetables with, 224; Salad with, 104; Sliced Tomatoes and Red, 126; Summer Soup with, 78; Tuareg use, 43, 44, 47, 49 ff.
Onoda, Hiro, 284
Opium, 14, 169, 170
Oral contraceptives, 307, 309, 311, 314. See also Estrogens
Orange juice, 293, 343
Oranges, 179, 213, 226, 243, 312; Cranberry Relish on Greens with, 154
Oregano, 245
Organ meats, 146, 275–76, 307, 309, 310, 317, 321. See also specific organs

Orientals (see also Chinese; Japanese): and milk, 41
Osteoporosis, 316–17, 325
Ostrich, 42, 43
Otami Indians, 232–33
Ovaries, sugar and, 280
Overweight. See Obesity
Oxalic acid, 305
Oxygen, 305, 312, 314, 346–47
Oysters, 320

Paak-kwo, 195
PABA, 308, 310
Pacific Coast. See Eskimos
Paint, lead in, 342
Pakistan, 65
Palm oil, 43, 47, 49
Pancreas, 320
Pangamic acid, 311
Pantothenic acid, 308, 309–10, 345
Papain, 242
Papayas, 227, 242, 282; Fruit Cocktail with, 25
Paprika, 37
Para-aminobenzoic acid (PABA), 308, 310
Parchment paper, 344
Parsley, 167, 212, 340; in Mixed Greens, 155
Parsnips, 302; in Couscous Dinner, 51
Passion fruit, 243
Pastries, Mexican, 283
Peaches, 63, 69, 179, 213, 226
Peanut butter, 134, 279, 290, 297, 301, 302; Candy, 133
Peanut oil, 174, 181, 185, 187, 209, 212
Peanuts (ground nuts), 109, 114, 119, 120, 124 ff., 128 ff., 133, 134, 288, 310, 311 (see also Peanut butter; Peanut oil); Sauce, Recipe for, 129; Stodge, Bean and, 133
Pears, 63, 69, 179, 213, 302
Peas, 116, 185, 189, 196, 224, 225, 269, 273, 318 (see also Snow peas); how to sprout, 81; Summer Soup with, 78
Peastarch noodles, 195
Pecan Nut Cake, 256
Pecans, 300
Pectin, 69, 70, 345, 347
Peeling foods, 321–22, 334
Peking, 163, 165–66
Peking Duck, 190–91
Pellagra, 238
Pemmican, 108
Pepper, 43, 318; peppercorns, Chinese, 167
Peppergrass, 98–99
Peppermint, 44
Peppers, 43, 44, 46, 47, 61, 69, 73, 166, 185, 188, 250, 253, 305, 312, 313

(see also Chiles); Colache with, 248; Eggplant Stew with, 52; Pickled Mixed Vegetables with, 224; Summer Soup with, 78; Tempura with, 222
Perch, 112, 116, 119
Pernicious anemia, 311
Peroxides, 314
Persimmons, 179, 210, 213
Pesticides (insecticides), 320, 329, 330, 334 ff., 344; Hunzas and, 62
Phillips, Roland L., 259
Phlebitis, 314
Phosphate, 233, 341, 343, 344
Phosphoric acid, 332
Phosphorus, 62, 206, 263, 273, 277, 316, 317, 320, 324; Digueños and, 100; Hunzas and, 71; Marquesans and, 16, 18, 21; Mexicans and, 244
Phytic acids, 305
Phytin, 267
Pickled foods, 210–11 (see also Fermented foods); Mixed Vegetables, 224; Mushrooms, 224
Pickles, 266
Pigeon eggs, 182
Pigs, 11, 21–22, 344. See also Pork
Pigs' feet, 180, 316; Recipe for Pickled, 193–94
Pike, 146
Pineapple, 179, 185, 188, 227, 243, 282; in Fruit Cocktail, 25; Rice Pudding, 29
Pine needles, 312
Pine nuts. See Piñon nuts
Pinole, 86, 91; Recipe for, 108–9
Piñon nuts (pine nuts), 85, 89, 93–94, 100, 102, 288; Date Balls with, 54; Sunflower Seed Cakes, 106
Pinto beans, 232, 233, 235; Refried, 249; Stodge, Peanut and, 133
Pizzas, 6–7
Plankton, 342
Plantain, 116
Plants (see also Fertilizers; Gardening; Soil; specific cultures, types): eating whole, 323; and oxygen, 345
Plastics, 345, 347
Plums, 179, 210, 213
Plum wine, 284
Pneumonia, 10, 16, 306
Poisons, 326–46. See also specific kinds
Polar bear, 149
Polio, 306
Pollution, 326–47
Polo, Marco, 57–58, 165
Polo (game), 58, 59
Polygamy, 110–11
Polyps, Gandans free from, 117
Polysiloxane, 338
Pomegranates, 243

Pork, 258–59, 308, 311, 318, 338–39 (see also Lard; Pigs; Pigs' feet); Carnitas, Recipe for, 250; Chinese and, 164, 165, 167, 174, 180, 284; Fish in Coconut Cream with, 27; Hunzas and, 63, 64; Jerky, 107–8; Marquesans and, 11, 21–22, 27, 272; Mexicans and, 232, 235, 244, 246, 247

Potato chips, artificial, 289

Potatoes, 3, 4, 6, 270, 273–74, 278, 318; Fish Soup with, 154; Hunza use, 61, 69, 72, 77, 268; Indian, 148; Kidney Stew with, 157; Mexican use, 227, 241; Winter Stew with, 77

Poultry (fowl), 174, 183, 196, 211, 244, 296, 297, 299, 307, 309, 317, 338–39 (see also Stews; specific fowl); in Squash Blossom Omelet, 253; in Szechwan Bean Curd, 193; Tamales with, 254

Pregnancy and childbirth, 60, 309 (see also Breast feeding); Chinese and, 180; Eskimos and, 271; Marquesans and, 15–16; Mexicans and, 230; miscarriage, 314, 339

Preparation, food, 321–23, 343–44

Preservation and storage, food, 262–64, 343–44. See also Preservatives

Preservatives, 265, 290, 305

Pressure-cooked foods, 298

Price, Weston A., 2, 117, 139, 141, 145, 287, 288, 293, 304, 306, 316, 319

Prickly pear cactus, 239, 243

Prince's plume, 99

Prostate, 98, 317, 320

Prostitution, 169, 170–71

Protein, 3 ff., 42 n, 65, 263 ff., 269, 272, 273, 275, 277, 280, 296–98, 299, 306, 307, 309 ff., 320, 322, 323, 333, 334, 345, 348, 354; in algae, wheat, beef, 234; chelated mineral tablets, 324; Chinese and, 168, 174–75, 180, 181, 183, 186, 187; cornmeal, kidney beans, beef compared, 240; Digueños and, 93 ff., 98, 99, 101, 103, 104; and early sexual maturity, 202–3; Eskimos and, 140, 146, 149, 152, 153; Gandans and, 113 ff., 120, 123, 124, 127, 128; grains vs. legumes, 68; Hunzas and, 64 ff., 74, 75, 286; insects vs. beef, 101; Japanese food and, 205, 209, 210, 212 ff., 217, 218; Marquesans and, 17, 20, 21, 24, 25; Mexicans and, 233, 234, 238, 240, 244, 245, 247, 248; milks vs. bean curd, 175; organ meats vs. beef, 276; sesame seeds vs. milk, 213; Tuareg and, 36, 40 ff., 48

Prothrombin, 313

Prussic acid, 115, 121

Ptarmigan, 144, 148

Puberty rites, 87–88

Pudding: Coconut, 29; Pineapple Rice, 29; Pumpkin, 106

Puerto Rico, 331

Puffin, 148

Pulque, 230, 236

Pumpkin (greens; seeds), 44, 102, 120, 311; Blossom Omelets, Stuffed, 252; Buckwheat Groats with Seeds, 103, 105; Marrow Paste with Seeds, 107; Pudding, 106; Squares, 103, 105

Purslane, 239

Pyorrhea, 287

Pyrethrum, 336

Pyridoxine. See Vitamin B_6

Quassia tree, 337

Quinoa, 113

Rabbit, 144; Barbecued, 105; Digueños and, 89, 93, 99, 100, 102, 104, 105

Radiation (radioactivity), 140, 205–6, 309, 313, 345–46. See also Light

Radishes, 61, 69, 73, 178; Japanese and, 218 (see also Daikon); Mexicans and, 235; sprouts, 81, 268

Raisins, 109, 285

Rats, 113, 123, 262, 328

Raw food, 268–70

Rectum, cancer of, 262

Red Dye 2, 338

Red peppers. See Peppers

Refrigeration of grain, 262

Reproductive organs, 320

Reservoirs, chemicals in, 330

Respiratory problems, 10, 205, 306, 325, 327–28; and breast feeding, 271

Rheumatism, 309

Rheumatoid arthritis, 243

Rhubarb, wild, 148

Riboflavin. See Vitamin B_2

Ricci, Father, 163

Rice, 68, 277, 292, 296–97, 308, 324; Boiled Brown, Recipes for, 190, 221; Chicken Soup with, 255–56; Chinese and, 161, 163 ff., 168, 170, 173 ff., 183, 185, 187; Fried, 225; gruel (see Congee); Hunza Breakfast with, 79; Japanese and, 177, 200–1, 202, 205, 208–9, 212, 214, 216, 218, 221, 223, 225, 309; Mexicans and, 232, 238, 245, 255–56; Pudding, Pineapple, 29; Sushi Recipe, 223; wine, 164, 177, 215, 284

Rickets, 136, 315

Ricotta cheese, 266; Curd Curry, 55

Rockefeller Foundation, 232, 241

Rodent poisons, 344

Roe, 137, 138, 145, 146, 287, 305, 315; Baked, 158
Romaine, 104, 155, 275
Roman Empire, and lead, 341–42
Roquefort cheese, 266
Ror, 23
Rose hips, 312, 324
Rotenone, 337
Russians, 135, 265, 311, 332
Rutin, 67
Ryania, 337
Rye, 67, 68, 267, 321; Bread, Recipe for, 155; how to sprout, 81; Hunza Breakfast with, 79; substituting flour, 292

Sabadilla, 337
Sage, 87. See also Chia
Sahara. See Tuareg
Sake (rice wine), 215, 284
Salad, 3 ff., 64, 102, 104, 242 (see also Greens); Bulgur, 53; Dressing (recipe for oil and vinegar), 104; Gazpacho, 252; with Marinated Scallops, 28
Saliva, 280, 318
Salmon, 138, 142, 143, 145–46, 159, 263, 287; Fish Soup with, 154
Salmonella, 306
Salsa, 249
Salt, 33, 43, 87, 121, 201, 203, 279, 318, 321
Salt Lake City, 336
San Diego. See Digueños
Saponin, 239
Sapote, 243
Sardines, 23, 30, 315
Sauerkraut, 177, 266
Saxena, K. M., 205
Scallops, 100; Cucumber-, 218–19; Marinated, 28; Tempura with, 222
Schistosomiasis, 170
Schizophrenia, 309
School cafeterias, 290, 292–94
Screw bean, 95–96
Screwworms, 336
Sculpin, 146
Scurvy, 35, 43, 312
Sea bass, 204–5
Sea cucumbers, 214
Seafood, 237, 297, 320, 321 (see also Fish; Shellfish; specific foods); Digueños and, 100, 102; Japanese and, 200, 201, 209; Marquesans and, 13, 17, 21; in Szechwan Bean Curd, 193
Seagulls, 336
Seal oil, 137, 139 ff., 146, 147, 152, 266, 269, 287
Seals, 140, 141, 147, 342
Sea mammals, 136, 140–41, 145, 146, 147, 287. See also specific animals, organs
Seasonings. See Spices and herbs
Seaweed, 311, 312 (see also Kelp); Chinese and, 181–82, 195, 204, 321; Japanese and, 200, 204–6, 211, 212, 214, 283, 284
Seeds, 267–68, 297, 298, 300, 302, 307, 311, 312, 314, 317 ff. (see also Oils; Sprouts; specific plants); Chinese and, 179 ff., 267; Digueño use, 87, 100, 102, 108, 109 (see also Atole); Eskimos and, 149; Gandans and, 121–22; Hunzas and, 69, 70, 267; Japanese and, 212–13; Mexicans and, 242, 244–45; Pemmican with, 108; soaking, 322–23; Toasted, 26; Tuareg and, 44, 267
Selenium, 320, 343, 344
Semen, 320
Semolina, Couscous with, 51
Sesame oil, 121, 126, 181, 209, 212, 218, 300
Sesame seed, 213, 297, 309, 316 (see also Sesame oil); Cakes, 133; Chinese use, 180, 185, 196; Dip, 52–53; Gandans and, 116, 121–22, 133; Granola with, 108; Japanese and, 212–13
Seven-spice, 182
Seventh-day Adventists, 258–60, 343
Sex and marriage (see also Sex hormones; Sexuality): Eskimos and, 144; Gandans and, 111 ff.; Hunzas and, 58, 61; Marquesans and, 9; Tuareg and, 34
Sex hormones, 309, 339. See also Estrogens
Sexuality: alcohol and, 333; protein and early maturity, 202–3; vitality and protein, 300; zinc and, 320
Shabu shabu, 205
Shangri-La, 72
Shark, 11, 162, 183, 200, 214
Shashimi, 214
Sheep, 336; Hunzas and, 57–58, 71; Tuareg and, 32, 37, 42
Shellfish, 12, 93, 166, 200, 259, 277, 320 (see also Seafood; specific shellfish); in Fish with Coconut Cream, 27; Tempura with, 222
Shepherd's purse, 99
Shortening, 279, 292, 300
Shoyu. See Soy sauce: Japanese use
Shrimp, 321; Chinese use, 185, 187, 188–89, 284; Custard, Main-Dish, with, 224–25; in Fish with Coconut Cream, 27; Japanese use, 205, 209, 214, 222, 224–25; Sweet and Sour, Recipe for, 188–89; Tempura with, 222

Sickle cell anemia, 117–18, 121
Siegal, Sanford, 200
Silicon, 67, 321
Sinus headaches, 234
Skin, 132, 280, 300, 306, 310, 344; freshener, papaya, 243; grafts, 314
Sleep, 235. See also Insomnia
Smallpox, 13, 14, 91, 135
Smelt, 146; Fried, 28
Smog, 305, 312, 328, 346
Smoke, 305, 312, 327; from burning newspapers, 342
Smoking. See Tobacco and smoking
Snacks, 282–94. See also specific cultures
Snakes, 99
Sneezing, 327
Snow blindness, 305
Snow peas (edible pod peas), 178, 192, 210, 222
Snowy owls, 148
Sodas. See Cola drinks; Soft drinks
Sodium, 71, 272, 273, 317–18, 319
Sodium acetate monoglyceride, 338
Sodium nitrate. See Nitrates
Sodium nitrite. See Nitrites
Soft drinks (carbonated beverages), 237, 284, 287, 290, 332. See also Cola drinks
Softeners, 265
Soil, 347. See also Fertilizers
Sole, 216
Sorghum, 118, 176, 312; Gandans and, 114 ff., 122; Tuareg and, 35, 40
Sorrel, 102, 140, 147
Soup, 148, 150 ff., 179, 183 ff., 201, 205, 214, 216, 218, 241; Chicken and Rice, 255–56; Fish (Eskimo), 154; Fish (Ugandan), 131; Summer, 78–79
Sour cream, 292, 300
Sourdock, 148
Sourdough bread, 152, 266, 267; Rye, Recipe for, 155; Starter, 155–56
Sourdough Hot Cakes, 156
Soybean curd. See Bean curd
Soybeans, 68, 301, 308, 310 ff., 315 (see also Bean curd; Soy . . .); Chinese and, 164, 168–69, 174 ff.; Hunzas and, 67, 68; Japanese and, 202, 209–10; roasted, 197
Soy flour, substituting, 292
Soy milk, 175
Soy nut, 197
Soy oil, 174 ff., 181
Soy sauce, 266; Chinese use, 168, 175–76, 184, 189 ff., 266; Japanese use (shoyu), 209 ff., 215, 216, 269, 309
Spaghetti, Sukiyaki with, 221
Spanish, 83, 89–90, 96, 227, 228
Spanish omelet, 241

Speke, John, 110, 111, 116
Sperm, 320, 333
Spices and herbs (seasonings) (see also specific foods): Chinese, 182; Digueño, 87; Hunza, 73; Japanese, 212; Mexican, 245; Tuareg, 37, 43, 46
Spinach, 270, 275, 321 (see also Lamb's quarters); Chinese use, 177, 185, 188; Curry, Recipe for, 75; Fish Soup with, 131; Gandan use, 120, 131; Hunza use, 61, 73, 75, 78; Japanese use, 210, 221, 222, 224; Mexican use, 242; Salad with, 104; Summer Soup with, 78; Tuareg use, 44
Spiny cactus, 84
Spleen, 276
Sports (athletics), 311, 314
Sprouts, 267–68, 270, 312, 340 (see also specific plants); Chinese and, 164, 176, 267; how to grow, 81; Hunzas and, 68, 81, 267; Tuareg and, 40, 44, 267, 286
Squab, 183
Squash, 44, 72, 302; Blossom Omelets, 253; Mexicans and (blossoms; seeds), 227, 228, 239, 245, 246, 248, 253; Pudding, 106; Squares, 104–5
Squash bug, 337
Squirrels, 99
Stanley, Henry, 115–16
Starch, 298–99. See also Carbohydrates
Starfish, 100
Stefansson, Vilhjalmur, 139, 141, 144
Stelae, 228
Stews, 4–5, 293. See also specific cultures, ingredients
Stickleback, 138, 144, 146
Stilbestrol, 339
Stock pot, 274
Stodges, 132–33
Stomach, 122, 205, 280, 311, 343 (see also Digestion; Gastric juices; Hydrochloric acid); contents, eating, 140, 141, 146, 312; in Eskimo diet, 147
Storage. See Preservation and storage
Strawberries, 179, 213
Straw mushrooms, 210
Stress, 307, 312, 345
Strontium poisoning, 205
Sugar, 119, 265, 267, 279–81, 289 ff., 298–99, 302, 303, 306–7, 331–32 (see also Blood sugar; Lactose; Sugar cane; specific foods); Digueños and mesquite, 95; Eskimos and, 140, 141; Hunzas and, 286; Japanese junk foods, 284; Mexicans and, 237, 283
Sugar cane, 16, 116, 281, 283, 285

Suimono, 216, 218
Sukiyaki, 202, 205, 211; Recipe, 221
Sulfa drugs, 307, 308, 313
Sulphur, 320
Sulphur dioxide, 327
Sumashi, 205
Summer Soup, 78–79
Sunburn, 310
Sunflower seeds, 109, 244, 245, 283, 308, 311, 315, 345; Buckwheat Groats with, 105; Cakes, Piñon Nut, 106; Granola with, 108; Marrow Paste with, 107; Pumpkin Pudding with, 106
Sung dynasty, 161
Sunglasses, 345
Sunlight, 37, 315, 345
Sunomono, 216, 218–19
Supplements, 324, 347
Sushi, 209, 226, 284; Recipe, 223
Sweating, 9, 318, 320
Sweeteners, 291. See also specific kinds
Sweet pea vine, 162
Sweet potato(es), 305; Eskimos and, 148; Fish Soup with, 131; Gandans and, 115, 116, 120, 122, 131, 133, 134, 288; Japanese use, 210, 222, 226, 283–84; Marquesans and, 20, 23, 30; Mexicans and, 227, 242; Paste, 226; Stodge, 133; Tempura with, 222
Swimming, 9, 10–11, 61, 296
Swiss chard. See Chard
Swordfish, 200, 214
Syphilis, 13, 91
Szechwan Bean Curd, 192–93
Szechwan cuisine, 165, 166–67

Taboos and prejudices, 272 ff., 274–77
Tai Chee, 173
Taiohae, 15
Tamales, 235–36, 238, 282–83; Recipe for Sweet or Regular, 254
Tangerines, 179
Tapeworm, 19
Tapioca, 121
Tar, tobacco, 329
Taro, 12, 15, 16, 18–19, 23
Taste powder, 182
Tea, 119, 258, 331 (see also Herb tea; Mint); Chinese and, 183, 284; Japanese and, 215, 216; Mormons and, 259; Tuareg and, 36, 43, 44, 46, 286
Teahouses, Chinese, 284
Teeth (and dental arch), 2, 16, 70, 279 ff., 283, 285, 293, 304, 315 ff., 321, 332; Chinese and, 284–85; Digueños and, 87, 90, 288; Eskimo, 141, 287; and flouride, 330–31; Gandans and, 117, 288; Hunzas and, 60; Japanese and, 204, 205, 285; Mar-

quesans and, 9, 10, 285; Mexicans and, 231, 232, 237, 283; and school cafeterias, 293, 294; Tuareg and, 37, 286
Television, 345
Tempura, 201, 204, 284; Recipe, 222–23
Termites, 114–15, 119, 124
Testes, 320
Theophylline, 332
Thiamine. See Vitamin B_1
Thiocyanate, 118, 121
Thousand Island dressing, 302
Thousand-year-old eggs, 182–83
Thrombosis, 229
Thurston, Emory, 201
Thyroid gland, 206
Tiger lilies, dried, 195
Tilapia, 112
Tissue repair, 312
Tleguil, 227, 230
Tobacco and smoking (cigarettes), 116, 258, 259, 312, 329, 337, 339, 347
Tofu (see also Bean curd; Japanese use): Sauce, Carrots and Kidney Beans in, 225
Tomatillos, 241
Tomatoes, 3, 4, 109, 312, 322, 343; Gandan use, 114, 116, 121, 122, 126, 129 ff.; Gazpacho, 252; Hunza use, 61, 73, 78; Mexican use, 227, 228, 235, 238, 242, 245, 246, 248, 249, 253; and Red Onions, 126; Summer Soup with, 78; Tuareg use, 44, 47, 49 ff.
Tomato paste, in pizza, 6–7
Tomato Sauce, 253
Tom cod, 146
Tongue, sore, 307
Toothpaste, 279, 342
Tortillas, 7, 231–32, 233, 235, 238 ff., 244 ff., 251, 257, 283, 316, 317; Recipe, 255
Toyon, 96
Trace elements, 335, 340–44. See also Trace minerals
Trace minerals, 320–21, 347
Trachoma, 91
Triglycerides, 301
Trout, 112, 146
Trowell, Hugh, 202–3
Tsukemono, 224
Tuareg, 1, 31–55, 266, 286, 303, 348 ff.
Tuba root, 337
Tuberculosis, 13, 90, 91, 135, 141–42, 306
Tule, 98
Tuna, 200, 320, 343
Tuna cactus, 85, 97

Turkey, 236, 244, 309; Mole Recipe, 251–52
Turnips (greens), 44, 69, 177, 210, 274

Udon, 221
Uganda. *See* Gandans
Ulcers, 201, 325, 332, 343, 345
Ultraviolet, 313 ff.
United States (America), 3–4 ff., 258–60, 289–94, 348 ff. (*see also* Pollution); and breast feeding, 271
Uric acid, 321
USDA, 336
Utah, 259

Vaginal cancer, 339
Vanilla, 227, 291
Varicose veins, 229, 262, 302, 314
Vascular disease. *See* Cardiovascular system
Vegetables, 258, 264, 290, 293, 297, 298, 302, 305, 307, 312, 314, 320, 322, 323, 334, 342 (*see also* Greens; Oils; specific vegetables); Chinese and, 164, 165, 169, 173–74, 177–78, 266, 284; Colache Recipe, 248; Curry Recipe, 49; Gandans and, 122, 125; Hunzas and, 61–62, 66, 68–69, 73, 77 ff., 268; Japanese and, 200, 201–2, 204, 205, 209, 210–12, 214, 224, 284 (*see also* specific vegetables); Mexicans and, 239–42, 245 ff.; Pickled Mixed, 224; Summer Soup, 78, 79; Tuareg and, 44, 47, 49 (*see also* Couscous); Winter Stew, 77
Vegetarians, 311
Vegetarian's Ten Varieties, 195–96
Venereal disease, 169, 171
Verdolagas, 239
Vinegar, 177, 266, 298, 324, 334
Vinyl chloride, 346
Violence, 309
Viruses, 122, 313
Vision. *See* Eyesight
Vitality, loss of, 344
Vitamin A, 3 ff., 272, 274 ff., 299, 305–6, 320, 324, 328 ff., 333, 334, 346, 347, 350, 354; and alcohol, sperm, 333; Chinese and, 174, 177, 178, 186, 187; Digueños and, 93, 97, 100, 103, 104; Eskimos and, 140, 141, 146, 147, 149, 152, 153; Gandan, 113, 115, 120, 122, 127, 128; Hunzas and, 66, 69, 70, 71, 74, 75; Japanese and, 203, 205, 209, 213, 214, 217, 218; Marquesans and, 13, 17, 19 ff., 24, 25; Mexicans and, 233, 235, 238, 242, 247, 248; Tuareg and, 35, 36, 40, 43, 44, 48, 49

Vitamin B (B complex), 262–63, 267 ff., 280, 281, 301, 306–12, 324, 328, 331–32 ff., 345, 347 (*see also* specific vitamins); Chinese and, 174, 177, 180, 181; Digueños and, 93; Eskimos and, 141; Gandans and, 123, 124; Hunzas and, 64, 67, 69 ff.; Japanese and, 205, 209, 210, 212; Mexicans and, 239, 242, 244, 245; Tuareg and, 41, 45
Vitamin B$_1$ (thiamine), 3 ff., 264, 273, 291, 308–9, 350, 354; Chinese and, 161, 174, 176, 178, 186, 187; cornmeal, kidney beans, beef compared, 240; Digueños and, 93, 94, 97, 101, 103, 104; Eskimos and, 141, 146, 152, 153; Gandans and, 120, 123, 127, 128; grains vs. legumes, 68; Hunzas and, 66 ff., 70, 74, 75; insects vs. beef, 101; Japanese and, 209, 210, 213, 217, 218; Marquesans and, 16, 17, 24, 25; Mexicans and, 236, 238, 240, 247, 248; organ meats vs. beef, 276; sesame seeds vs. milk, 213; Tuareg and, 40, 44, 48, 49
Vitamin B$_2$ (riboflavin), 3 ff., 264, 273, 291, 308, 309, 351, 354; Chinese and, 174, 186, 187; in cornmeal, kidney beans, beef, 240; Digueños and, 93, 97, 101, 103, 104; Eskimos and, 146, 152, 153; Gandans and, 120, 127, 128; grains vs. legumes, 68; Hunzas and, 66, 68, 74, 75; insects vs. beef, 101; Japanese and, 209, 213, 217, 218; Marquesans and, 16, 17, 24, 25; Mexicans and, 238, 240, 247, 248; organ meats vs. beef, 276; sesame seeds vs. milk, 213; Tuareg and, 40, 48, 49
Vitamin B$_6$, 309, 310, 345
Vitamin B$_{12}$, 68, 71, 98, 175, 308, 310–11, 312, 321
Vitamin B$_{15}$, 311
Vitamin B$_{17}$ (nitrilosides), 41, 64, 67, 121, 123, 211–12
Vitamin C (ascorbic acid), 3 ff., 268, 272 ff., 312–13, 319, 321, 324, 328, 331, 334, 339, 342, 344, 345, 347, 352, 354 (*see also* Bioflavonoids); Chinese and, 163, 174, 177, 178, 186, 187; Digueños and, 93, 97, 99, 103, 104; Eskimos and, 146, 149, 152, 153; Gandans and, 115, 120 ff., 127, 128; Hunzas and, 66, 69, 74, 75; Japanese food and, 205, 209, 213, 217, 218; Marquesans and, 16, 17, 19, 20, 24, 25; Mexicans and, 233, 235, 236, 239, 241 ff., 247, 248; Tuareg and, 35, 40, 42, 44, 48, 49
Vitamin D, 277, 299, 301, 306, 315, 316, 324; Chinese and, 181;

Digueños and, 98; Eskimos and, 141, 146, 148, 149; Gandans and, 124; Hunzas and, 70, 71; Japanese and, 210; Marquesans and, 19; Mexicans and, 231, 245; Tuareg and, 37, 45, 286

Vitamin E, 175, 263, 264, 268, 272, 299, 306, 313–15, 320, 324, 328, 329, 334, 346, 347; Hunzas and, 67, 69, 70; Marquesans and, 16; Mexicans and, 242; Tuareg and, 44

Vitamin F, 300

Vitamin K, 71, 267, 299, 313

Vitamins, 65, 265, 266, 269, 287, 300, 304–15, 323–24, 347

Vomiting, 318. *See also* Nausea

Wakame, 211

Walnuts, 64, 70, 212, 285, 300; Date Balls with, 54; Fruit and Nut Snack, 80; Hunza Breakfast with, 79

Walking, 65, 296

Walrus, 140, 141, 147

Walsh, Michael, 231

Waste matter, and longevity, 37

Water, 206, 303–4, 318, 330–31, 342–43; Hunzas and, 60, 62, 64, 66, 69, 72, 303; retention, 302; Tuareg and, 46

Water chestnuts, 178, 224

Watercress, 177, 340; Mixed Greens with, 155; Salad with, 104; Summer Soup with, 78

Water hyacinth, 121

Watermelon, 121, 213, 302

Waterpipes, 342

Water sedge, 148

Webworm, 337

Weizen Factor, 269

Whales, 144, 147

Wheat, 68, 234, 268, 292, 313 (*see also* Bulgur; Wheat germ; specific products); Chinese and, 165, 176; Hunza Breakfast with, 79; Hunza use, 61, 63, 66–67, 68, 79; Stew, Lentil and, 53; structure of grain; nutrients, 263; Tuareg and, 35, 40

Wheat germ, 292, 296–97, 300, 302, 307, 310, 311, 314, 317, 319, 324; Granola with, 108; oil, 300, 324; Toasted, 26

Whey, 63, 70 ff.

White, Ellen, 258

White, Paul Dudley, 60, 173

Whitefish, 138, 146, 237

Wickiups, 101

Williams, Roger J., 301

Willow leaves, 148

Window glass, 345

Wine, 266, 298, 324, 339; Chinese rice, 164, 177; Hunza, 58–59, 273, 286; Japanese rice (sake), 215, 284

Winter melon, 179

Winter Stew, 77

Woks, 184, 215

Wonton, 284

Wood preservatives, 344

Woolly lousewort, 148

Worms, 95, 234, 243–44; garlic for intestinal, 167

Worry, 312

Wounds, 205, 312, 320

Wu, Madame, 161

X-rays, 345

Yaks, 71

Yambean root. *See* Jicama

Yams, 20, 111, 114 ff., 118, 122, 210

Yellow River, 163

Yogurt, 41, 160, 266, 267, 324; Carrots and Kidney Beans in, 225; Hunza use, 63, 70, 73, 75 ff.; Recipe, 54–55; substituting for sour cream, 292; Tuareg and, 35 ff., 42, 46, 47, 49, 50, 54–55

Yosenabi, 205

Yucca, 85, 96, 239

Zinc, 320, 347; alcohol and, 332; and cadmium, 341; and coil, 335

Zucchini, 270, 340; in Eggplant Stew, 52; Mexican use, 246, 248